This book belongs to

___

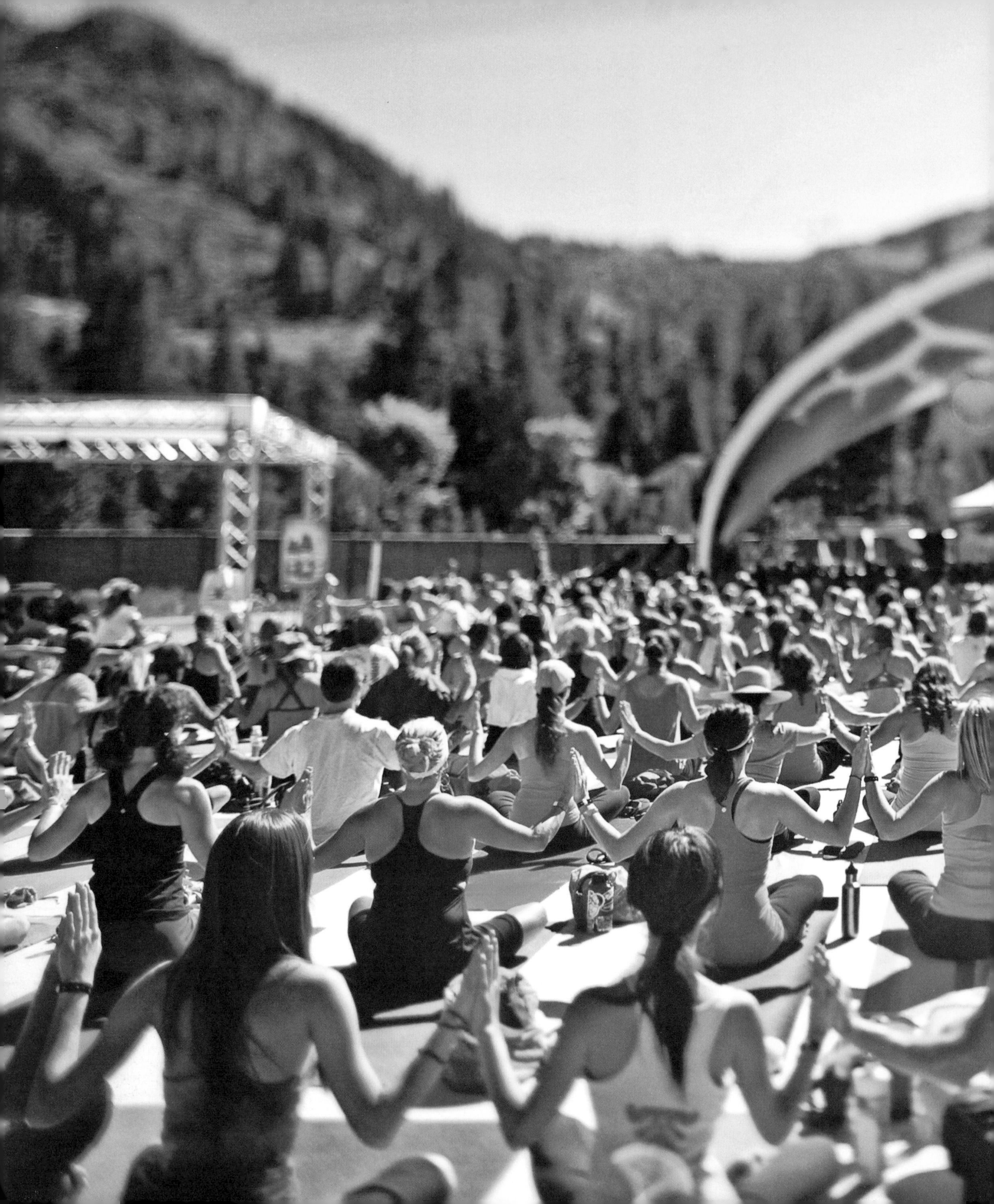

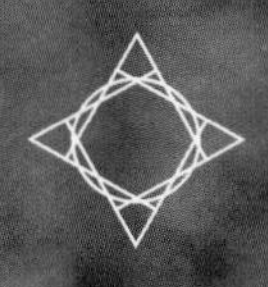

wanderlust

an irrepressible desire to . . .

travel the world

practice yoga

eat locally

live sustainably

consume ethically

be creative

and build community around mindful living

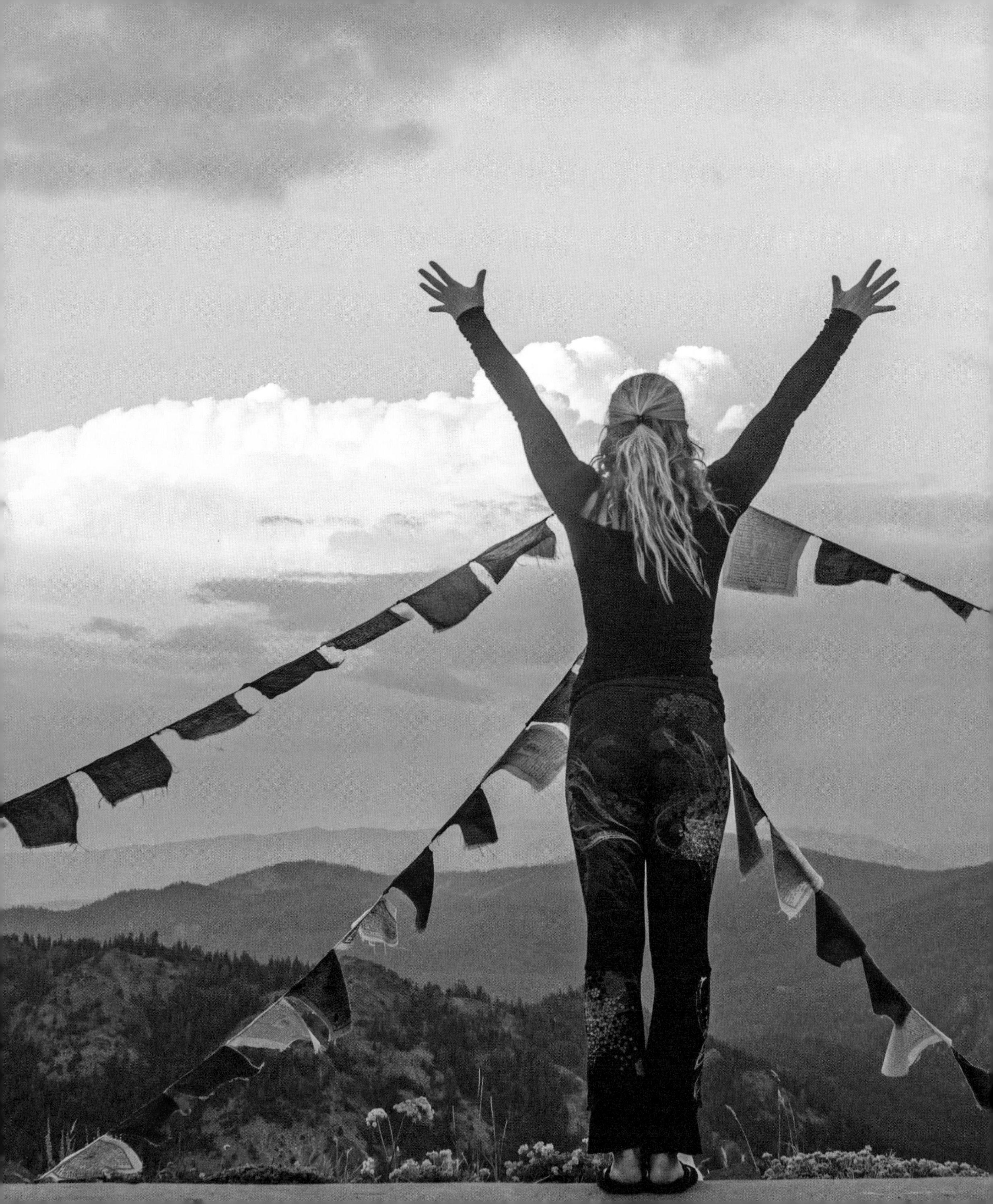

WANDERLUST

A Modern Yogi's Guide to Discovering Your Best Self

JEFF KRASNO

with SARAH HERRINGTON
& NICOLE LINDSTROM

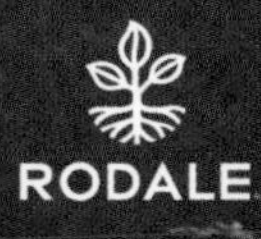

RODALE

Rodale books may be purchased for business or promotional use or for special sales. For information, please write to:

Special Markets Department, Rodale Inc., 733 Third Avenue, New York, NY 10017

Printed in China

Rodale Inc. makes every effort to use acid-free ♾, recycled paper ♻.

Design and illustration by Erica Jago
Principal photography by Ali Kaukas and Sasha Juliard
For additional photography credits, see page 286.

Library of Congress Cataloging-in-Publication Data is on file with the publisher.

ISBN 978-1-62336-350-5 paperback

Distributed to the trade by Macmillan

2 4 6 8 10 9 7 5 3 paperback

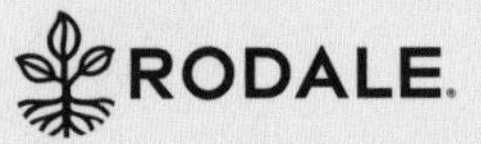

We inspire and enable people to improve their lives and the world around them.

www.rodalebooks.com

For my love, Schuyler,
who, by example,
shows me the best way to live
and then
graciously
leaves the rest to me

Contents

Introduction

What do a meditating congressman from Ohio, a free-range farmer from Virginia, a yoga instructor from New Jersey, and a vegan DJ from LA have in common?

As I sit in my Brooklyn office on a crisp fall day in 2013, the answer is Wanderlust. I scrawl my to-do list: Track down Congressman Ryan, Joel Salatin, Seane Corn, Moby. I am programming next summer's festivals.

Five years earlier, in 2008, my best friend, Sean, and I embarked on the first of many bumpy trips in the name of yoga. My wife, Schuyler, was leading a yoga retreat to Costa Rica and we tagged along. It was here, deep in the rain forest of the Osa Peninsula, practicing yoga, eating from the garden, surfing, dancing, and drinking with friends, that we envisioned the world's largest yoga retreat.

If you are reading this, you likely have an incurable case of wanderlust. I do. The dictionary describes *wanderlust* as an innate desire to travel. This yearning to explore and understand the world beats restlessly in our hearts. Far-flung adventures are the passionate fancy of many a daydream, and, sometimes, they happen.

Inextricably connected to this craving is the longing to know and actualize our true and best self. Alongside our physical exploration, we are also spiritual seekers—searching for a happy, enlightened, and purpose-driven life. Our geographic pilgrimage is mirrored by an inner journey.

The intention of this book is to provide guidance along your trek. We chose *Wanderlust*'s principal image, a compass, with a clear purpose. *Wanderlust* is a base camp for ideas and practices from master teachers, provocative thinkers, mind/body experts, cutting-edge artists, and conscious business leaders that set the coordinates for your journey. And the hope is for you to discover gems of wisdom and inspiration to help navigate life's challenges and cultivate your own best self—to *find your true north*.

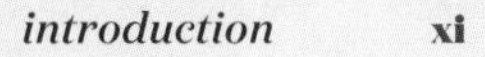

The lens for our journey is yoga: asana, meditation, breath, and philosophy. It is dedicated, daily practice that will keep you on course.

We also see *Wanderlust* as a bridge connecting yoga, the practice, with yoga, the lifestyle. Are you happiest in nature, eating healthy food and listening to great music? Do you seek a good life that is also good for those around you and for the Earth? If so, even if you cannot hold a handstand, you may already be a yogi. It is this wider definition of yoga that creates the possibility for Tim, Joel, Seane, and Moby to gel seamlessly, as our sherpas, under one tent. *Wanderlust* provides a broader way to understand yoga—not just as something you do in class, but an overarching principle for living.

Lastly, yoga literally means union (to yoke)—union with your higher self. Baked into the core of the practice is self-actualization—realizing your capacity for limitless transformation in the service of this best self.

This book guides you from the simplest of daily practices to techniques for manifesting yourself as a leader in the world. But it just scratches the surface. I have often described Wanderlust as a gateway drug for yoga. We hook you and hope you dive deeper. Like the festival, this book is an invitation to *take a sip*. The artists, scholars, and teachers that contribute to *Wanderlust* are the true experts. If something in this book sparks your interest, pursue it. The voyage is life long. This book gets you just out of the harbor. You must scull ahead.

I hope this book lives in your life. It's a cookbook with recipes for living. And like a cookbook, a source of inspiration and experimentation. A pinch more of this. A dash more of that. Just don't let it languish on your coffee table; better to spill coffee on it. Some days, a tablespoon of tadasana will be enough. Other days, you will want to pull all the ingredients off the shelf and start from scratch with everything you've got.

It is said that the hardest part of any journey is taking the first step.

Take a deep breath. Step forward.

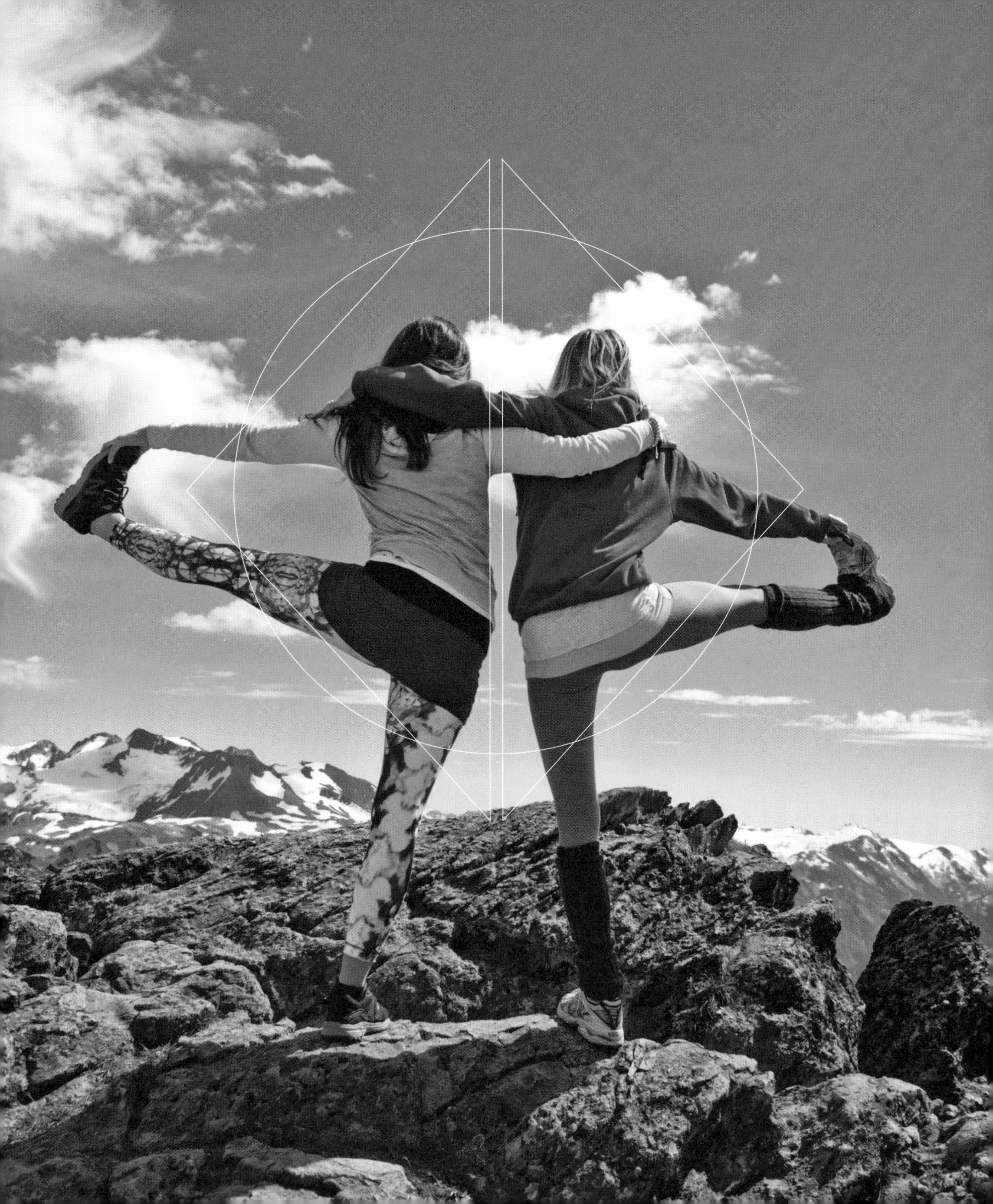

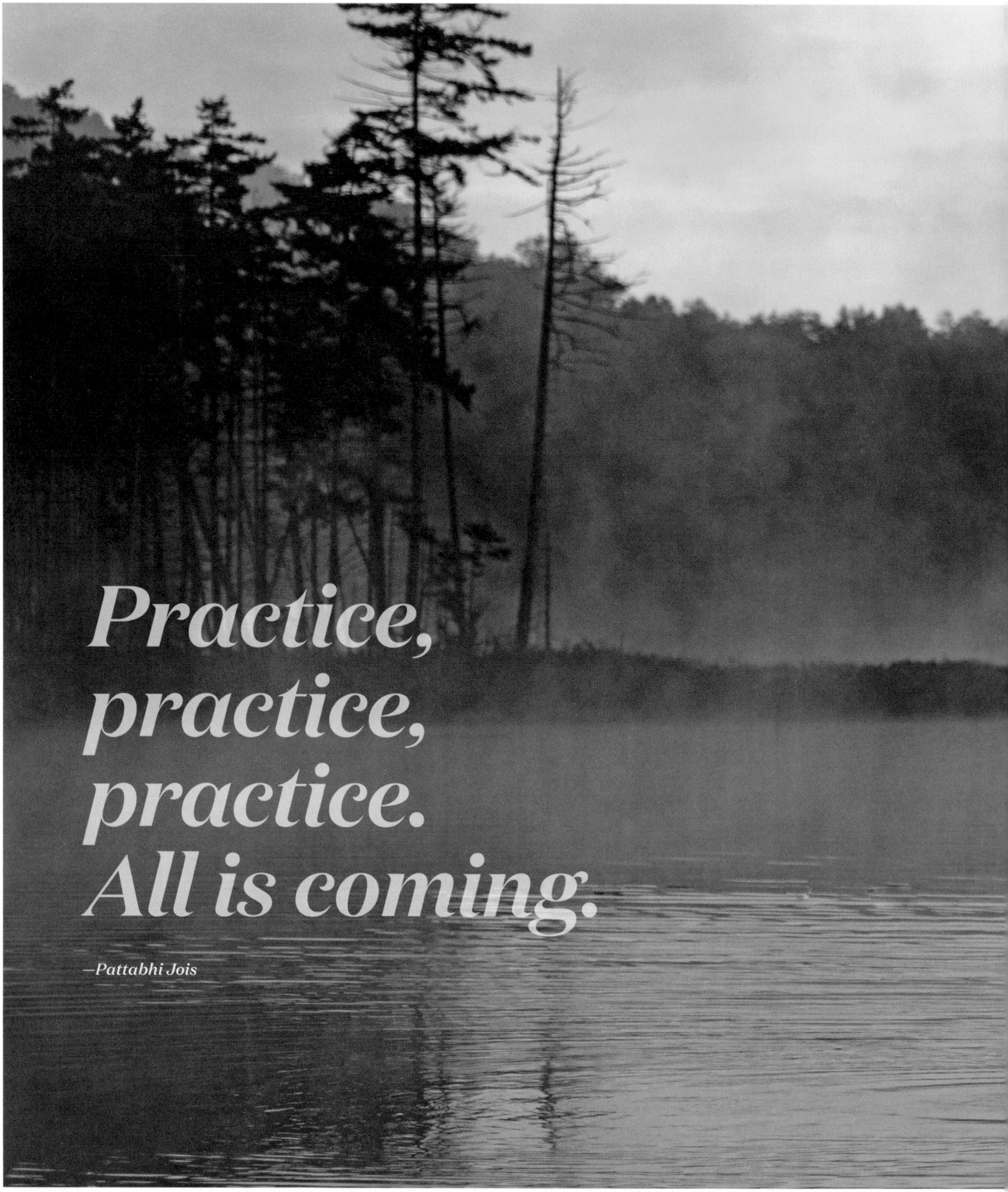

Practice, practice, practice. All is coming.

—Pattabhi Jois

CHAPTER 1

find your practice

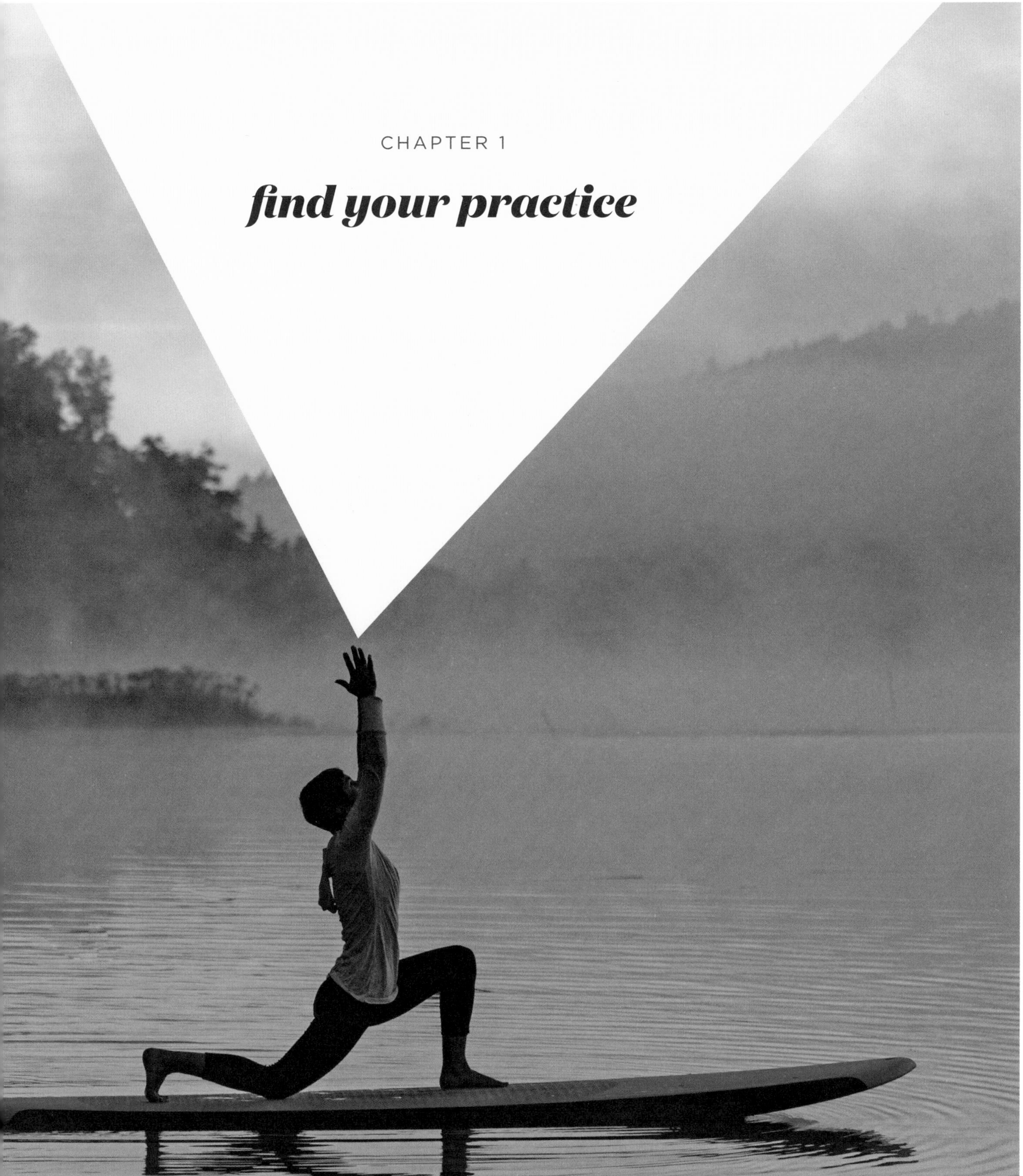

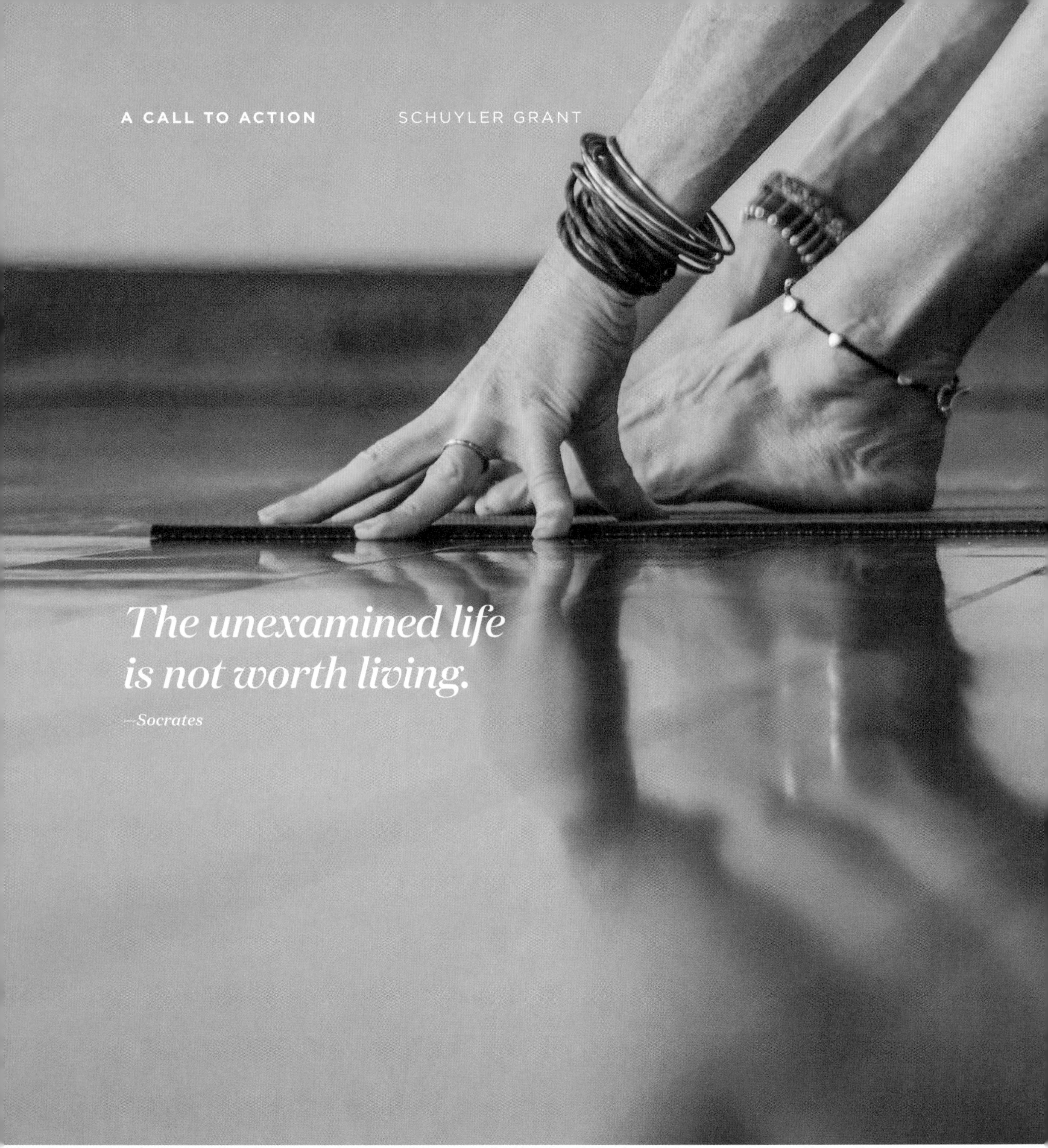

The unexamined life is not worth living.

—Socrates

This is the threshold. To plow through life, seeking pleasures, avoiding pain, rejecting dissonance, reveling in success, and cursing the vicissitudes of fortune. Or to pursue a life of inquiry, simultaneously nonattached and deeply immersed. To experience yourself as both the center of the universe and a dust mote on the filament of history. To choose to have a practice—a daily discipline of yoking your heart to your mind, your mind to your breath, your breath to your body, your body to the earth and the rest of humanity—is to pass this threshold into the examined, mindful life.

The exact way in which you engage in that yoking (in Sanskrit, the yoga) will change. Should change. The course of your relationships, your career, and your health will inevitably shift; the only constant is change. Likewise, your asana practice and other mind/body pursuits will, should shape-shift over a lifetime.

Passion, depression, contentment, injury, exaltation, loss. Will you engage or will you deflect? Will you be immersed or consumed? Like anything substantial, to live a mindful life isn't easy. It takes attention and skill. It takes beginning where you are, as you are now, yoking this larger intention to the present moment. It takes practice.

Let's begin.

OM

SARAH HERRINGTON

Sit tall

Place hands mindfully open
or at heart center

Close your eyes

The focus of this moment is resonance: OM. Like the ringing of a bell. Like an elliptical sound that begins and ends in full silence.

Breathe into the space
behind your chest

While OM is often written with just two letters, it is said to be made of four sounds: A, U, M, and the silence afterward. Together these sounds invoke a sense of wholeness, and of cycles. When we sing OM, we touch each part of our mouth's palate, from the front behind the teeth to the top peak, the inside of our mouth, to the depths of the throat, guttural. The sound moves in a wave this way, with a beginning, middle, and end, and then the after-effect: a feeling of shifted energy in the room, a vibration in the core of our chest.

Heart open

Back strong

Empty all of your air
and take a deep breath

OM

OM is a sacred syllable that represents a very specific yet indescribable conception of the Absolute, of All. In the East, many prayers and powerful mantras start with OM. Here in the West, OM is often found at the beginning and end of a yoga class, opening the practice and sealing up the energy at the end like sonic bookends.

Sing from your guts,
your heart,
your throat

Sing from your spirit and
your body

Said to be the sound of the universe, OM reminds us of interdependence: We are connected to the universe, and it is expressing itself through us. We are connected to each other in the room, and beyond the room. When we chant OM, we consciously join our intentions and attentions and expand our thoughts universally. The vibration flows strongly through the body and penetrates the center, resonating deep within us the feeling of yoga, union, with all.

Sit for a moment in quiet,
be the fourth part,
the full silence

Feel the shift you've created
with your own voice

The arch and the circle,
the ringing, the reminder,
the calling toward home

ॐ

OM is the one eternal syllable of which all that exists is but the development. The past, the present, and the future are all included in this one sound, and all that exists beyond the three forms of time is also implied in it.

—Mandukya Upanishad

MMMMMMMMMMM

YOGA ASKS US TO ACT: THE EIGHT LIMBS

It's safe to say that as human beings wandering this planet, we share a common desire to be happy. Individually, what fulfills that desire is as unique as our fingerprints or the color of our eyes. But if we look at the grand unifiers, we see a universal longing to create meaning in our lives, the desire to be content and to be free from suffering. It's what this book and the phrase "find your true north" are all about.

Cultural conditioning suggests we can find relief through objects like new clothes, cars, or the latest device. Ironically, this way of thinking may translate to yoga as well. We might be sure that once we nail that elusive posture all will be well. As most of us will agree, this is simply not the case. Learning to do a perfect-looking headstand doesn't equal lasting contentment.

There must be more.

Contemplating this might be enough to take you on a lifelong journey. Fortunately, if that sort of heady pursuit is not your thing, the system of yoga has an eightfold path that provides experiential suggestions to help you find your way. This is a path we walk not just by considering and thinking about, but by doing. Yoga asks us to act.

The Yoga Sutras of Patanjali, a text roughly two thousand years old, presents this eightfold path as scaffolding for the hugely transformational endeavor of calming the mind and opening the core of the heart. The eight limbs are a blueprint for self-discovery and are intended to be studied and engaged with over a lifetime.

Yama

Ethical practices often referred to as "restraints" that pertain to the way one interacts with the world.

Niyama

Practices that the yogi employs to refine the relationship with one's internal world.

Asana

Physical postures the yogi practices in order to create steadiness and ease in the body and mind.

Pranayama

Liberation or extension of the life force through practice with the breath.

Samadhi

Absorption in the experience of supreme consciousness.

Dhyana

Outcome of long-held concentration on a single point or experience: absorption.

Dharana

Practice of concentration.

Pratyahara

Practice of turning the power of one's senses inward.

KEVIN COURTNEY

The Yamas

These moral principles can be likened to the basic tenets in almost all spiritual traditions, as they provide the foundation for living a conscientious life, from one's relationship to others to one's relationship with self.

AHIMSA: Nonviolence, compassion, kindness.

SATYA: Truth, truthfulness, honesty.

ASTEYA: Nonstealing.

BRAHMACHARYA: Often translated as celibacy, it is more broadly defined as the conservation of vital energy in order to direct one's attention toward divine pursuits and self-knowledge.

APARIGRAHA: Nongreed, or nonhoarding.

The Niyamas

The niyamas are observances that the yogi employs to refine the relationship with one's internal world.

SAUCHA: Cleanliness, inside and out.

SANTOSA: The practice of being happy for no particular reason at all.

TAPAS: Self-discipline, austerity; literally translated as "to burn." To purify through power and heat of intentional practices such as asana and pranayama.

SVHADYAYA: Self-study.

ISVARA PRANIDHANA: Surrender to the supreme, devotion to the divine, recognizing the divine essence in all beings.

Asana

In one aspect, it's a preparatory practice that enables one to sit for extended periods in order to study and experience one's internal state through meditation. As the practitioner's attention is drawn toward the physical sensations and energetic shifts that occur throughout the body, the ability to concentrate is refined, and the mind is made ready for a similar course of study on more subtle aspects of being.

Pranayama

Here, prana means life force, but also breath. Ayama can be interpreted as "with restraint," and also suggests length or expansion. Thus, pranayama is the practice of working with the breath to regulate, extend, or restrain it, in order to affect the flow of vital life force in one's being.

Pratyahara

Unregulated, the senses of touch, taste, sight, sound, and smell, and the desires they produce, can control one's actions, thoughts, and behaviors. Through the powerful push and pull of raga and duesha (attraction and repulsion), the impact of the senses, like a wild horse, can lead an unstudied individual to follow every whim and visceral impulse with abandon. It is thus imperative to retrain one's mind to gain control over these aspects, if one wishes to lead a steady and conscientious life. The ability to witness stimuli, and the feelings they produce, without feeling the need to act or respond to them, tones the yogi's mind.

Dharana

An initial step toward meditation, the practitioner simply fixes attention on a single point or experience, such as the body, breath, an object, or mantra. An example is candle gazing. The practitioner's focus steadies on the flame while taking notice of all the thoughts, feelings, and sensations that arise. The intention of dharana is to build the muscle of focus and objective observation.

Dhyana

Dhyana can be understood when we consider that to concentrate the mind initially takes effort (dharana). Sustained concentration, cultivated with consistent practice and sincere effort, eventually transitions into an effortless flow. It's as if a type of inwardly directed momentum takes over and all effort falls away. This is dhyana.

Samadhi

Samadhi is absorption in the experience of supreme consciousness, and is the direct result of continued practice in the meditative state. As one becomes absorbed in the object or experience one focuses on, an experience of beingness is achieved. Eventually, even that original object falls away, and one feels that beingness expand to all things, allowing the practitioner to merge with the heart of consciousness itself. This ecstatic state is beyond the confines of language or regular mental understanding, and so it is often described as neti neti: not this, not this.

Thirty-Day Challenge

The practices and philosophies presented in the eight limbs are not meant for us blindly to accept as truth. The teachings are intended to be put into practice, chewed on, and wrestled with over the course of time.

What you put into it is what you get out.

The following is a very practical and effective method for helping integrate principles like compassion, contentment, and self-study into everyday life. Commit to thirty days of this practice to start.

First:

Create a comfortable place to sit and read through each of the yama and niyama.

Feel which one attracts or compels you in some way.

Choose that one to work with for the month of this exercise.

Second:

Write the chosen yama or niyama on sticky notes and place them throughout your home in places that you visit on a regular basis (entrance, refrigerator, bathroom, nightstand). Another good idea is to change your passcode on your phone to the Sanskrit word.

Once the sticky notes are in place, they act as spontaneous check-in points. Over the course of the month, as you come across a note, reflect on your current state and how it relates to the quality you're aiming to cultivate.

It's within that moment of reflection that insights come and awareness of yourself begins to increase.

Watch out for:

JUDGMENT: A crucial component to this exercise is the offering of nonjudgmental awareness to yourself. This is a time of learning and self-exploration.

One of my favorite teachers, Don Stapleton, likes to say, **"IT TAKES THE TIME IT TAKES."**

Be patient; honor and respect the process. This is in part how we cultivate a healthy, insightful, and ultimately loving relationship with ourselves. And it's from this place of love and deep connection that we experience the courage and strength to step into the world and truly follow our hearts.

track your daily progress

1	2	3	4	5	6	7	8	9	10	11	12	13	14	15
16	17	18	19	20	21	22	23	24	25	26	27	28	29	30

SHINE BRIGHT: SUN SAL A

MC YOGI AND
SARAH HERRINGTON

Look behind the mind
And you will find
The place inside
Where the sun shines
Feel it shine like a star
Inside your heart
Sun light shine bright
Wash away the dark

—"Sun Light" from the album Pilgrimage *by MC YOGI*

Walk into any yoga class and you're bound to meet Sun Salutation A, aka Surya Namaskara. By linking movement with breath in a continual dance, warm up the body like the sun warms up the earth in a full expression of gratitude. Take this opportunity to give thanks for body, breath, and world around you. Check in. Together let's get ready to move into deeper asana and ignite our practice.
ROLL OUT YOUR MAT, LET'S RISE.

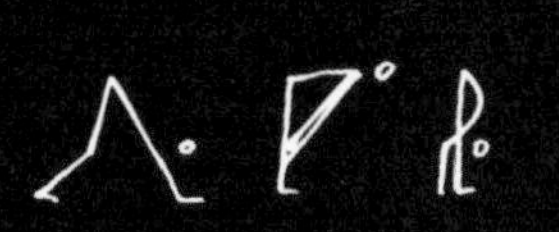

Let devotion rise within like the sun
in a happy humbling of spirit

You cannot step in the same river twice.

—Heraclitus (500 BCE)

Please take out a timer now to mark your time reading this section on meditation. We'll talk about why later on.

Meditation, despite its mystical connotations, is first and foremost a practical perspective-taking exercise: a tool to get to know your own mind and that part of you that is eternal. Over time, long-term yogi meditators not only feel strong and flexible, but also more confident and clear-minded.

During most of our waking hours, we are so engaged with our thoughts and perceptions that we don't have an awareness of the filter through which we receive them. When you sit in meditation, you step back from the activity of analyzing/processing/creating and witness as these mental processes unfold.

Much as rivers are always shifting, all things, including the mind, are constantly changing. As you become adept at watching the ephemeral nature of the mind, you start to get rooted in that which is constant, unchanging, and always present. *The Yoga Sutras of Patanjali* calls this purusha: the part of you that is the witness. This gravitational shift in consciousness is the great promise of meditation.

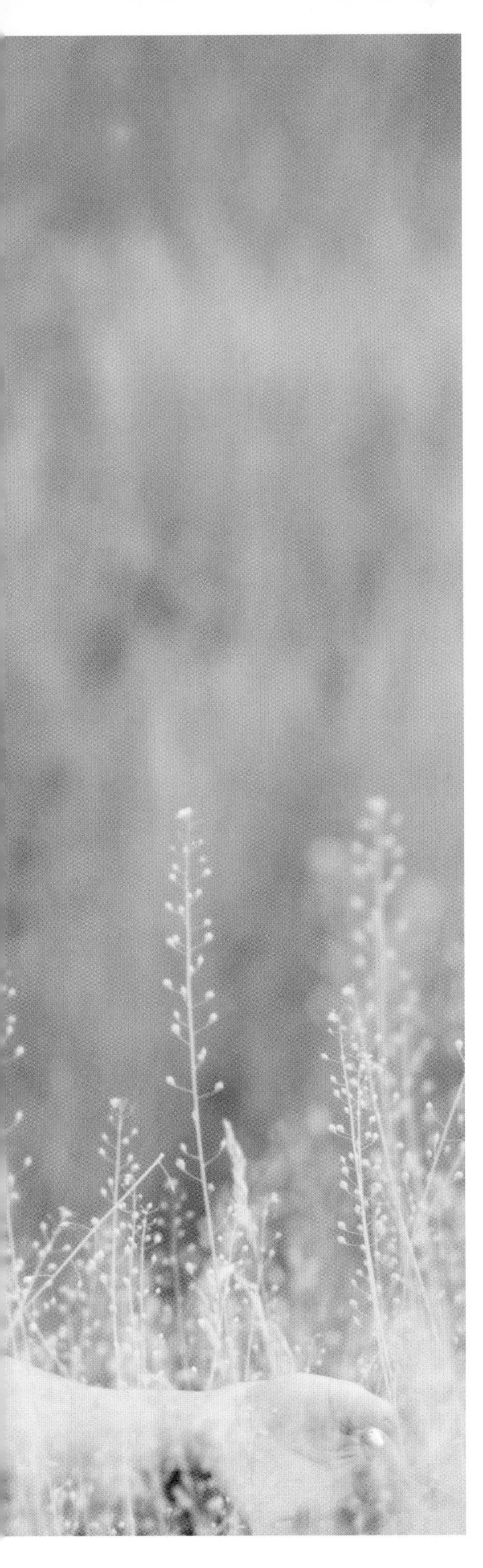

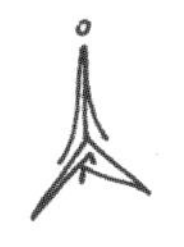

All meditation practice starts with observing.

1. AFFIRM TO YOURSELF THAT YOU WILL TRY MEDITATING. RIGHT NOW.

Ask just about anyone if they'd like to incorporate meditation into their daily routine, and nearly everyone will say yes! However, the leap between acknowledging the value of the practice and actually doing it is particularly wide. Why is that?

Meditation may appear serene, but it can actually be quite strenuous. When we sit, we are asking ourselves to peel away the multi-layered defense of conditioning. Most of us have created a highly functional personality around our insecurities, wounds, and losses, creating a self-image that projects health, happiness, and confidence, both to others and to ourselves. In meditation, there is no one to impress or hide from. You come face-to-face (so to speak) with your raw, unguarded self.

It's not always comfortable to engage at this deeply honest level. We often avoid practices of introspection. Consider that the immediate benefits of meditation practice are not as obvious as a yoga practice. Nobody can see whether you're a good meditator or not. But with sustained effort, most practitioners discover very quickly that they are less reactive and come out of anger and other states more quickly than before. Why not commit to trying it?

At the moment of commitment, the entire universe conspires to assist you.

—Goethe

Benefits of Meditation

- Meditating is linked to stress reduction, and stress is widely acknowledged as a primary cause of disease.
- It makes you smarter. Studies show that meditating facilitates neuroplasticity, or your brain's ability to build new pathways of understanding.
- Research is showing that meditators develop greater emotional intelligence. Practitioners have a greater ability to perceive their own thoughts and feelings; to harness those thoughts and feelings for high-level problem solving and other cognitive tasks; to work with complicated relationships; and to harness emotions for the greater good.

2. GET COMFORTABLE.

Practically speaking, we exist in two dimensions: **time and space.** When preparing to meditate, you want to be as relaxed as possible in both of these dimensions.

Time

Decide a length of time to sit for—it could be five minutes, twenty minutes, or longer. Five minutes may not sound long, but it's a good place to start, and you can always increase your sit time tomorrow. More important than the duration is the commitment. A timer can be very helpful. Let the timer manage this dimension for you.

There is no wrong time to meditate.

Many prefer to sit in the morning, but if a midday sit or evening practice works better for you, sit then. As you fall in love with the practice, you may find yourself rearranging your day for it! Also, reaching stillness is often easier after a yoga practice, so you may find a postyoga sit just the thing for you.

Space

Meditators are often instructed to find a comfortable seat, but the truth is, no seat will be perfectly comfortable, especially at the beginning. The good news is: It doesn't need to be. It just needs to be comfortable enough that you stay still and unbothered for your designated period of time.

Some ideal characteristics of your comfortable-enough seat:

Spine straight

Hips relaxed

Arms supported

Gaze level with the horizon

Jaw soft

Breath moving easily

Try an elevated cross-legged position. Sit high enough so that your hips are above your knees. If the knees are higher than the hips, the hip flexor muscles are engaged and this will tire you out. Try sitting on a folded blanket or cushion.

If this is not comfortable, sitting on the front edge of a chair is a good option. Place both feet on the floor, and think of having a tall, straight spine. A gentle alertness in the body will lead to a gentle alertness in the mind.

Whether you're on a cushion or a chair, aim to center yourself over your sit bones, so that the spine is leaning neither forward nor back, left nor right, and the shoulder blades are moving easily down the back.

Place your hands either face up or down gently on the thighs. Palms up bring energy to practice, palms down can ground you. Pay attention to which feels right each time you sit. No two sits are alike.

Check your chin and lift it slightly so that your gaze is comfortably toward the horizon. Relax your jaw and let the tip of the tongue rest gently behind the front teeth.

Once settled, gently close your eyes or keep them ever so slightly cracked open. Up to you.

3. STAY IN YOUR SEAT.

This is actually one of the more challenging instructions. As soon as we find a position and close our eyes, inevitably our nose will itch, back will need to crack, hair will need to be redone, you name it. This is the nature of the mind: It is never satisfied. When we ask the body to slow down and be still, we notice how habituated we are to unconsciously seeking new, and presumably better, experiences all the time.

Tell yourself that this seat is good enough. Let this seat be fine as it is.

Each time you indulge the urge to fidget, you draw your awareness away from the breath.

4. BE WITH YOUR BREATH.

We are always breathing, but how often do we really pay attention to it?

The breath functions very well as what meditation teachers will call the "object of meditation," meaning: the focal point for your mind as you sit. The mind needs something to land on: an object. The breath works well as an object because it is ever present. You don't need to conjure it up; it's always there.

Feel your inhales and your exhales. You can even label "inhale" and "exhale" silently, inside, to help you observe when you are beginning. The mind is unlikely to be satisfied with just watching breath. It will prefer to wander off and find things to think about. To have a mind that wanders does not make you a bad meditator. Actually, there's no such thing as a bad sit! Your job is to notice, and when the mind does wander away, see if you can use the feeling of breath in the body to bring it back. This is a process that will happen again and again. These moments of drifting and regathering attention are part of your quest to know the mind.

Eventually, the duration of your experiences of presence will increase. It is in this place of stillness and presence that we access what yoga calls the purusha, the inner witness, the intuitive knower, the inner guide, or, in Wanderlust parlance, true north.

Check the timer you set when you began reading this section. How long has it been? Many of us will spend far longer reading about meditation than we will actually meditating. No author's thoughts on the practice, however, will do you much good unless you put them to use.

Treat your mind with the same regard you give—or are doing your best to give—to others, following Patanjali's advice from **YOGA SUTRA 1.33: MAITRI KARUNA MUDHITA UPEKSHANAM.** Be kind, be compassionate, rejoice, and move on.

Yantras are mystical diagrams, symbols of cosmic unity. Roughly translated from Sanskrit, yantra *means tool, device, or liberation support. There are many types, from curving, looping diagrams that almost look like handwriting to complex symmetrical forms made from layers of overlapping geometric shapes.*

The yantra featured here is from the North Indian tradition of Harish Johari and is for invoking the power of deities. It is said to be a blessing simply to see one.

Beautiful examples of sacred geometry, yantras elegantly illustrate the relationship between consciousness and manifestation. Each of the shapes represents a different element. We begin at the outside with the densest element, earth, represented with a square shape. We move inward toward the most subtle, space, represented by the center dot. Here we abide in a state of complete unity. Yantras may be used as a focal point for eyes-open meditation, Trataka. They may be placed on an altar or hung on a wall.

Yantras are similar to mandalas in appearance, and there is some overlap in function. Mandalas are a "circle" of beings, or illustrate a relationship between many items.

Yantras are usually more specific, belonging to one divine being, concept, or action. According to Swami Satyananda, mandalas have the energy of creation, and yantras of dissolution. "Dissolution" in this context means dissolution of attachments and a focus on unity rather than diversity.

Yantra Meditation Practice

Place this yantra just above eye level.

Sit comfortably with the spine straight.

Gaze at the center point with a soft but steady gaze that includes the entire form.

Blink when needed. Try counting the breath; calm the heart and settle the mind.

Inhale for a count of six, exhale for a count of six.

Once the body is steady, try silently chanting a mantra such as "OM."

Sit as long as desired without straining.

By meditating regularly on a yantra, our consciousness is repatterned into a more harmonious, enlightened state.

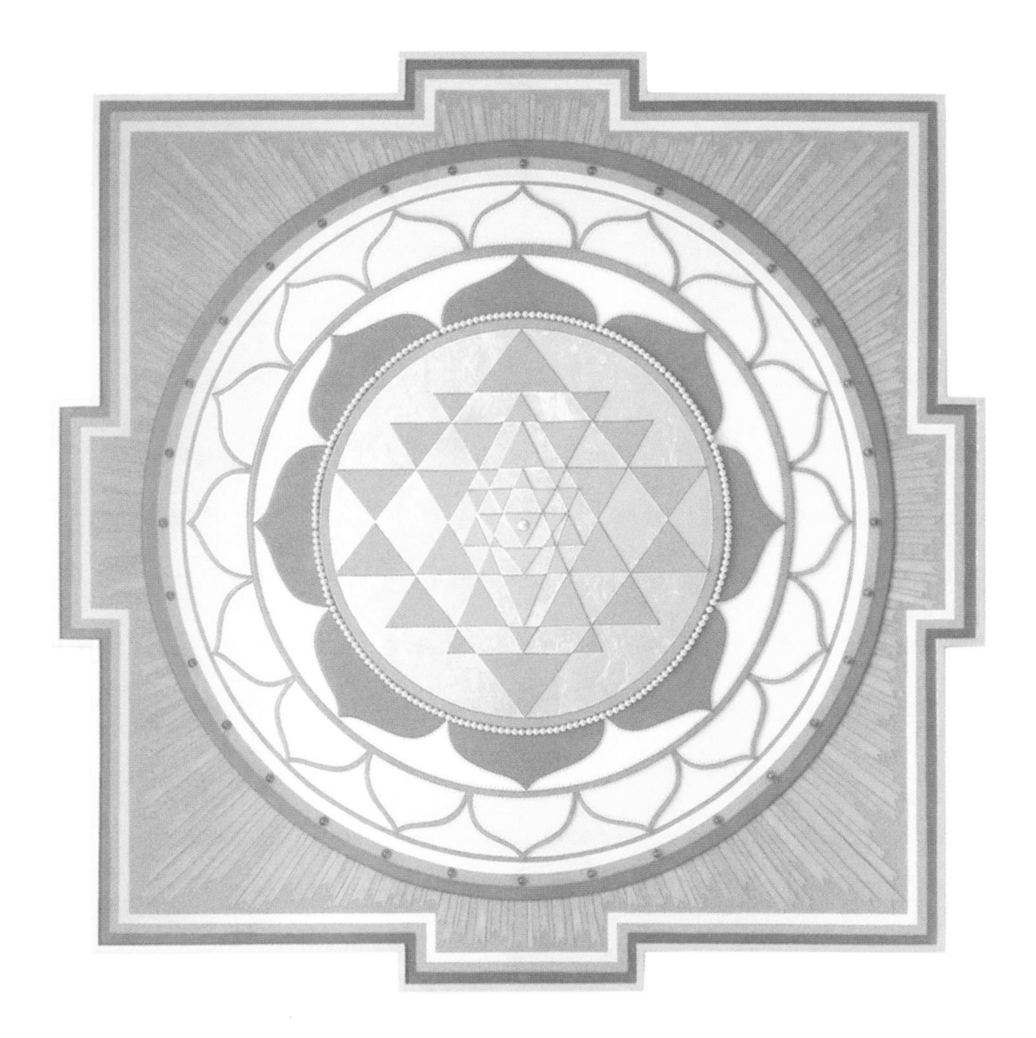

"What can I do?"

It's perhaps the most common question people ask me when I'm speaking and teaching about farming and the food system today. It's a simple request filled with angst and hidden perceptions. Often a sigh accompanies the question. In that sigh lives a sense of powerlessness, the kind of a resignation of a single person fighting city hall. When we look at the Monsantos, the Archer Daniels Midlands, the McDonald's from our little household vantage points, it can surely take the wind out of our sails. "What can I, just little I, do?

But consider this. Whatever exists now is a cumulative manifestation of all the individual decisions made by the majority of the people in the culture for a period of time. For example, when a 1950s mother decided breast-feeding was archaic, barbaric, and Neanderthal, that decision set in motion a host of results. Infamil and Similac flew off the shelves. We now see this led to increased risk for asthma. Today, many studies link breast cancer risk to a lack of breast-feeding. Dependency on formula rather than self-reliance on breast-feeding—always available, always the right temperature—catalyzed a nation of disempowerment. We were literally looking outside of ourselves for nourishment—quick, easy, prepackaged nourishment. You could say this grew into fast-food and industrial-food customers. And this is only one example.

The point is that our decisions are not made in a vacuum. We are all interconnected and, moment by moment, building a future world. The micro affects the macro. When we decide that participating in the soccer league is more important for the children than eating a locally sourced, home-cooked meal around the dinner table, we build a certain kind of farm and food system. When lots of people do that, it changes the face of food, rural economies, farm families, wellness, and familial cohesion. It might even affect our children's attitudes toward aging parents—sending them to the old folks' leagues rather than fixing up the back bedroom for elder care.

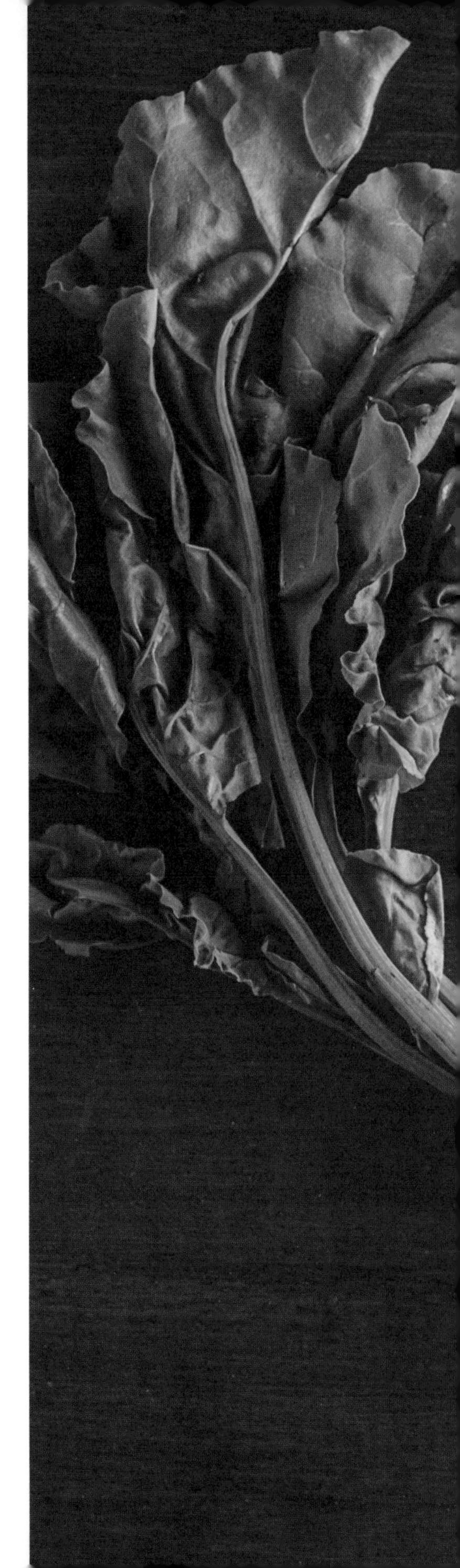

JOEL SALATIN

"What can I do?" is such a pregnant question that whenever someone asks it, I have a hard time pinning down what she's really asking. Is she asking for information? Help? Is it a general cry of frustration? Many times, today's epidemic of domestic culinary ignorance intimidates would-be food connectors from even trying to fix something from scratch. A beet grown in the garden or purchased at the farmers' market does not look like the Harvard beets in the microwavable heat-n-eat meal package. When that real unprocessed beet looks at you, "what can I do?" takes on new meaning.

So what can you do?

You can participate. You can connect. You can get actively involved in the process of turning that beet into Harvard beets. You can turn off the TV. You can cancel the cruise vacation and buy bushels of tomatoes to can or turn into salsa. You can get some pots and grow a pot garden of vegetables. You can put a beehive on the roof of your house, two chickens in the foyer instead of that aquarium or parakeet cage.

Just like today—whatever today looks like—is the manifestation of billions of individual decisions accumulated over time, tomorrow will be too. And if you, I, we don't start making different decisions, we will end up where we're headed, only it may be worse because we'll be farther down the wrong road.

I wish I could snap my fingers and things would be different. Farms would grow soil instead of depleting it. Food would be nutrient dense instead of deficient. People would fall in love again with domestic culinary arts. Domestic larders would supplant the entertainment center as focal points for domestic tranquility and security. But that doesn't happen when I snap my fingers. That happens when you, you, you, and you—and I—begin making different decisions.

What can we all do? Stop incessant victimhood mentality. Somebody else will not fix things. Somebody else will not make us healthy; somebody else will not make us happy. These things are our responsibility. Not the neighbor's, not the government's, not the church's or civic club's.

If I don't know what to do with a beet, I need to find out. Knowing what to do with a beet begins a long chain of events that ends up creating a soil in which earthworms happily procreate.

And that is a good thing.

FEAST: BEET RECIPE

SARAH COPELAND

As someone who became a gardener in the concrete jungle of New York City, I say, if we can do it here, you really can do it anywhere. Growing food makes sense of so many things; it quiets the mind, it creates a richness and rhythm that affects your whole life and, of course, makes it more delicious.

Most of what I plant comes up easily—good soil, sun, and water make easy work of pea, bean, squash, radish, carrot, and leafy greens seeds. But year after year, I fail at growing beets. Sure, there are books upon books where I could learn to do it right, but I'm happy to hop over to the farmers' market and buy a bunch of sweet baby beets (red, or yellow) and toss them with my own homegrown carrots, radishes, and arugula in this hearty salad, complemented with toasted hazelnuts and creamy chive dressing. Give it a shot. Roast some beets, invite some friends over, and, you know, participate. You just may feed a revolution.

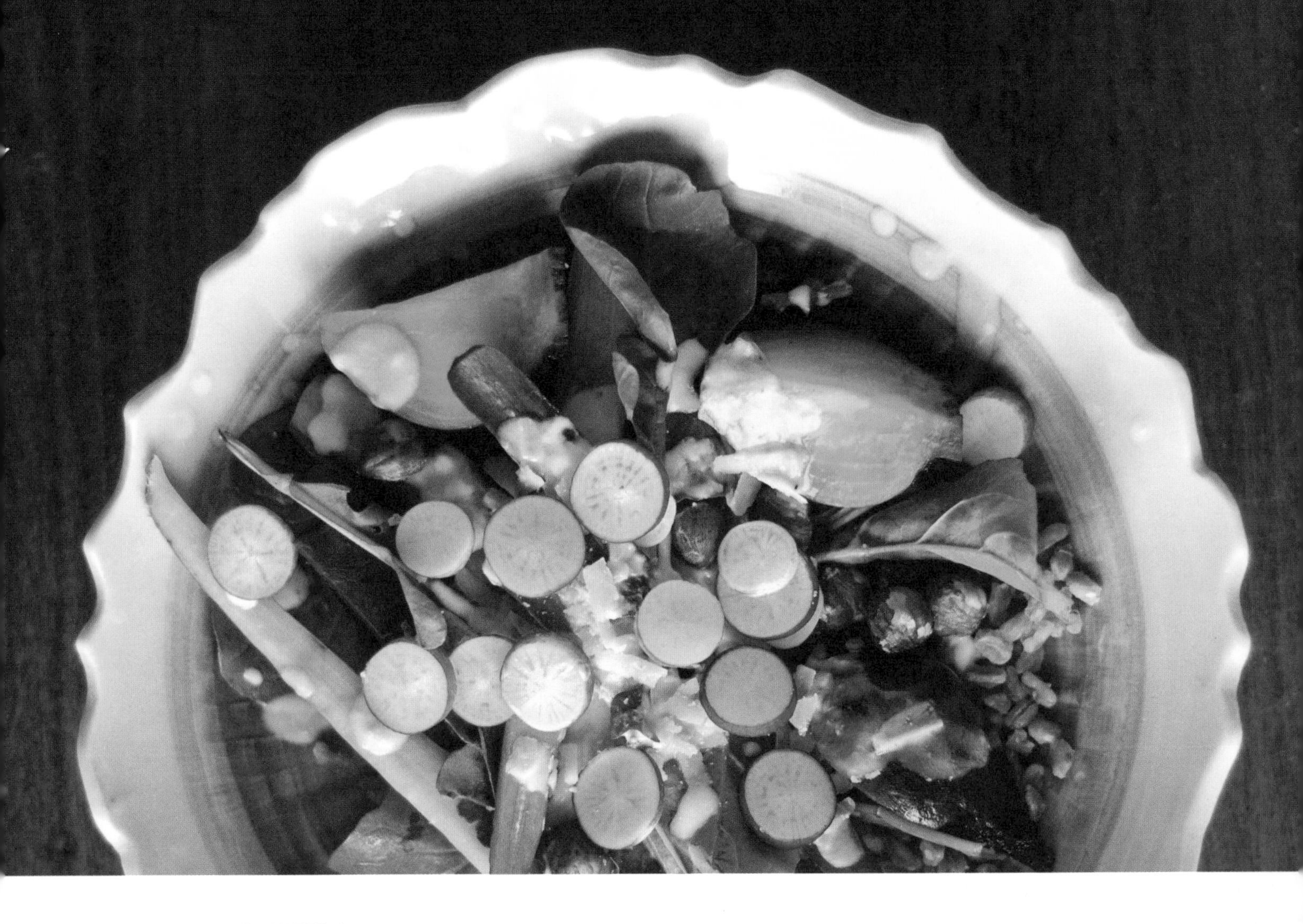

Roasted Root Vegetable and Farro Salad

SERVES 4

8 red or yellow baby beets, scrubbed and trimmed

¼ cup plus 2 tablespoons extra-virgin olive oil

Sea salt and freshly ground pepper

6 young heirloom carrots or baby turnips, scrubbed, trimmed, and halved lengthwise

1 tablespoon honey

1 sprig fresh thyme

8 ounces farro

6 radishes

DRESSING

¼ cup full-fat plain yogurt

Juice of ½ lime, plus more as needed

2 tablespoons finely chopped assorted fresh herbs

1 tablespoon hazelnut oil

1 tablespoon extra-virgin olive oil

Fine sea salt and freshly ground pepper

2 heaping handfuls arugula or baby leaf lettuce

Small handful toasted hazelnuts

Flaked sea salt

3 ounces aged Parmigiano-Reggiano or pecorino cheese

Preheat the oven to 400°F. Drizzle the beets with the olive oil and season with salt and pepper. Wrap them tightly in aluminum foil and roast until they can easily be pierced with a fork, about 20 minutes. Remove from the oven and cool in the foil.

Combine the carrots, honey, thyme, and 1 cup water in a medium skillet over medium heat. Bring to a simmer and cook until the vegetables are fork-tender and the broth has reduced to a glaze, about 25 minutes. Remove from the heat and keep warm.

Meanwhile, put the farro in a medium pot and add enough water to cover by about 2 inches. Bring to a boil over medium-high heat, reduce to low heat, and simmer until tender, about 20 minutes. Drain.

When the beets are cool enough to handle, peel the skins with a paring knife and quarter. Slice the radishes as thinly as possible with a mandoline or a very sharp knife.

To make the dressing: Whisk together the yogurt, lime juice, herbs, hazelnut oil, olive oil, ¼ teaspoon salt, and ¼ teaspoon pepper in a medium bowl. Taste with a leaf of arugula; adjust the salt, pepper, or lime juice as needed.

Divide the farro among shallow bowls. Drain the carrots. Combine the beets, carrots, and arugula in a large bowl; toss together; and arrange over the farro. Top with the radishes, drizzle with the dressing, and sprinkle with hazelnuts and flaky salt. Generously grate or shave Parmigiano-Reggiano over the top with a vegetable peeler. Serve warm.

It helps to know why you're practicing.

I remember learning the term *daily practice*. I had fallen in love with yoga, but I was a little ways off from fully integrating my practice. As I enrolled in my first teacher training, I had a touch of the fraud complex.

I was a tough-and-stubborn, early-years yoga practitioner. My favorite yoga teachers floated soundlessly on their mats and had studied with a member of the Jois family.

I was also living my dream: experimental rock violinist in two touring bands, seeing the world one dirty rock club at a time. I was happily at the mercy of a crazy schedule and less happily at the mercy of my hard-swinging emotions.

The yoga mat morphed from trainer to therapist. I was becoming seasoned with tour cycles and with my own cyclical patterns. I was full of optimism and adventure and I couldn't shake the feeling that the bottom might drop out at any minute. This could be the last tour, the last record, the last wave of creativity, of luck, etc.

My enrollment in teacher training was more than a career backup plan, though; it was a bonding to my yoga practice. I sensed that it was keeping me tethered to a subtle solidity, and I was grasping for more.

I ramped up my practice in the year leading up to teacher training with so much gusto I gave myself a wrist injury. I devoured the lectures and the readings and the practice teaching like a hungry sleepless child, and arrived back from training to tour, glowing with purpose. I had the sense that all of this work would override my flaws as a human; that with enough practice, and now with teaching, my old behavior patterns and reactivity would cease to exist. I muscled my way through those first years of teaching, completely voracious, taking in as much reading and additional trainings as time permitted.

By this time, a daily practice felt natural and attainable, and I was seeing something subtle shift on the inside. I first noticed the shift on a European Bell Orchestre tour in 2009. I had committed myself to practicing yoga every day on tour, no matter what the circumstance. And that was just it: no matter what the circumstance. My own practice, given that parameter, started to shift and soften.

A Bell Orchestre tour had less free time and more heavy lifting than an Arcade Fire tour post-2005. We drove ourselves country to country in a cramped van, loaded in gear, sound checked, performed, sold our records, loaded out, and drove on.

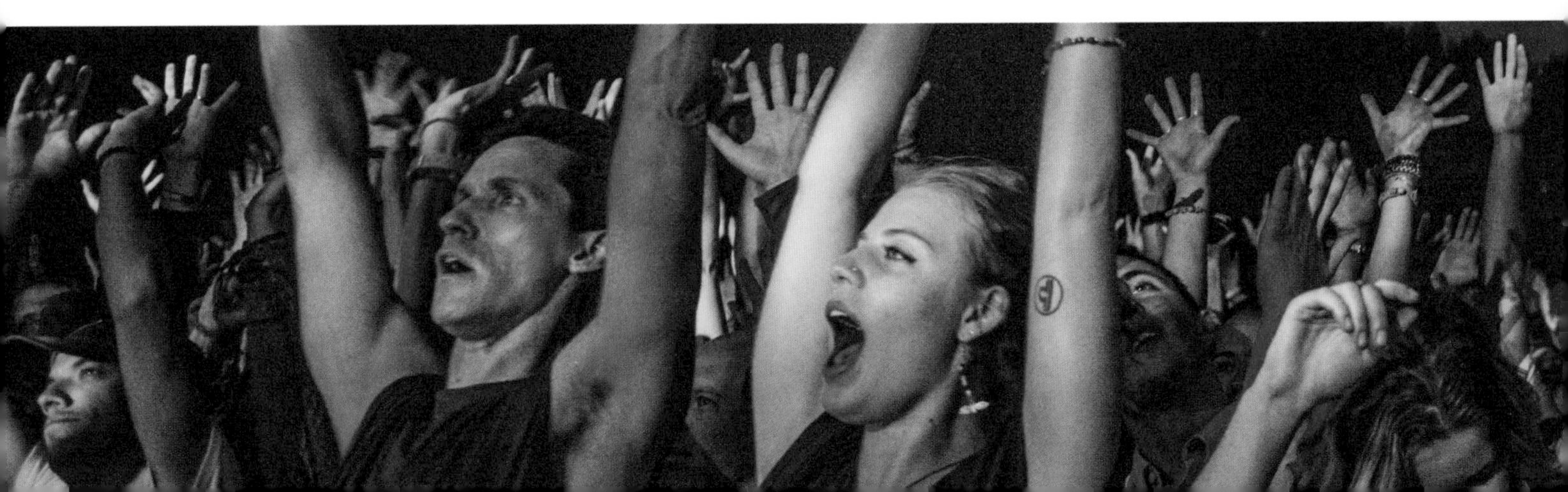

I would gently assess the daily schedule and its particular set of obstacles, knowing that I would practice at least half an hour no matter what. I'd often find myself rolling out my mat while the drums set up and sound checked. What was once an impatient waiting game was now a practice opportunity. Sometimes I'd wind up downward dog in a beer-soaked alley, a bathroom, or a crowded public place. It was easy to keep it up once I started. The reason being that I always felt better after.

When I gave in to the varying circumstances life presented every day and still found a way to practice, my practice became more rooted in the present. Less about forcing a style, length, or duration of time on myself, it became a reflection of what was intelligent and possible at that moment.

Over the years, that approach has stuck with me, especially as pranayama and meditation took root.

In a perfect world, I'd wake up early after a good night's sleep, roll onto the cushion for half an hour, then a good hour of asana. And I wouldn't fantasize about coffee for a second!

In reality, I've often performed the night before, gotten to a nervy sleep at 2:00 a.m., and woken up with just enough time to get completely freaked out on coffee and Internet and make it out the door without forgetting my passport. On those days, I might do pranayama and meditation sitting in a van or an airplane, and perhaps my muscles are sore and jangly and I opt for some Yin poses and a bath instead of the usual chaturangas.

I don't always practice as much as I'd like; sometimes I fall off my meditation for days at a time, but the approach that I've adapted to is about being flexible with myself. I'm able to maintain physical and contemplative practices over the long term because I've figured out how to meet myself where I truly am, and letting that guide the way I practice.

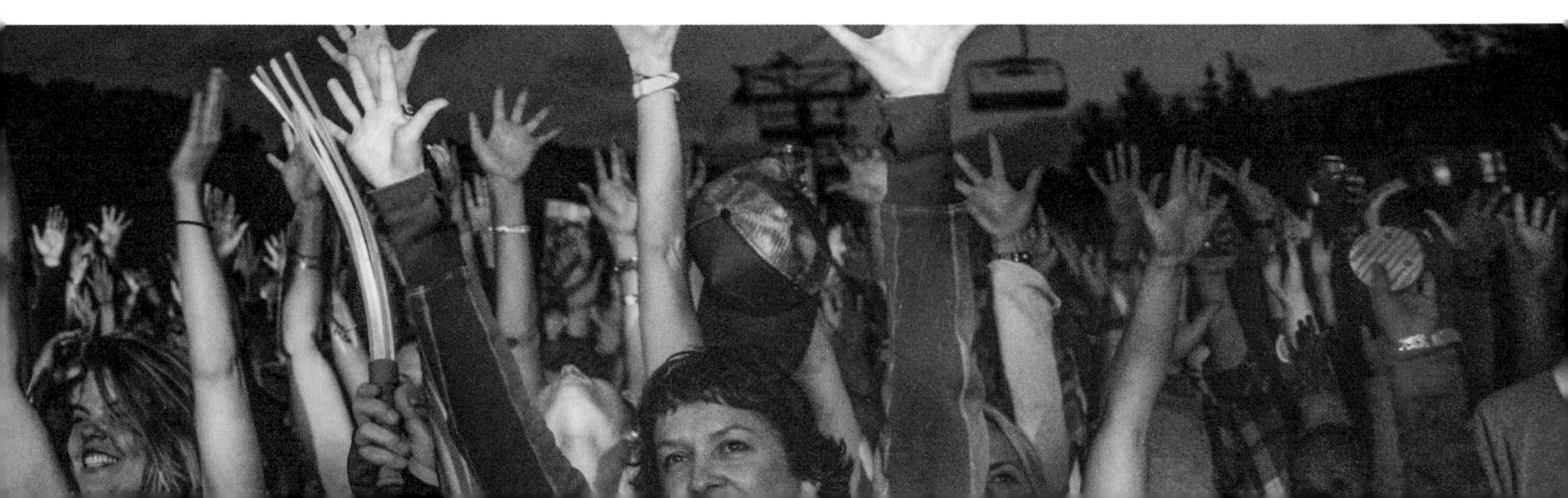

find your practice

SARAH NEUFELD

wave one *check in*

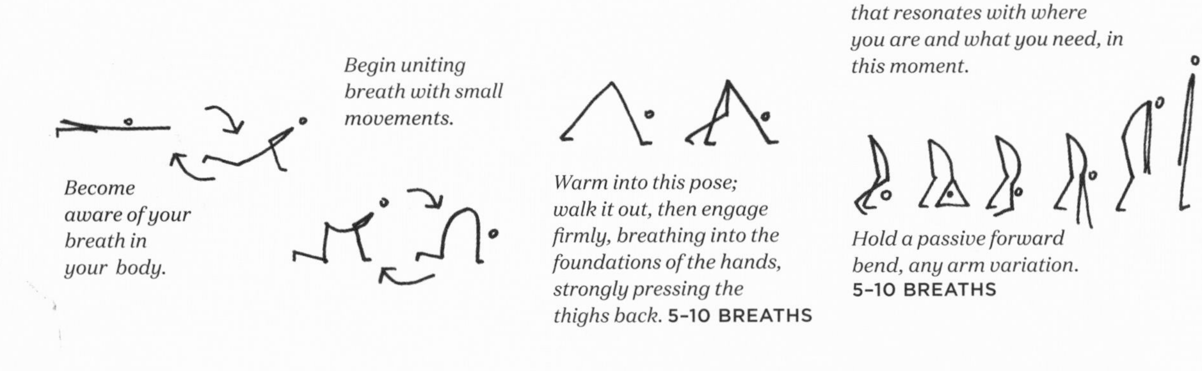

Become aware of your breath in your body.

Begin uniting breath with small movements.

Warm into this pose; walk it out, then engage firmly, breathing into the foundations of the hands, strongly pressing the thighs back. 5–10 BREATHS

In TADASANA, *set an intention that resonates with where you are and what you need, in this moment.*

Hold a passive forward bend, any arm variation. 5–10 BREATHS

wave two *get the blood moving*

No matter what your surroundings, relish in this moment.

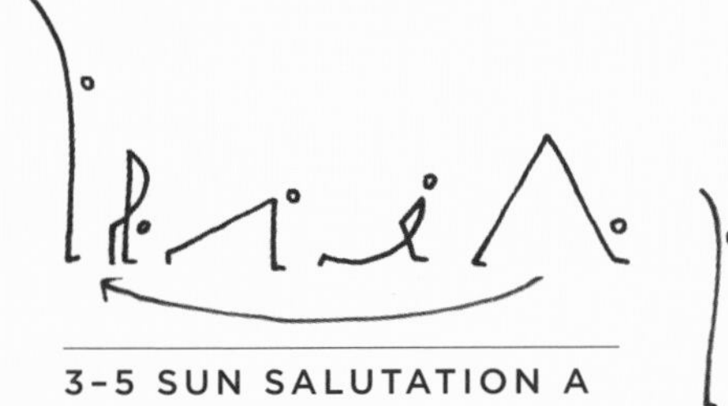

3–5 SUN SALUTATION A

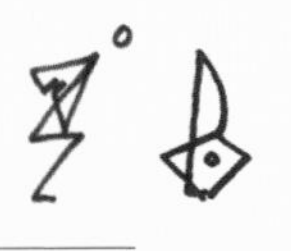

Both left and right sides

Feel how fantastic it is to be alive in your body!

3–5 SUN SALUTATION B

WARRIOR SEQUENCE

Challenge yourself to keep the breath slow and steady. Stay rooted in the inner and outer edges of the feet.

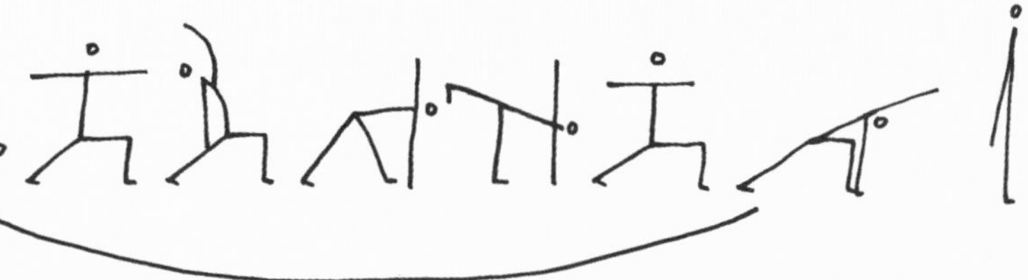

End in TADASANA.

Hold each pose in this sequence, as well as the final downward dog for 3–5 BREATHS.

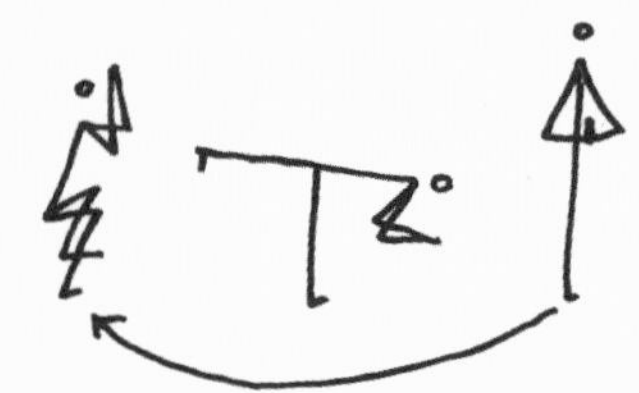

LIZARD POSE

Lean back for an optional twist and thigh opener.

Balance expression with containment.

DANCER'S POSE *Drop the hip of the lifted leg, and stay lifted through the standing leg/hip.* **5 BREATHS**

OR **STANDING FIGURE FOUR POSE**

1 MINUTE *with any arm variation*

wave three *ground down*

Pulse between **NAVASANA** *and* **ARDHA NAVASANA** **10X** *and lower to the floor.*

5 BREATHS
Repeat **2X.**

WINDSHIELD WIPER LEGS

THREAD THE NEEDLE

Both left and right sides

PASCHIMOTTANASANA
Feel the effort in the legs more than the upper body. Root the thigh bones into your body.

Both left and right sides

Choose third eye or heart as point of focus to watch the breath.

Practice Playlist
compiled by Sarah Neufeld

- **Saku**—*Susumu Yokota*
- **Peacock Tail**—*Boards of Canada*
- **Xtal**—*Aphex Twin*
- **Nine Black Alps**—*Helios*
- **Familiar**—*Nils Frahm*
- **Dungtitled (In A Major)**—*Stars of the Lid*
- **All Farewells Are Sudden**—*A Winged Victory for the Sullen*

Just as the explorers of old documented their experiences and discoveries, keeping a journal on your practice and life will allow you to capture pivotal moments of change and discovery. This will support and enhance your yoga practice and illuminate your voyage in hindsight.

Journal to track your trip while building a self-made souvenir of your journey to reflect on later.

Journaling is the act of tapping into your stream of consciousness—where there is no right or wrong—just find your flow.

Your Journal Pages

DURATION
Anytime

LOCATION
Anywhere

MINDSET
Exploratory

TOOLS
This book or a separate journal + muse (aka you)

STEPS

1. Use the page here to track your thoughts, dreams, insights. If you need more room, you can also go out and hunt for a journal you love. Make a day trip to bookstores, paperies, and shops to find a hidden gem. Go on instinct: Seek out the colors, textures, and sizes that speak to you. (If you're not 100 percent in love with how it looks, decorate it!) If you're using our journal page here, feel free to write outside the given lines.

2. Commit to writing in your journal for five minutes every morning and after your yoga practice. Notice how yoga practice can change your mindset. Designate time for writing but also keep your book with you in case inspiration hits randomly, while you're stuck in traffic or grabbing coffee.

SOME THINGS TO CONSIDER

- You are mapping your journey, so include as many details as possible, like writing down quotes that speak to you, or make a collage of pictures, business cards, flyers, or magazine clippings that catch your eye. You can also draw, paint, paste, or press plants: Record and remember the details of your journey that burn bright.

- Be consistent and persistent!

- Keep track of your progress and pitfalls in all honesty, without censor.

This is a practice in self-expression that will capture the essence of the journey you have just started. Within the pages of your travel log you will find clarity and insight, so trust your intuitive voice, unlock your creativity, and play!

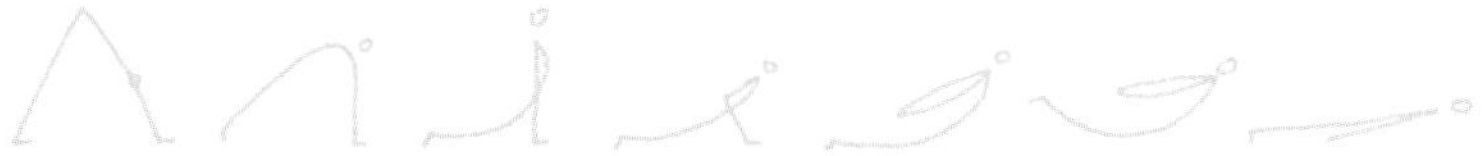

In the long run men hit only what they aim at.

—Henry David Thoreau

CHAPTER 2

find your direction

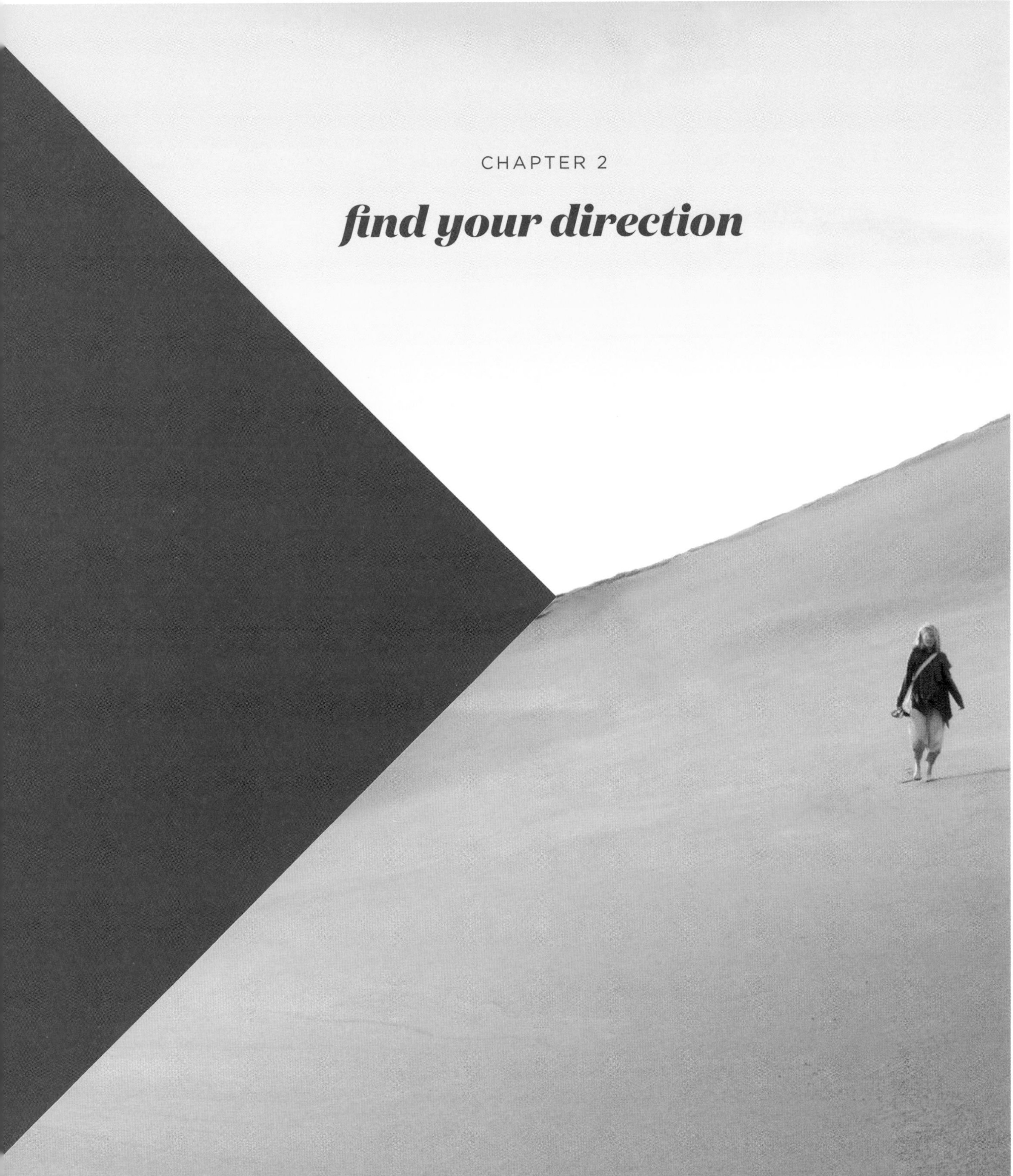

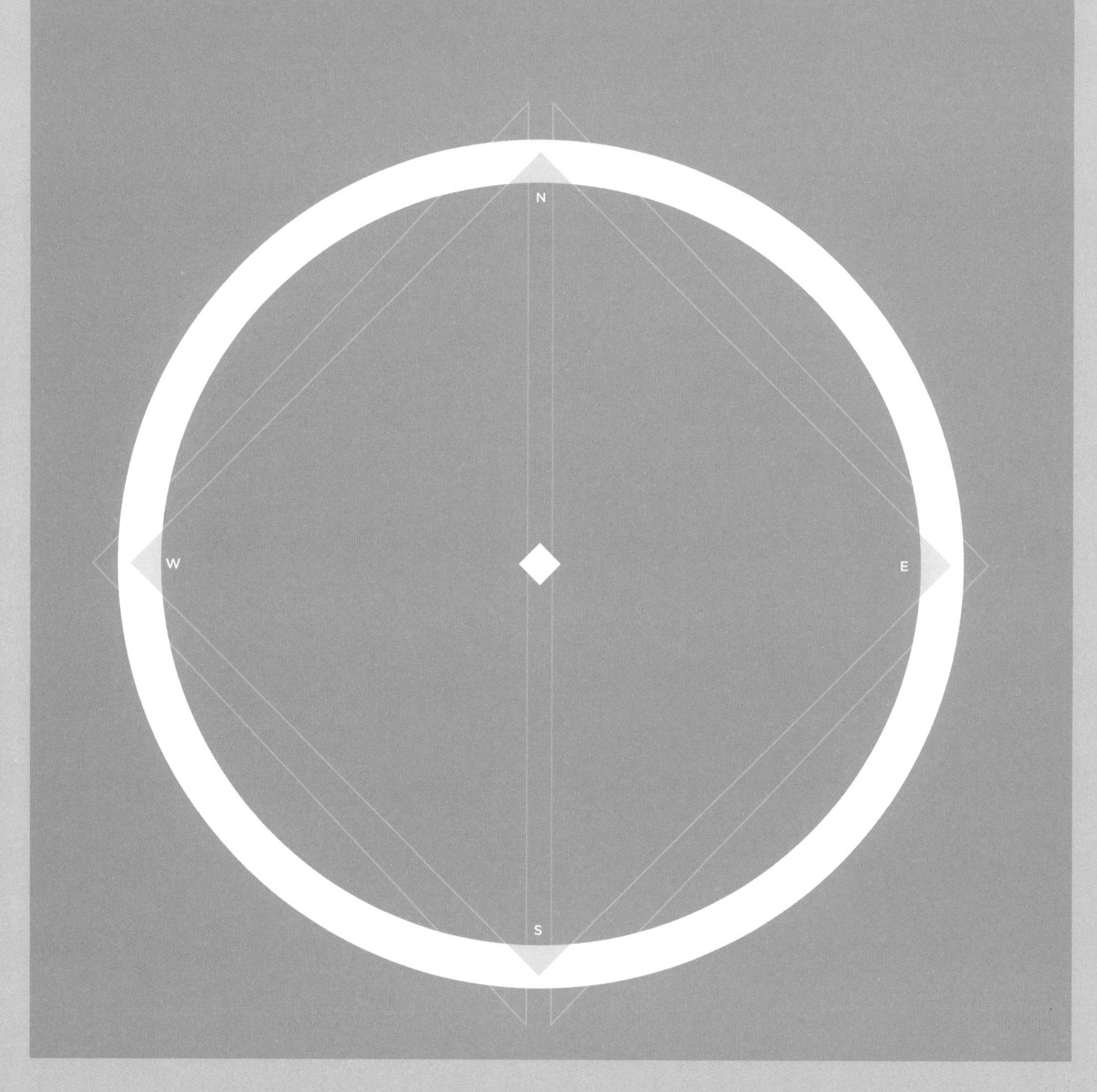
CHECK YOUR COMPASS
SARAH HERRINGTON
N
W
E
S

Start where you are, take a good look around, then explore. Radiate outward, with love and curiosity. Face your fears—don't be afraid to fall or look foolish. Know that going within is just as much a journey as climbing Mount Everest. Yogis are, above all, seekers, using the map of the body, the wisdom-gift of the breath, the lineage of texts that came before us as guideposts along the trail to truth. When you get into the spirit, finding a "right" direction becomes less important than yielding to the Wanderlust, the joy of the travel that is life.

Here, teachers are guides, introducing us to the maps within and without, in the present moment via the breath and the past in ancient texts. We call forth what we desire through manifestation and what qualities we need symbolized by the deities. We explore what is tight and what is loose and aim to find a balance in mind, body, and spirit.

On a journey, question unfolds unto question, in the mountains or in the heart.

When you get into the spirit, adventure becomes more important than any set answer. And, often, as soon as you let go of the utter need to know your destination and begin to enjoy the ride, poof! There, you've found it, your center, your unpuzzling, what you were hoping and loving toward all along.

So get your symbolic hiking shoes on, your nonperishable snacks, your inner-self flashlights: We're going on an adventure of supreme discovery within.

Here you are, at the beginning. Within five years your life could be unimaginably different. You will still be you. You will still be recognizable, but everything can be vastly unlike what it is today. You want to be sure you're moving in the direction you desire.

It takes time to change. But know that here, right now, is the place to start.

Let's use three questions as guides toward creating the future:

WHAT DO YOU WANT?

It is a question that is asked to us forty thousand times a day by marketers in advertisements, and another 565 times every time we scroll through our online feeds. It encompasses feelings, as well as things, moments, and relationships. It captures every possible desire. What is your next purchase? What do you want your home to look and feel like? How much money do you want to make? What kind of relationship do you want to have? What do the perfect moments with your friends, family, and partner involve?

The question of what do you want is at the center of Western civilization and we know it well. It is inescapable but it is also powerful.

Don't try to want less right now. Often we feel like we aren't allowed to want because of what it would mean to get it, and who we would have to be. I give you permission right now to ignore that voice.

Give in for a few minutes. Let yourself want everything.

So what do you want? What inspires you? When did you last feel envy for something or someone? What are things that you imagine will bring you moments of happiness?

Write it all down.

If you build a life after only asking this one question, you could easily be misguided; but with these next two questions we will move toward true north.

The second question is important but rarely asked with as much depth as the first question:

WHAT PATH DO YOU WALK?

If you don't ask this question, your path will choose itself based solely on your answers to "What do you want?" The path that chooses itself is often the one that seems quickest or that we have heard about or seen others take. If your desire is endless money, then the path that is easiest or most visible is that of the banker or businessperson running around frenetically, stressed, sacrificing family, time, and happiness for money. This is the easiest and most visible path, but it does not mean it is the only one. You end up on this path because money is on your want list but you didn't ask the question, What path do you want to walk?

So I invite you to reflect. What path do you want to walk? What does the process of your life look like? How long are your days? What do you spend your time thinking about? What are your home and work space like? How do you spend your time? How does creativity fit into your days? What role do your relationships have in your daily routine and when things are challenging?

These questions will help bring color and detail to the path you want to live. We use tools like Facebook, Pinterest, and our journals or scrapbooks to visualize our wants, but rarely do we use them to visualize our path. They work for both. Choose the tool you use currently to help you visualize your wants and apply it to the path you want to walk.

The third and final question is:

HOW CAN OUR CHOSEN PATH HELP US GET WHAT WE WANT?

The human mind can't help but put disparate ideas together. It intuitively finds commonalities and has the capacity to bring two competing interests into synergy. Trust that your mind can find the connection toward your goal and the path you specifically need to get there.

On your path, you will face obstacles, initially. The critical voice in your head will say, “Well, that is not reality, reality works like X, not like Y.” That voice is showing you the easiest and most visible path, the path that you would default to if you didn’t ask all three questions. Challenge yourself. Begin searching for answers out in the world. Look for models and mentors that typify just one piece of your united path/want list. As you begin to search, you will start to build a portfolio of real stories, real people, and real experiences that prove to you it is possible.

It is possible to get the things that you want and walk the path that provides happiness along the way. It takes time and it starts now. Here you are, at the beginning.

WHAT DO YOU WANT?

WHAT PATH DO YOU WANT TO WALK?

HOW CAN OUR CHOSEN PATH HELP US GET WHAT WE WANT?

KEVIN COURTNEY

The Five Sheaths

Human beingness, the yogis discovered, is a multidimensional, multisensory experience. Contained within our physical forms is a richly layered landscape that interrelates to make us who we are. Yogis called these layers of beingness "koshas" or sheaths. They were described in part in the Taittiriya Upanishad around the sixth century BCE.

ANNAMAYA KOSHA

Physical Sheath

The most obvious aspect of our being is the physical body. It is no surprise, then, that this is where the yogic exploration began. As students of the body, ancient yogis practiced asana to tone, strengthen, and detoxify the physical layer in order to prepare it for sustained periods of concentration and reflection. What we eat, drink, read, and watch becomes increasingly important as the yoga process unfolds. As the yogis examined the physical self, all of the other layers begin to reveal themselves.

PRANAMAYA KOSHA

Energetic Sheath

Even a brief study of the physical body will reveal that there is more to it than what is on the surface. Although our bones, flesh, and vital fluids are all essential aspects of the physical sheath, there is another essential part of our makeup that is indisputable. If you study the body of one who is living, and compare it to one who is dead, it becomes clear there is something beyond just the physical trappings that animates us into being. This vital energy, this life force, is often understood and visualized as the breath. Those who practice pranayama (which translates to extension/control of the life force, or prana, through breathing practices) can experience for themselves the profundity of this sheath, as altered states of awareness and physical sensations arise. Yes, you are made of the physical body, but also the pranic (energetic) body.

VIJNANAMAYA KOSHA

Witness Sheath

Through self-study, it becomes evident that there is an aspect of our being that is simply awareness itself. This is the self that watches. The ability to observe our physical, mental, and emotional selves, as we do in reflection, meditation, or asana practice, implies this faculty of attention. This sheath is the seat of our witness consciousness, the discerning body that is beyond the power of thought found in the previous sheath. It is an unwavering flame that can be used to illuminate all of the others.

MANAMAYA KOSHA

Mental/Emotional Sheath

This sheath describes our mental and emotional selves, encompassing our ego/personality and all of our fluctuations of thoughts and feelings. Without objective awareness of this layer of our being, this sheath has perhaps the most control over our lives. It is the seat of the small "I," the self an unrealized individual believes himself or herself to be.

Any stimuli from the first two sheaths will most likely be noticed by the manamaya kosha; commented upon, judged, and processed; and then stored somewhere in our consciousness, helping us further define our own identity. ("I am a dog-lover; a tomato-hater; a person who is afraid of heights; someone who seeks adventure," and so on, and on, ad infinitum.)

Although an unexamined manamaya kosha can be a pitfall in one's spiritual development, when one does turn the light of awareness onto this sheath, the ability to witness patterns, thoughts, and deep emotions can lead to an increase of understanding, self-knowledge, and personal growth that allows one to live a more joyful and liberated life.

ANANDAMAYA KOSHA

Bliss Sheath

As a manifestation of pure consciousness itself, the core of our being is understood to be bliss. Although bliss is our underlying, innate nature, most of us in this lifetime must extend effort to observe, experience, and harmonize all of our other sheaths in order to return to the profundity of this essential state.

TO FIND OUR TRUE NORTH, WE MUST SALUTE THE SOUTH

SARA ELIZABETH IVANHOE

Sometimes we want to get out of our head and just practice our yoga. Other times we want to study and learn what is behind it.

"Where did yoga come from? Why was this pose invented? How has the practice changed over time? How might I do it better?"

It is helpful to see what others have done in the past, and to build on their knowledge. As we cook up yoga's future, it is helpful to see what is in the recipes of the past.

The first evidence we have of yoga was found in the Indus River Valley in northwestern India and dates back several thousands of years BCE.

The oldest yogic texts are called the *vedas* (meaning "knowledge"). These texts have a disputed date of 3000 BCE and were passed on through oral tradition for years until the written word was invented. Not only are the vedas the earliest recorded yoga text, they are some of the oldest written words—period.

Following the *vedas* are the *Upanishads,* which are a series of stories in the form of the "teacher-to-student" dialogue. These are where we get our first comprehensible definition of the word *yoga*.

"Tat twam asi 'Thou art That' (Union between the individual soul [Atman] and the Infinite [Brahman])"

—Chandogya Upanishad

The individual merging into the Infinite is best described as a wave in the ocean. The wave is born, and all it sees are other waves and feels these other waves are separate. But things are not as they seem. The wave is simply the ocean in *specific expression.* Once the life of the wave is over, it goes back to being the ocean. It was *always* the ocean. The Upanishads teach us that we are all ocean *(Brahman)* in specific expression *(Atman).* As yogis, it is our job to see past the obvious—to remember this true nature.

Several thousands of years later, we get the more popular definition of yoga.

YOGAS CHITTA VRITTA NIRODHANA

"Yoga is the cessation of the fluctuations of the mind."

—Patanjali's "Yoga Sutras" 1.2

The system of *Raja* (Royal) yoga had been practiced for many years, but it wasn't until Patanjali recorded his yoga sutras (disputed 400 BCE–300 CE), that the practice was canonized.

Hundreds of years later, *asana* emerged as its own path called *Hatha* yoga. Roughly one hundred years ago, yoga came to America. In the last forty to fifty years, yoga has spread across major cities as a form of healthy lifestyle. In the last twenty years, yoga has begun to explode into a practice done by millions of people of every race, religion, and gender—in every country, every sport, every business, and every type of educational institution. It is only about 20 years ago that the Internet was even created and only a little more than 10 years ago that social media was invented—and then dominated.

It's not really possible to do justice to more than five thousand years of yoga history. But as we step into being trailblazers of the future, we can gather valuable tools by observing our past. As you embark on your journey to find your true north—take a moment to salute the south.

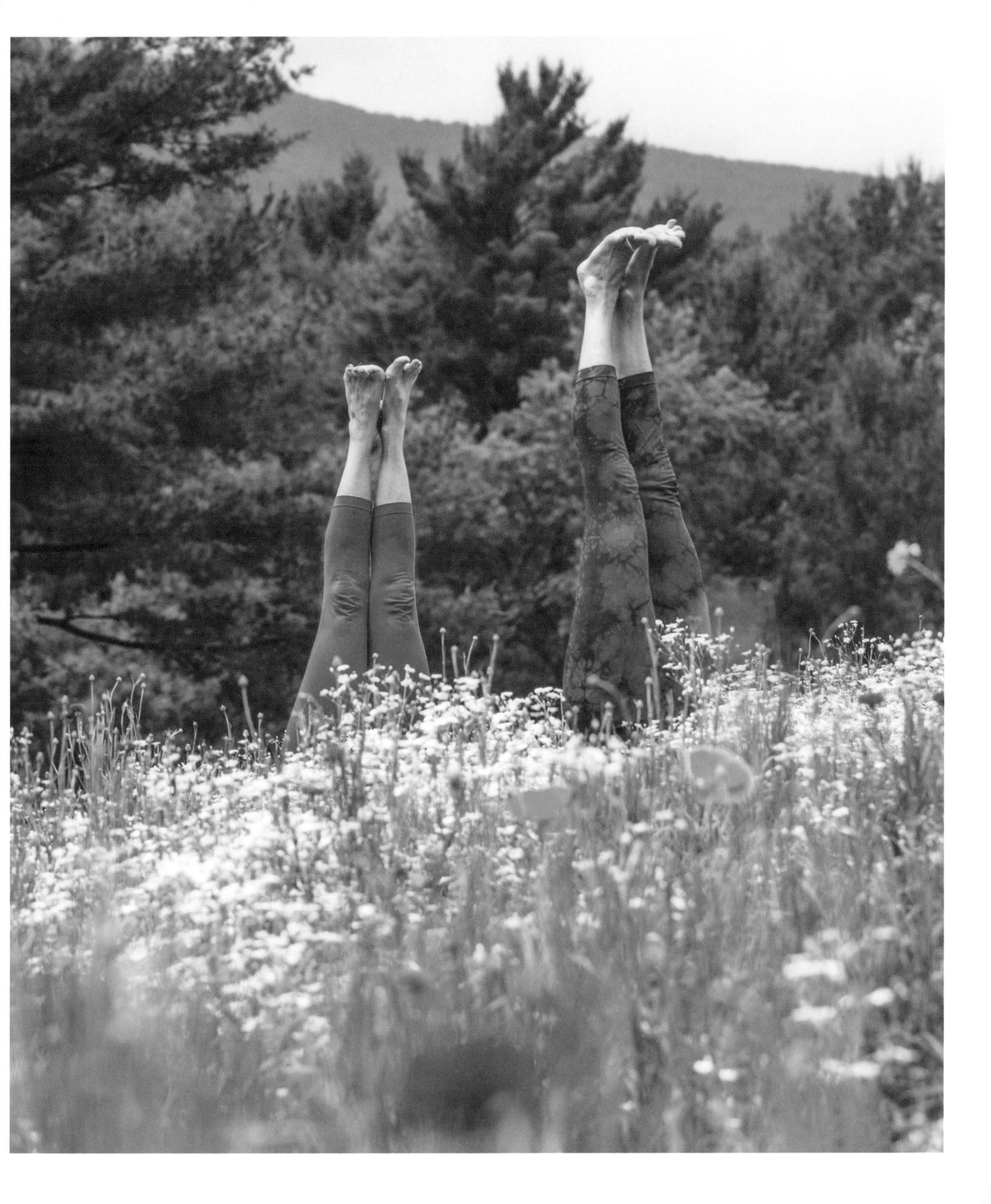

THE FOUR MARGAS: A MAP OF THE ROAD

You don't have to do yoga poses to be a yogi! There are four traditional paths (margas) *that lead to* **moksha**, *or liberation. You may find that while the physical practice supports your physical health, the other methods speak to your heart, your curiosity, or your morality. Can we really say that a nurse is not a yogi? A farmer? A musician? A creator of breakthrough technology? Yoga itself is flexible.*

The word ***karma*** comes from the Sanskrit root "kri" which means "action." *Karma* yoga is the path of selfless service and doing good work without attachment to the result of your action.

KARMA

JŇANA

moksha

RAJA

HATHA

BHAKTI

The word ***jňana*** means "wisdom" or "learning." *Jňana* yoga is experiencing union through a course of study (like what you are doing right now—reading!).

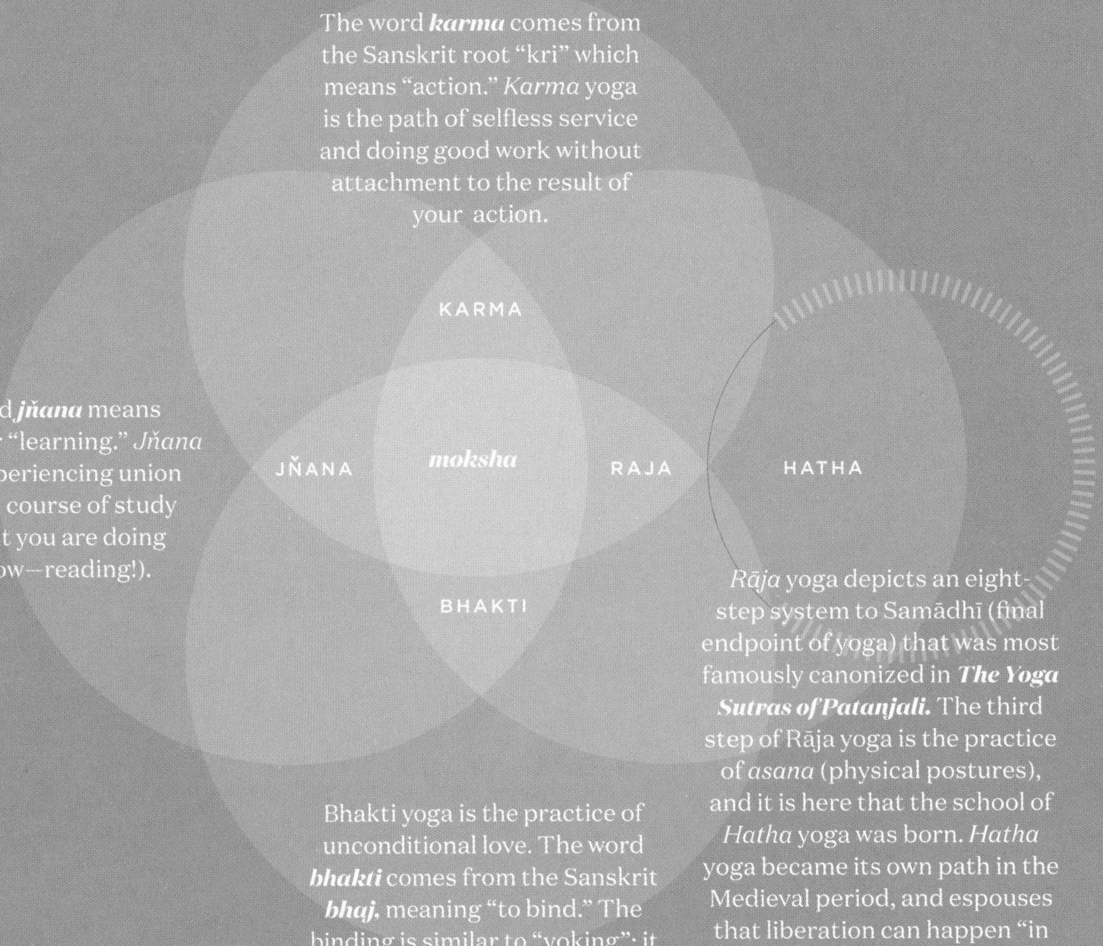

Rāja yoga depicts an eight-step system to Samādhī (final endpoint of yoga) that was most famously canonized in ***The Yoga Sutras of Patanjali.*** The third step of Rāja yoga is the practice of *asana* (physical postures), and it is here that the school of *Hatha* yoga was born. *Hatha* yoga became its own path in the Medieval period, and espouses that liberation can happen "in this body, in this lifetime."

Bhakti yoga is the practice of unconditional love. The word ***bhakti*** comes from the Sanskrit ***bhaj,*** meaning "to bind." The binding is similar to "yoking"; it refers to coming together and focuses on using unconditional love as a tool for liberation.

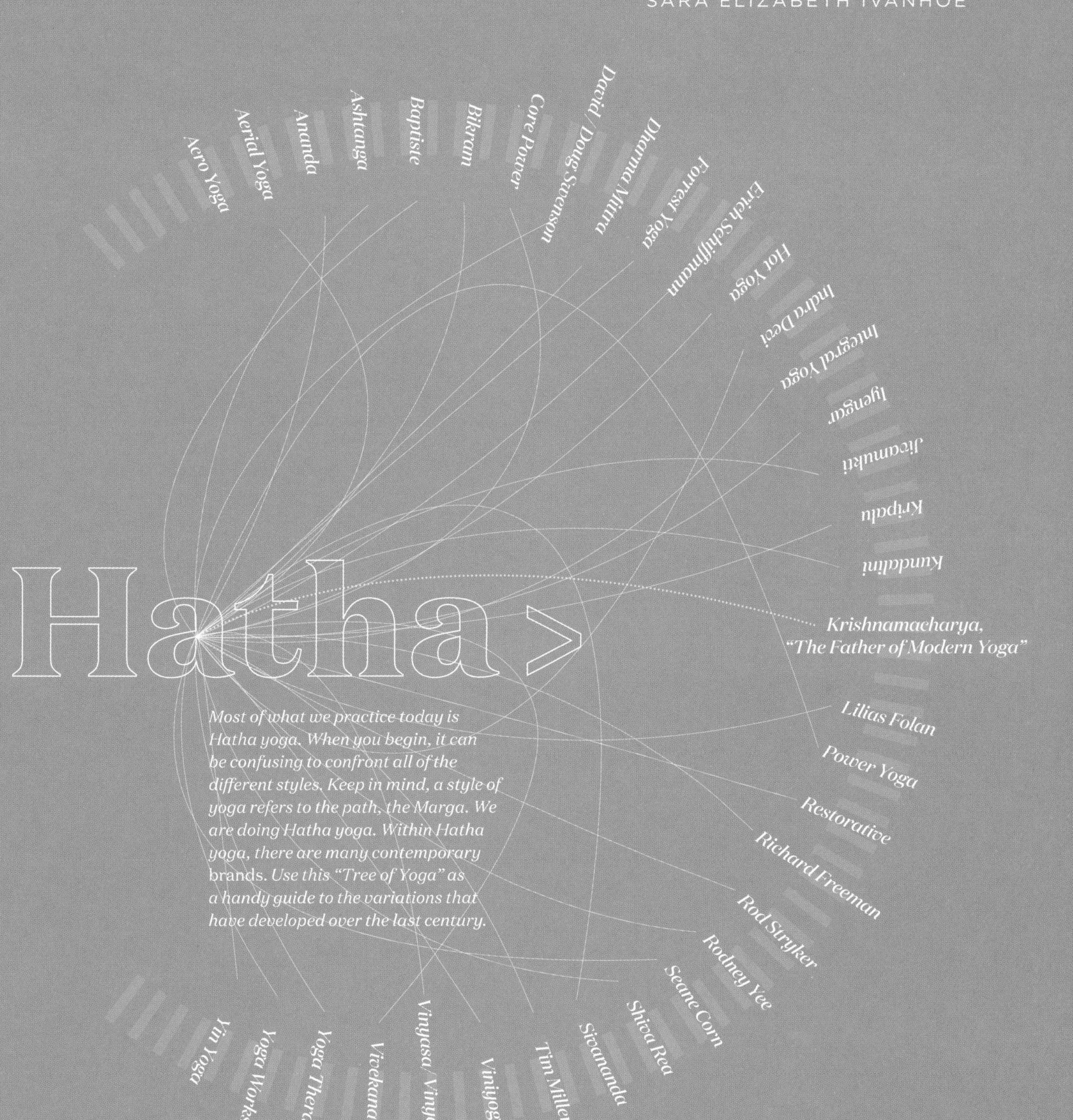

Most of what we practice today is Hatha yoga. When you begin, it can be confusing to confront all of the different styles. Keep in mind, a style of yoga refers to the path, the Marga. We are doing Hatha yoga. Within Hatha yoga, there are many contemporary brands. Use this "Tree of Yoga" as a handy guide to the variations that have developed over the last century.

SALUTING THE LINEAGE: "THE FATHER OF MODERN YOGA" TIRUMALAI KRISHNAMACHARYA

Krishnamacharya

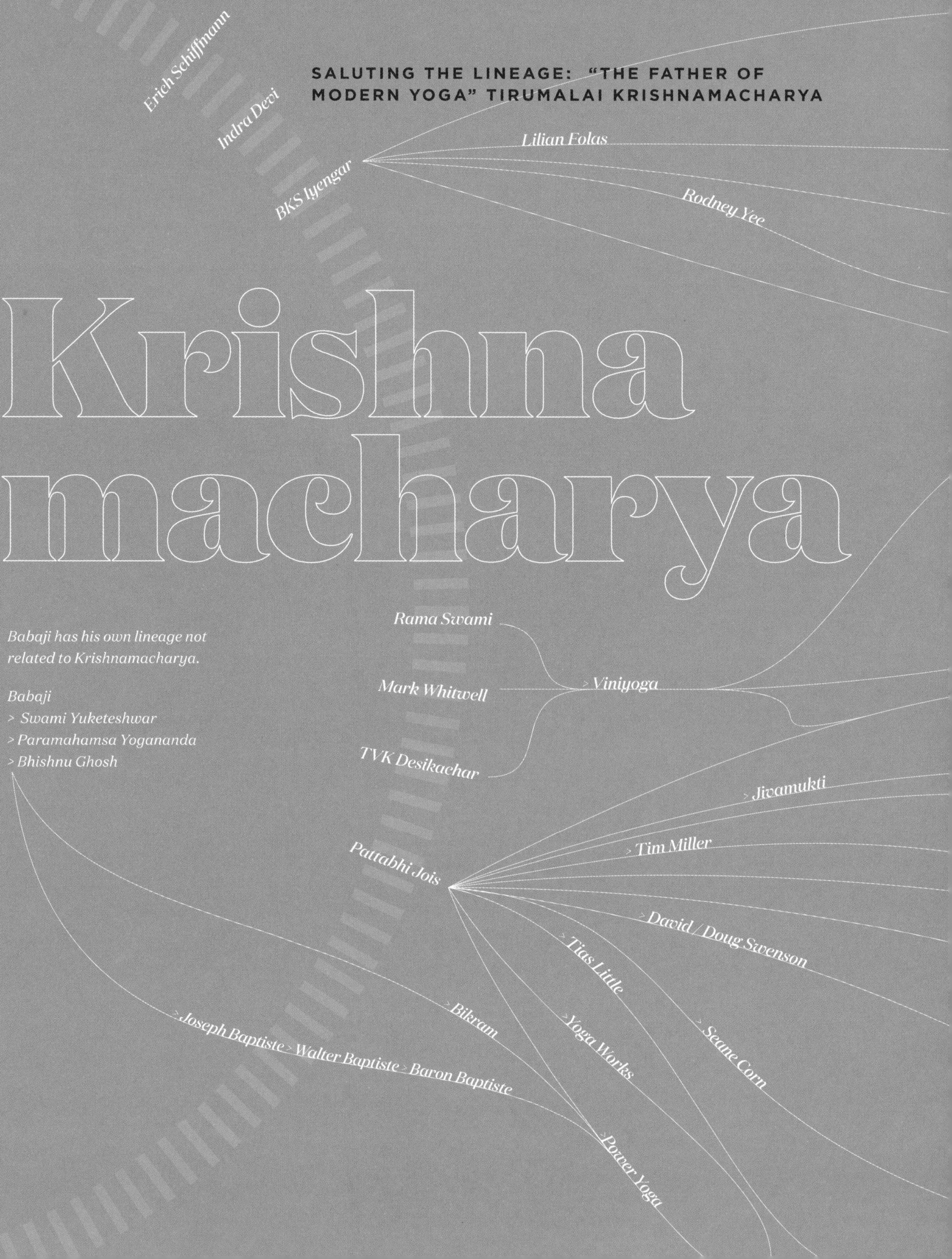

Erich Schiffmann

Indra Devi

BKS Iyengar

Lilian Folas

Rodney Yee

Rama Swami

Mark Whitwell

TVK Desikachar

> Viniyoga

Babaji has his own lineage not related to Krishnamacharya.

Babaji
> Swami Yuketeshwar
> Paramahamsa Yogananda
> Bhishnu Ghosh

Pattabhi Jois

> Jivamukti

> Tim Miller

> David / Doug Swenson

> Tias Little

> Seane Corn

> Yoga Works

> Bikram

> Joseph Baptiste > Walter Baptiste > Baron Baptiste

> Power Yoga

Bernard Rishi

SARA ELIZABETH IVANHOE

Restorative

> Yoga Therapy > Larry Payne

> Gary Kraftkow

> Vinyasaa / Vinyasa Flow

> Bryan / Johnny Kest

> Core Power

> Shiva Rea

Born on November 18, 1888, Krishnamacharya is thought by many to be the reason that we practice yoga today. His teachings have spread throughout the entire world, and many modern forms of yoga can ultimately be traced back to him through his various students, including the now well-known and widely respected teachers T. K. V. Desikachar, B. K. S. Iyengar, Pattabhi Jois, Indra Devi, Erich Schiffman, Mark Whitwell, and Ramaswami.

Krishnamacharya focused on tailoring the practice of yoga to each student individually and encouraged his students to honor their own perception of *Isvara* (God). He refused to be called a "Yoga Master," and referred to himself only as a student, emphasizing the focus on continued learning.

The significance of Krishnamacharya reminds us that we are part of a vast tradition that has been in existence for thousands of years and will be around long after we are gone.

If you have learnt something really well, then the way you express it will not be the same way you learned it.

—Krishnamacharya

THE SUTRA COMPASS

The yoga sutras were written down by Patanjali, a sage who is said to have lived in India 1,700 years ago. While yoga certainly existed before him, he was the first to codify it in this way, in a four-chapter book made up of 195 aphorisms, or sutras. In a thoughtfully systematic and concise way, the text offers insight into the goal of yoga, its many practices, and the time-tested results practitioners can expect when they dedicate themselves with sincerity and devotion to the practice.

The sutras sit at the center of an entire school of yoga called raja yoga. *Raja* translates to "royal union" and focuses on the cultivation of the mind. Raja yoga is concerned with philosophy, meditation, and contemplation while hatha yoga often takes a more physical approach, with the asanas as a technology unto themselves designed to open up fields of awareness. In raja yoga, texts and teachings show us the way.

It's important to notice that nowhere in yoga are we asked to blindly accept teachings as truth. We have the compass from those who came before, but walk the path on our own, in our way.

SUTRA 1.1

Atha Yoga Nushasanam

Now the Exposition on Yoga Begins

The entire Yoga Sutra text begins with the word *now*.

"Now" implies that we have finally arrived; that here we are, ready to begin. But it also alludes to the complexity of what it's like to actually come into the present moment.

To be present requires tuning in to the current state of the mind, feeling into the physiological state of the body, and sensing the emotional condition of the heart.

The present moment is filled with limitless feedback that moves us in so many directions. As soon as we tune in, we may be pulled away! The five senses, which are tools, can also distract. A smell, for example, can evoke many memories. Even if you stopped reading to look around right now, you'd notice so many things that make you think and feel other things.

But "now" is the gateway to the heart.

Right away the text asks us to become more receptive, more awake to what's actually going on inside ourselves (not what we wish were happening but what actually is). This can be intimidating. You never know what may come up, anything from traumas to blissful memories. To sit quietly, relax, and breathe into the present moment is one of the strongest gateways to understanding and revealing what truly lies at the core of one's own being.

SUTRA 1.2

Yoga Chitta Vritti Nirodha

Yoga Is the Stilling of the Movements of the Mind

Yoga is the means and the end. This is to say that we use the practices of yoga to experience the state of yoga. To establish the quiet state of mind necessary for insight to naturally arise in the present moment, we must create the right conditions. In the second sutra, those conditions are explained.

Sutra 1.2 says:

As the mind calms and the sway of the ego subsides, with the intellect becoming like a steady unwavering candle, a state of stillness emerges and a state of union with all the aspects of our being is experienced.

Obviously, quieting the mind is no small task, but the rest of the yoga sutra is loaded with clues, insights, and ways to approach the practice and achieve this state of being. And if you go back to the original inquiry into finding your true north, take note that presented in these first two sutras are essential tools for finding it: coming into the now and stilling the noise of the mind.

You may sit with these first two sutras for a long time, returning to them time and again. Their meaning will unfold differently each time you read them, as with each reading you are a slightly different person in a different place or situation in life.

When you are ready for more, the text goes on to describe what we can expect as we go inward, and presents several practical tools, philosophies, and ideas that can help the yoga practice bear fruit.

And just as a knife is sharpened by rubbing against stone, so too is the mind of the practitioner who engages with the teachings presented in *The Yoga Sutras of Patanjali.*

Love as Travel Companion:

Even with such a wonderful guide as the sutras, for an easeful journey inward we need something else: an agreement with ourselves to respond with kindness and respect to what we will find. This agreement is between you and you, and will immediately start revealing deep aspects of how you relate to yourself.

While yoga is a path toward union of body, mind, and spirit, it also remains a direct path to love. Love radiates out from the core of our being when unobstructed, and the practices of yoga remove the obstruction.

WHERE DO YOU WANT TO GO?

ROLF GATES

In my work, I regularly ask people to get clear about who they want to be and what kind of experience they want to have. I challenge people to use their imagination and to take responsibility for creating a future they are excited to live into. I believe that it is only by connecting to an authentic vision that we can access our true potential. But this invariably brings up the following questions:

HOW WE CAN EXPRESS OR EMBODY AN INTENTION WITHOUT FALLING INTO THE TRAP OF ATTACHMENT?

WHAT DOES IT LOOK LIKE WHEN WE BALANCE THE PRACTICE OF MINDFULNESS WITH THE PRACTICE DESCRIBED IN THE YOGA SUTRAS AS AN ORIENTATION TOWARD AN IDEAL?

I once watched two men play racquetball. One worked diligently to make the game happen; the other knew the game was happening and sought only to find his place in it. The first man played very hard and lost most points. The second man played smooth and easy and won most points while appearing to enjoy himself immensely. The second man was embodying the dual practices of mindfulness and intention. He stepped onto the court with a clear intention of who he wanted to be and what kind of experience he wanted to have. He then rested in a state of non-attached enjoyment, finding fulfillment in the game the way a river finds fulfillment vanishing into the ocean.

Yoga teaches us to step into life like this second man, clear about who we wish to be and what kind of experience we want to have while trusting in and vanishing into life's unfolding.

HOW TO FIND YOUR SHERPA

Traditionally, yoga was passed down via word of mouth from teacher to student. The essence of lessons was found not only within the poses but within the teacher/student exchange as well. A good teacher could pay attention to the deep individuality of the student and act as a sort of physician to her or him.

Nowadays, especially in the West, we often have a different approach to learning yoga. Today's teachers often address a whole class of students at once. We can also learn from nontraditional "teachers": books, the Internet, even Skype, or online classes. Some students do seek out one-on-one private sessions.

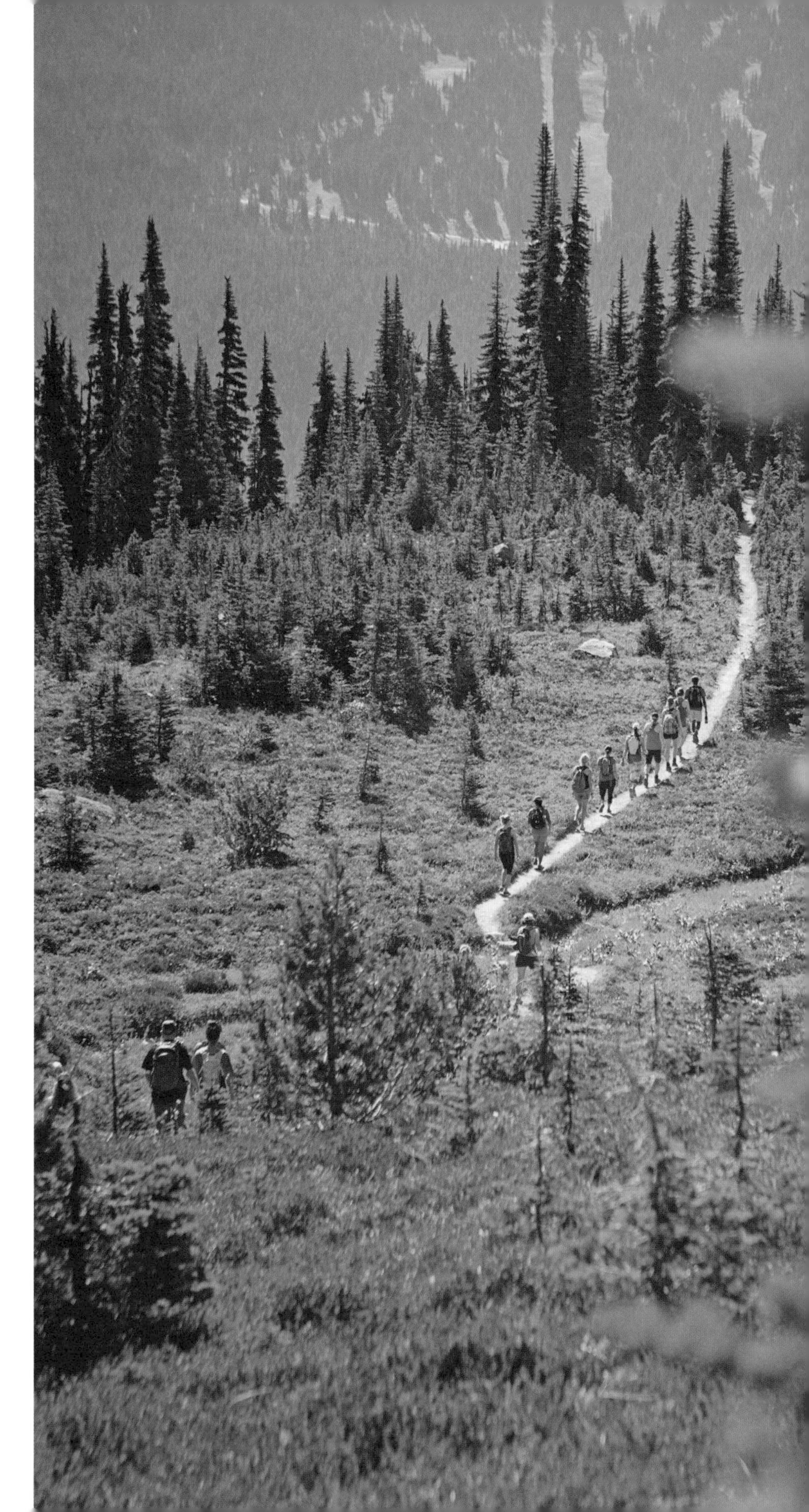

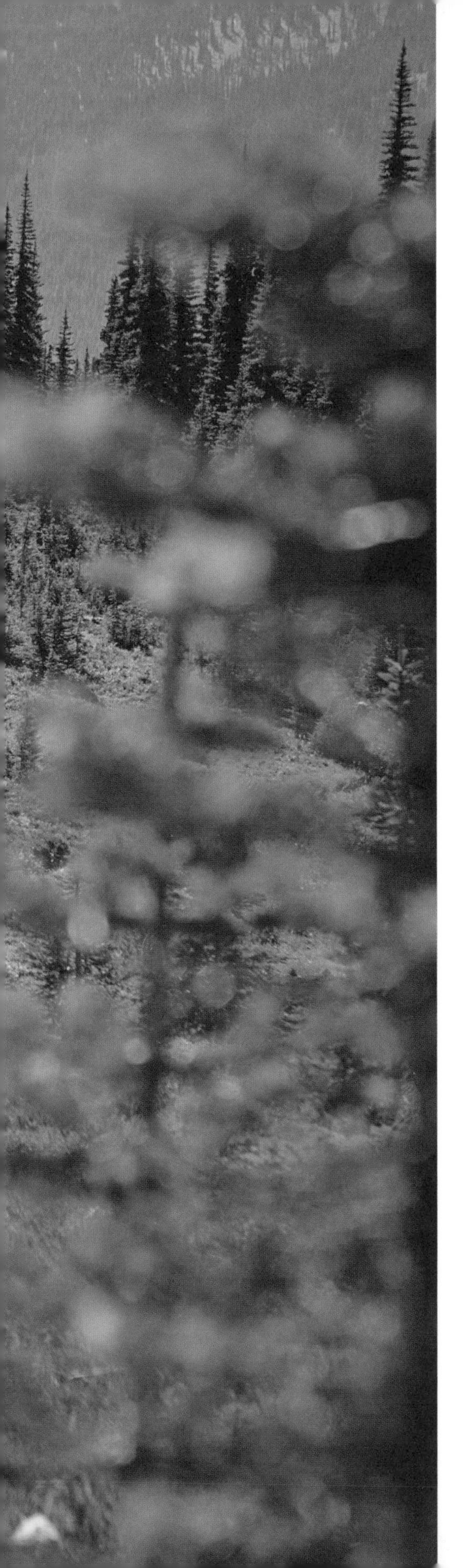

TIFFANY CRUIKSHANK
AND SARAH HERRINGTON

So how do we find someone who resonates with us?

1. **THINK ABOUT YOUR STYLE:**

   Check out the yoga tree and consider what kind of yoga you're hoping to learn right now. And when I say "consider," I mean check in with your mind AND your intuition. Yoga is a practice of listening to the body, after all, and if something inside you is telling you to try Iyengar (even though your mind doesn't know why), listen to it! Seek out a teacher who shares yoga in the style you're drawn toward.

2. **SHE KNOWS AND LIVES BY HER STUFF:**

   Look for someone who is well trained and continues to learn at every opportunity with trainings and workshops. And someone who teaches from her own life and practice is great. Again, yoga doesn't live in the mind but in experience. You want someone who has put in the time on the mat, the meditation cushion, and inside herself. Someone with heart-and-soul experience as well as training.

3. **RESPECT AND LISTENING:**

   Because yoga is a vulnerable practice in many ways (you may feel silly when you first start in the new poses, and you may be out of your comfort zone with things like breath work), you want someone who is respectful, a great listener, and someone you can trust. You want to feel comfortable going to your yoga teacher with all kinds of questions. Yes, you'll be listening a lot when you are the student, but a teacher who really listens will know how to direct and share and be there for you. You also want someone who respects the student/teacher boundary and works to make this a safe, loving, and fun space for you, keeping the focus on what will benefit you in your journey, always being professional. You should feel safe with your teacher, and respect and good boundaries can help with that.

[inhale]

Prāṇāyāma = Sanskrit for "extension of the prāṇa/ life force or breath"

"When breathing in, know that you are breathing in. When breathing out, know that you are breathing out."

These are among the first instructions given to students of mindfulness meditation dating back thousands of years to the Buddha himself.

If you are looking for an entry point to the here-and-now, breath is it. It's always happening in real time. And it carries with it lots of hints and information. Breath reveals our true state or underlying state: If it's short and choppy, you are likely feeling anxious, disturbed. If it's long and deep, you are likely feeling relaxed, calm. In this way, the breath is a mirror of the mind.

The great news is, we can flip the mirror and shift our energy and state of consciousness at will. By changing breath, we can shift mind and emotions. It's a tool, always with us, ever powerful.

Even if you can change nothing else in your circumstance, you can shift the way you're breathing through it.

Be

Notice.

Take a moment now to feel the constant wave of it moving your body, filling you, then emptying out.

It all starts with just observing the breath. Stay focused on the sensation itself and notice that often just by watching closely, we can move toward more peace and stillness. We sense what the great Indian poet Kabir calls "The breath within the breath," in other words, the energy that is moving through us. We are all filled with this prana. We are not separate from the totality of life.

Try

After observing, we can also learn to change the breath. My experience with the following breath practices has taught me that, as yogis, we have the power to change our energy at will. Think of these as devices intended to help you manage your energy and balance your mind. I keep them in my toolbox for optimal living.

Start practicing each breath for three minutes and gradually increase up to eleven minutes or more. Keep a daily journal of the practice so you can record your experiences.

Slow It Down

LONG, DEEP BREATHING: We breathe an average of sixteen to twenty-two times per minute. When consciously breathing deeply, we can do as few as four breaths or less. The deeper we breathe, the more relaxed we get.

Inhale through the nose, expanding first the lower lungs and abdominal cavity, then the midchest area, and finally the clavicle and upper chest in a smooth sequence. Exhale and empty the lungs in reverse, first the clavicle and upper chest, then the midchest, and then the lower lungs. This is also sometimes called "Three-Part Breath."

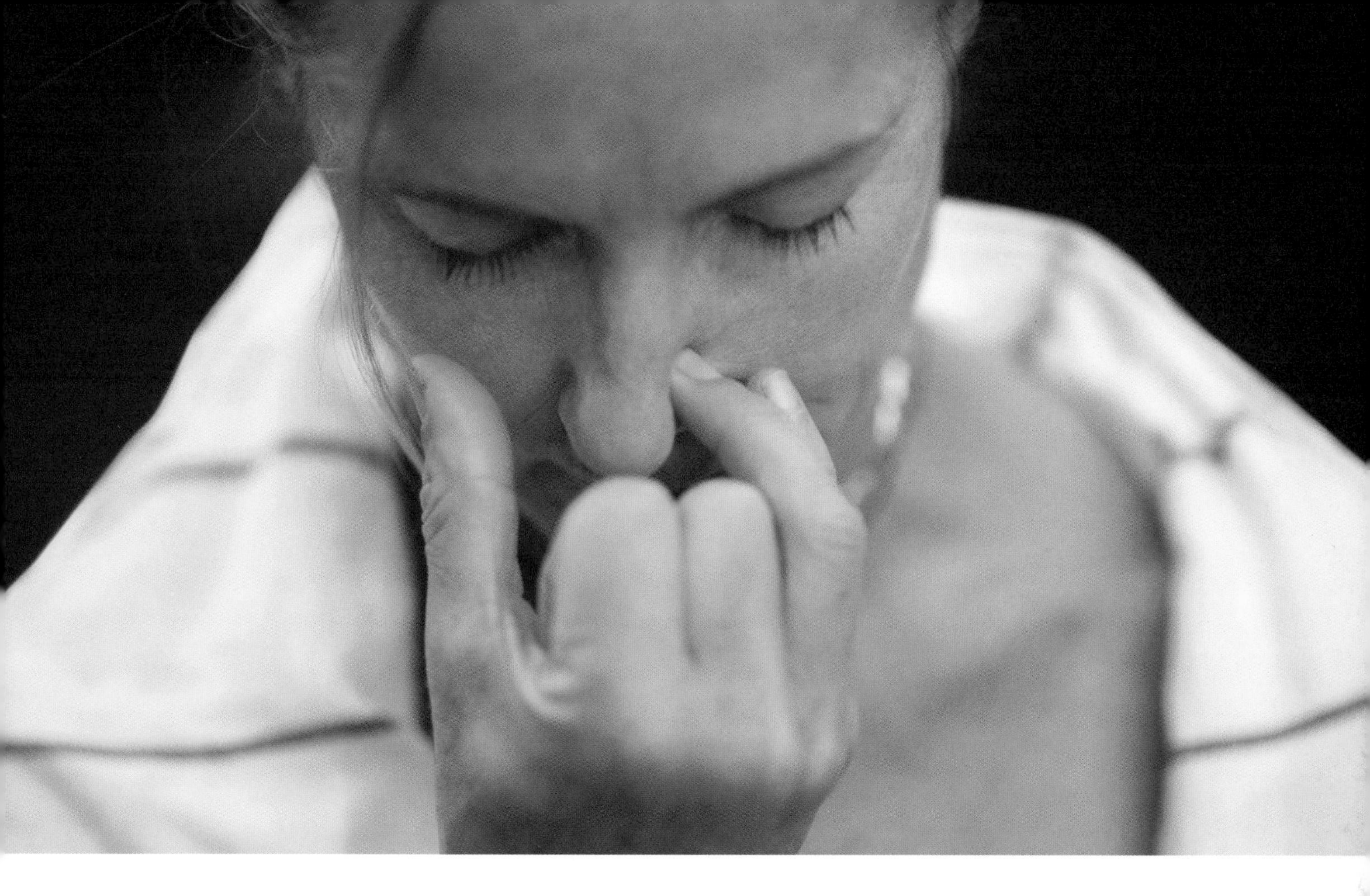

CHOOSE: You can try breathing through one nostril at a time for certain effects.

LEFT NOSTRIL BREATHING: Sit in easy pose. Block the right nostril with the thumb of the right hand, and take twenty-six long, deep breaths through the left nostril. This breath helps to reduce anxiety and nervousness and takes you out of an overly analytical state to a more creative right-brain space. It also helps to reduce cravings in your life and is great for periods when you need rejuvenation.

RIGHT NOSTRIL BREATHING: Sit in easy pose. Block the left nostril with the thumb of the right hand, and take twenty-six long, deep breaths through the right nostril. This breath helps to energize, revitalize, and become focused.

Better Than Coffee

BREATH FOR ENERGY: This breath involves inhaling and exhaling in strokes (sniffs) through the nose. It is a great way to build energy. Inhale in four strokes, exhale in four strokes. When you are done, take some time to sit quietly and integrate the energy you have cultivated.

Fire It Up

BREATH OF FIRE—AGNI PRASANA: I have found this breathing exercise to be the most powerful agent of change in my life, helping to eliminate old ways of being and behaving, and establishing a new inner dynamic of health and radiance.

This breath is created with short, fast breaths of equal length through the nose. Draw the navel point in and up on the exhale. The inhale is passive.

This breath will put you more in sync on every level. It purifies the blood and increases circulation (supplying an aerobic effect while allowing the heart to stay relaxed). It helps to balance the nervous system, remagnetizes the cells, and creates an optimum brain-wave balance.

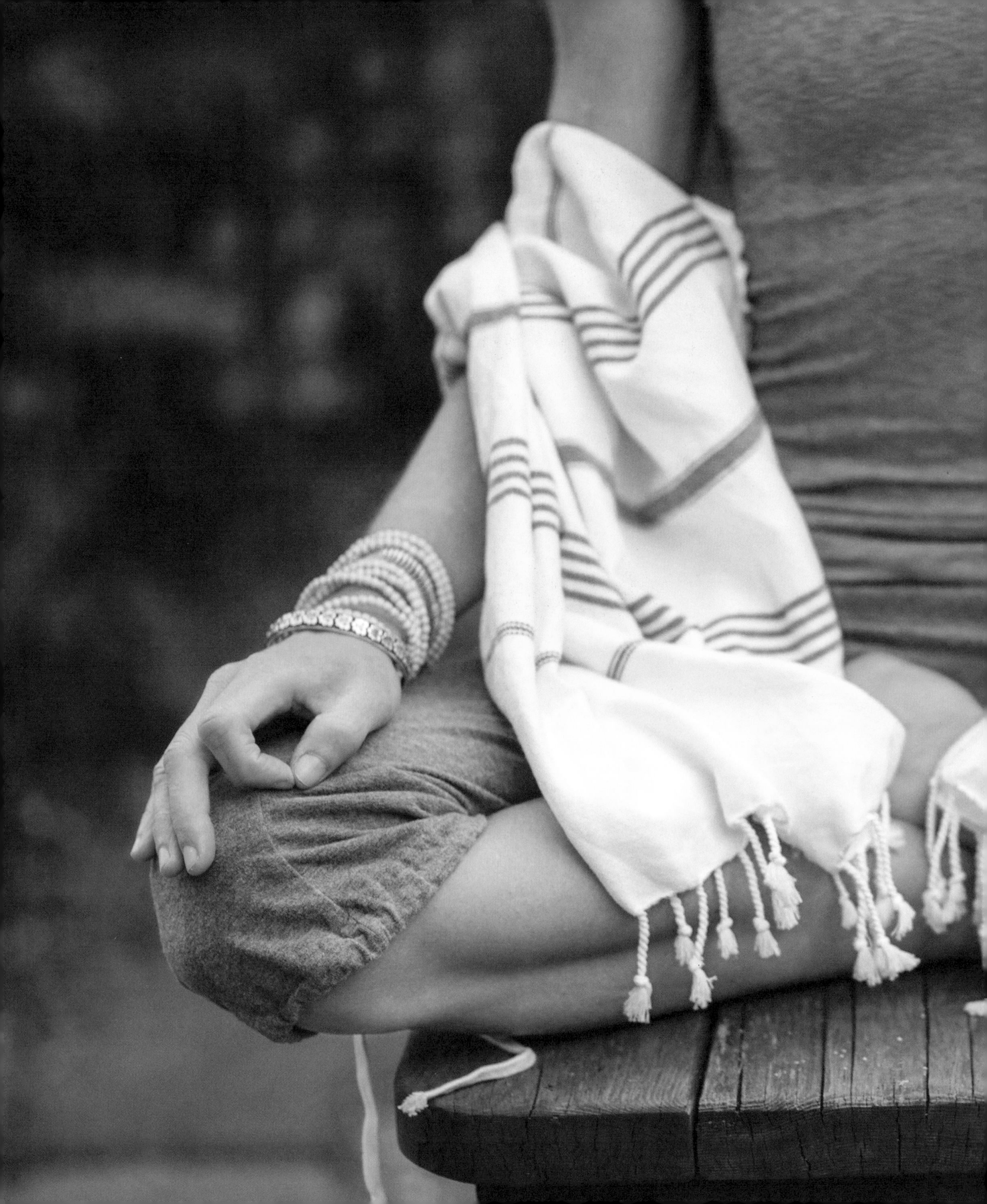

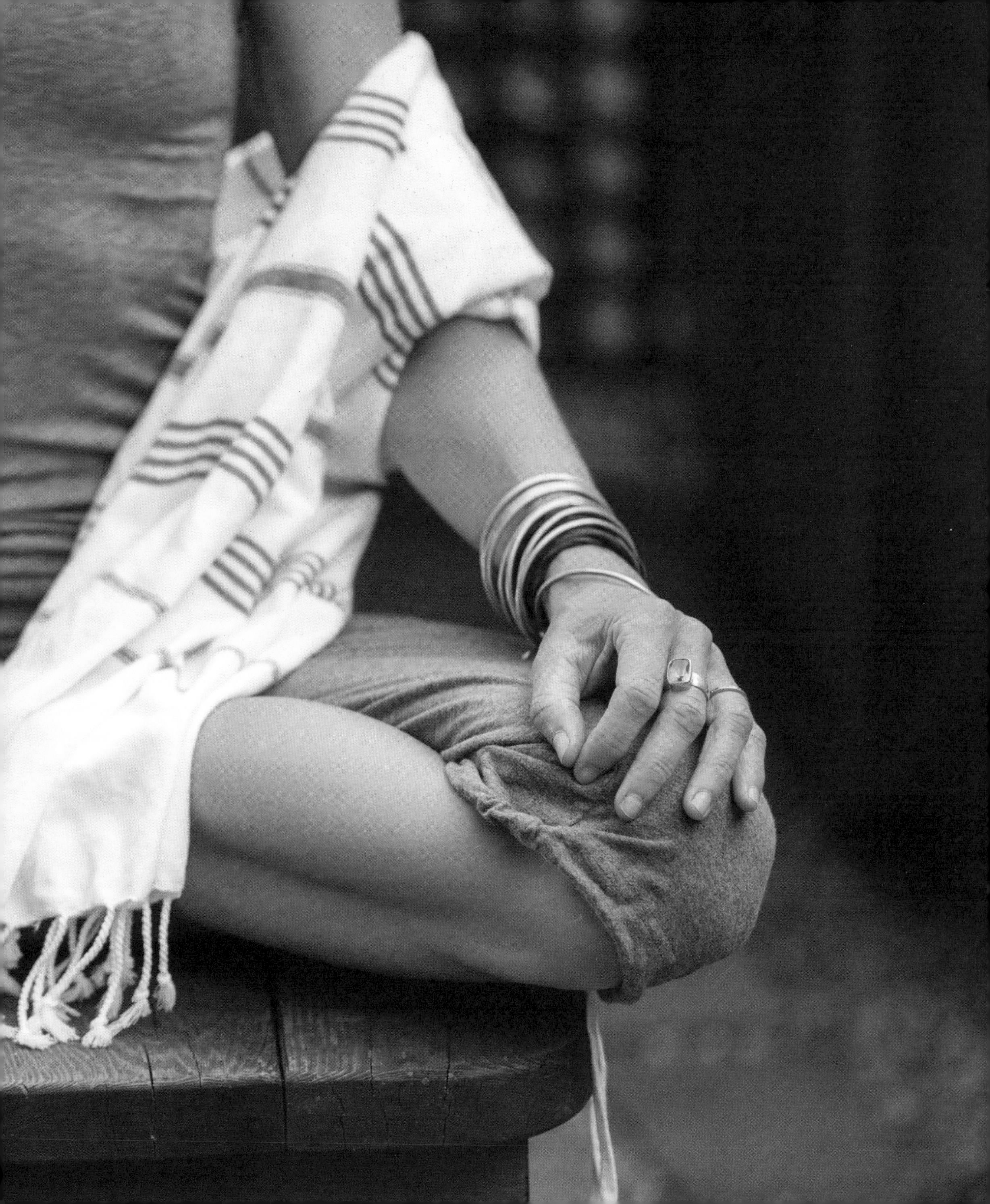

Pranayama can take us almost all the way to settling the mind into silence. With Pranayama, we are directly controlling the **prana***—the life force energy that animates the entire universe.*

Traditionally, after one becomes established in keeping the Ethical Rules (Yama) and the Yogic Observances (Niyama), and the practice of the physical exercises (Asana), one is ready for the breathing exercises.

There are many different sorts of breathing exercises that address many types of conditions. If you feel negative, you can do energizing breathing to feel more positive. If you feel cold or droopy you can do Bhastrika, or bellows breath, to warm up and get energized.

Pranayama is usually done while seated, although there are some breathing exercises done while standing or in poses. If you are sitting, it doesn't matter what position you assume, just that it is one you can sit comfortably in for a while with the spine straight and perpendicular to the ground.

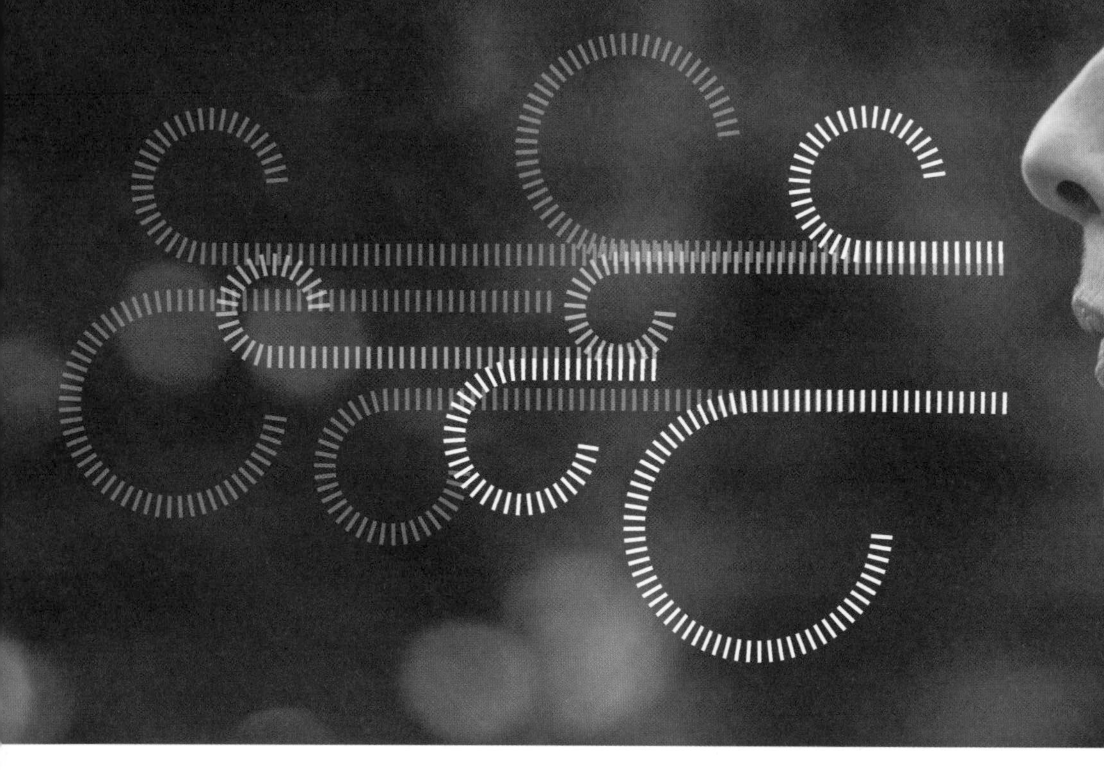

Try

NADI SODHANA PRANAYAMA (ALTERNATE NOSTRIL BREATHING): I recommend alternate-nostril breathing for everyone, every day for at least ten minutes, to turn the focus inward and calm the mind. The right hand assumes Vishnu Mudra and the left hand in Jnana Mudra.

- Inhale slowly through the left nostril according to your capacity.
- Close the left nostril with the ring finger and immediately open the right nostril by releasing the thumb.
- Exhale and inhale through the right, then close the right nostril and exhale through the left.

This is one complete cycle of Nadi Sodhana Pranayama. To make the exercise more powerful, visualize and watch the air enter the nostril and descend to the base of the spine while inhaling and watch it in reverse—up and out through the other nostril during exhalation. This is an excellent breathing exercise for those with heart problems and the elderly.

BREATH MEDICINE: Next time you feel stuck in a negative mind loop, or need to make a big decision, take some time to sit still and breathe consciously. This will help clear the mind and open you to your own inner source of inspiration and truth.

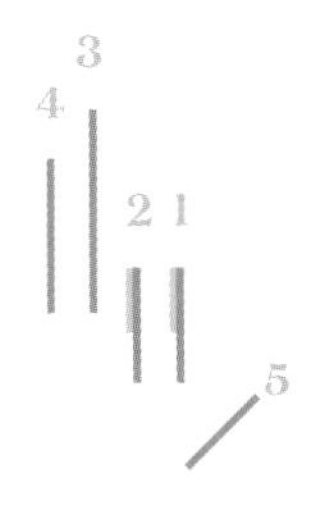

Vishnu Mudra

index and middle fingers are folded into the palm; the other fingers are extended

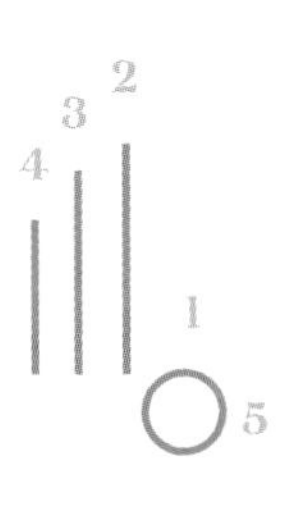

Jnana Mudra

making a complete circle with the index finger and thumb with the other fingers extended

[exhale]

When you visit a Wanderlust festival, yoga studio, or just about anywhere in India, you see Hindu deities such as Ganesh, Shiva, Lakshmi, and Durga. How can you relate to these deities, especially when you didn't grow up with them? An interesting way is to see them as your personal archetype. An archetype is a collectively inherited symbol or form.

You can ask yourself who your archetype is, whom you are called toward. You will find yourself gravitating toward one or two, and they might change in your lifetime because you change! Are you more of an elephant or a monkey? Who speaks to you? Think about how to consciously incorporate the ideas the archetype symbolizes into your life. They remind us of the grander ideals we can all live for.

Ganesh

Ganesh is considered to be the remover of obstacles. He is the ruler of thresholds. Ganesh is often called upon for new endeavors, such as a new job, teacher training, or even a birthday. He brings protection. Ultimately, he leads you to enlightenment.

[On a scale from 1 to 10, give yourself a Ganesh score. How much of an elephant are you right now in your life?]

① ② ③ ④ ⑤ ⑥ ⑦ ⑧ ⑨ ⑩

Ganesh usually is shown with a mouse at his feet. (If the Ganesh statue or picture doesn't come with a mouse, then your mind is the mouse and you make Ganesh complete!). The mouse symbolizes our minds, which wander all over the place the way the mouse scampers around. By riding on the mouse, Ganesh controls the mouse. He therefore controls our minds, helping to still them. Ganesh thus gets you in a state called "practicing samadhi" where the thought patterns in your mind are uniform. In that state, you do not experience any obstacle. So the obstacles we face in our lives are not outside us but inside our mind as ***vrittis*** (thought fluctuations).

That is the secret of how Ganesh removes obstacles by giving you an inner calmness.

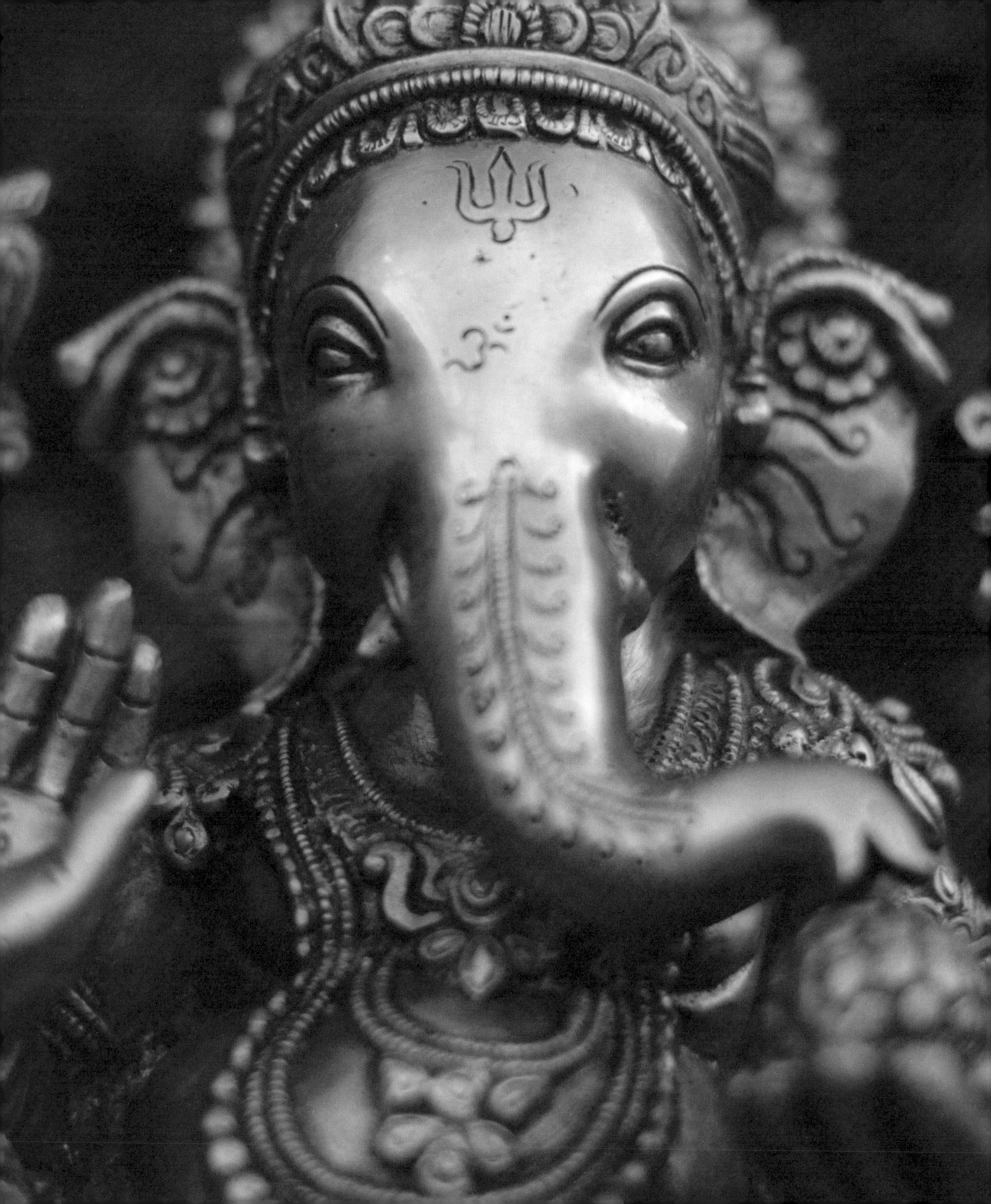

Dancing Shiva (Nataraja)

Life is uncertain. Anything can happen anytime to any one of us. The real question is, how does one live such a life of uncertainty with certainty?

By embracing the dancer, the Shiva Nataraja, we can learn to embrace life with joy and wonder. This dance reminds us of the constant flow of creation and destruction in life. Shiva helps us move with a balance of effort and grace through the ups and downs. Shiva helps us to know what to let go of and to surrender while moving with beauty to change what we can. Many people feel aligned with Shiva when undergoing more radical life changes.

Shiva tells us that life is a dance. It's inherently chaotic; engage with it, create, destroy. Do not, however, make the dance into a drama. Know who you are: You are pure Consciousness, the stillness that is never born and never dies.

[Your Shiva score] ①②③④⑤⑥⑦⑧⑨⑩

Durga

Goddess Durga is goodness in fierce form. She removes negative energies that don't serve us: both within as well as without.

Durga is able to kill the demons that plague us. She cleans out the patterns of repetitive behavior that hold us back and attenuates the effects of the ***samskaras*** (imprints left on the mind by experience) that can lead to addictions. She gives us inner strength and outer compassion so we can help people while having an inner firmness.

The lion she rides on is like a dream lion that pounces on you and, in fright, you are awakened into a higher state.

[What's your Durga score right now?] ①②③④⑤⑥⑦⑧⑨⑩

Lakshmi

Lakshmi teaches us to embrace life with abundance: both material and spiritual. She is the embodiment of beauty and fortune. There are many kinds of wealth and Lakshmi invites us to be open to all of them. She is also the goddess of shri: that which gives you luminosity and enables you to create beauty in every aspect of your life.

The abundance she grants is universal abundance in which everything in the universe is part of you. Every moment in life, be it good or bad, is embraced wholeheartedly.

The worldly goddess Lakshmi teaches us to be Grihastha yogis, to follow the path of the householder. She teaches us to bring the ashram home.

[Your Lakshmi score] ①②③④⑤⑥⑦⑧⑨⑩

Saraswati

Saraswati is the goddess of knowledge, speech, intuitive wisdom, music, dance, and creativity. Saraswati literally means *flow,* and it is said she was a river in ancient India five thousand years ago at the time when the Vedic civilization existed. Everything flows with her grace. She says the way to awakening is twofold. One way is through the scriptures; the other path is through the heart, represented by the sitar she holds. Chanting opens the heart chakra. Great insights can happen when the heart chakra is opened. In this age of darkness, where greed, jealousy, and wars predominate, the way of the heart is what she recommends.

The flow of intuition Saraswati grants you is of the highest kind, where you become so good at what you do that eloquence flows naturally from a source of deep wisdom. This flow leads to great creative advancements in knowledge, music, dance, and the arts. Saraswati gives the highest power of creative energy, access to what is behind the letters that make up words.

The swan's head is shown on one end of the sitar. The swan metaphorically represents *viveka,* the key quality of discernment a spiritual seeker should possess. Discernment is key in separating reality from illusion. The swan also glides gracefully through water without water sticking to it, as great sages might glide through life without events sticking to them. But under the water, the swan paddles furiously. This means the great sages do sadhana (spiritual practice) in order to seem to move effortlessly through events.

[Your Saraswati score] ①②③④⑤⑥⑦⑧⑨⑩

Buddha

The Buddha is a teacher of compassion healing, and liberation. The Buddha brings us to an awareness of calm, peace of mind, and, ultimately, spiritual awakening.

Buddha means the awakened one. He awoke from this living dream, got enlightened, and achieved *moksha* (release from the cycle of birth and death). The name Buddha comes from the root *buddhi,* the intellect. Thus Buddha means the intellect has awakened to the self. The buddhi is the closest mental faculty we have to the self.

The bodhi tree was the tree under which Buddha sat for forty-nine days until he attained nirvana. The peacocks represent the universality and abundance of spirit just the way the peacocks spread their feathers in the spring.

[Your Buddha score] ①②③④⑤⑥⑦⑧⑨⑩

Tara

Tara is the goddess of compassion and healing, and the bringer of people to liberation.

Going up the mountain for internal and external peace is a metaphor for the spiritual path. That is what Buddha did: He retreated from society, meditated, and went within. But goddess Tara descended down the mountain into this world of chaos and uncertainty so she could help people with love, healing, and ultimately moksha (liberation). Motivated by compassion, she is said to have been reincarnated as a *bodhisattva* (enlightened being) on Earth to help us all out.

Tara is similar to Kwan Yin in the sense they are both bodhisattvas, the difference being that Tara comes from a Nepal/Tibet/India tradition while Kwan Yin comes from the tradition of China and the Far East.

In our daily lives, Tara appears as an archetype in people who are great healers and/or serve selflessly. Prominent examples are Mother Teresa and Mahatma Gandhi. They never get tired because they are aligned with the divine energy. The tiredness comes when there is a selfish ego-based intention: And when that intention is not fulfilled, the mind generates static.

[Your Tara score] ①②③④⑤⑥⑦⑧⑨⑩

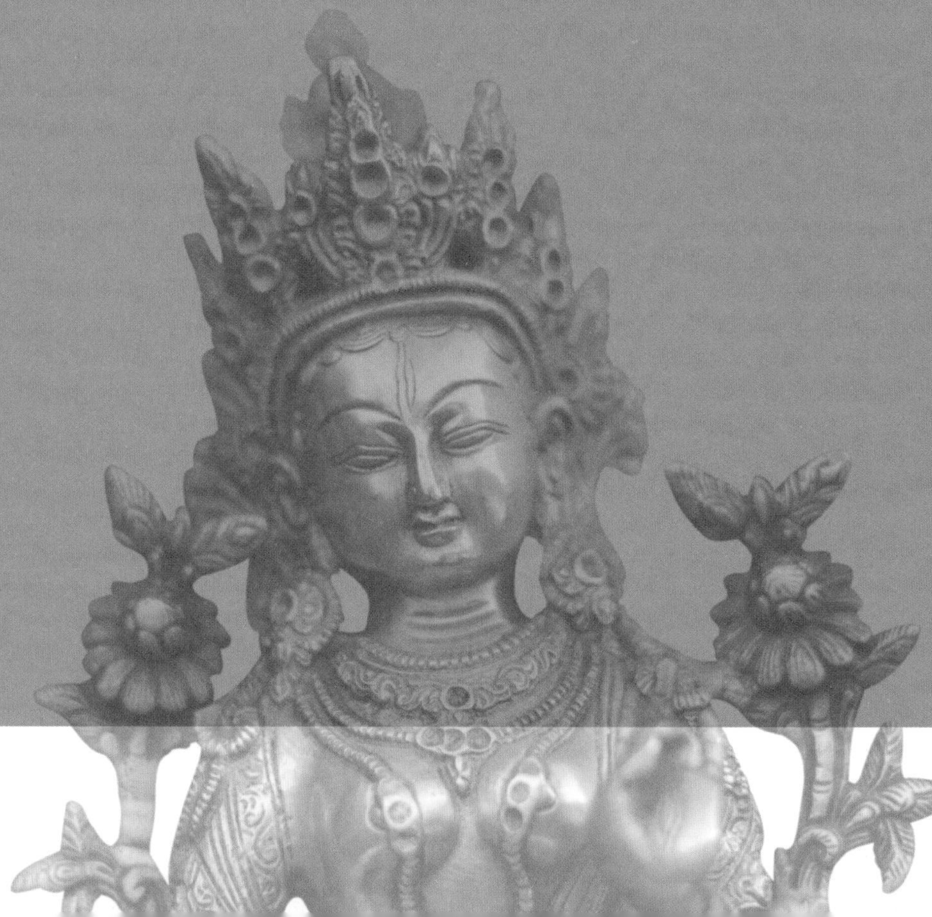

Hanuman

Hanuman represents superhuman strength and superhuman intellect with a high degree of devotion. He resides in the heart chakra. Hanuman is the ultimate superhero.

This is a little-known story: Hanuman is actually an incarnation of Shiva and Shakti. Shiva was meditating on Mount Kailash one day and came to a realization that he shared with his wife Shakti. He said Lord Ram is the main ruler of the universe. Shakti said, "What are you saying? You are the main man!" Lord Shiva replied, "No, things have changed. People are living too much in their heads, and excessive egotism has led to divisiveness, jealousy, and war. So I'm going to incarnate as a lowly monkey so people will take me for granted. Through my selfless service, I'm going to show everyone the power of devotion and living from the heart." Shakti replied, "In that case, I'm going to incarnate as your tail so we will always be together." So Hanuman is Shiva and his tail represents the Kundalini Shakti.

[Your Hanuman score] ①②③④⑤⑥⑦⑧⑨⑩

Kali

Goddess Kali is goodness in a fierce form. She removes the negative energies that don't serve us: both those within and those directed toward us.

She is naked because Maya (the world of Illusion) doesn't cover her. She is dark, the nearest there is to pure consciousness.

Kali chops off the hands of the demons and makes a skirt. Hands represent karmic actions (we do karmas with our hands), so she removes the effects of karma that bind us. She chops off all the heads of the demon clones and makes a garland. This way she eliminates all the negative patterns (samskaras) that bind us down. She wears a garland of fifty-four skulls representing the fifty-four letters of the Sanskrit alphabet. These skulls represent the samskaras, the addictive patterns that demonize our lives.

Goddess Kali cleans out the patterns of repetitive behavior that hold us back. She cleans out the samskaras that can lead to addiction. She gives us inner strength and outer compassion so we can help people while having an inner firmness.

[Your Kali score] ①②③④⑤⑥⑦⑧⑨⑩

We are always manifesting. Each thought we have creates an energy flow within and around our physical being. This energy attracts its likeness. So if you're thinking, "I suck," then your energy kinda, well, sucks—and you attract sucky experiences.

The opposite experience occurs when you think high-level thoughts like, "I rock!" When you think and feel, "I rock," you exude an energy of confidence and in turn attract great experiences into your life. Each thought you have informs your energy, and your energy manifests into your experiences. Your thoughts and energy create your reality.

MANIFESTING MISHAPS

Manifestation has become a buzzword lately. Though it's totally awesome that the Law of Attraction is now trendy, it also can be misleading for folks who are unwilling to do heavy lifting. If you truly want to use your energetic power to manifest greatness, you must clear all that blocks you from believing in your greatness.

A Course in Miracles teaches that, on some level, you've asked for everything that happens in your life. Your intentions create your reality. There's no need to beat yourself up: Simply recognizing how negative or unskillful thoughts affect your life is the first powerful step toward changing your experiences. Begin your manifesting process by getting honest about how your low-level thoughts, energy, and feelings of disbelief block you from receiving what you desire. Once you get clear about the blocks, you can begin to clean them up to make space for positive manifestations to occur.

Many people, when trying to manifest, focus too much on the outside form rather than the internal condition. What's important is our internal experience: whether we choose to experience love or fear. When we commit to our internal experience of love, we begin to attract more love. Many people approach manifestation from a place of "How can I get something to feel better?" Instead, the focus should be: "How can I feel better and therefore be an energetic match for attracting more greatness into my life?" The emphasis must be placed on healing the internal condition.

THE FIVE PRINCIPLES FOR MANIFESTING YOUR DESIRES

When practicing these steps, make sure to stay committed to the goal of feeling good first and attracting stuff second. Remind yourself that when you feel good, you energetically attract goodness into your life. Plus, when your primary function is to be happy, then whatever comes to you is irrelevant. Happiness is your true manifestation.

Principle One: Clear Space

Before you begin the manifestation process, you must take the necessary time to release any disbelief in your power to be happy. One of the best ways to clear the blocks is to pray for release. Begin a daily prayer practice of asking the universe to set you free from all the limiting beliefs that block you from your greatness. Stay open to signs from the universe and show up for the assignments that are brought to you. Universal assignments come in many forms. Maybe you're guided to the relationship that brings up all your shit so that you have to finally heal your fear. Or maybe you lose your job so that you can learn the lessons of self-reliance and strengthen your self-love. Trust that these assignments, however tough, are incredible opportunities for you to clean your energy and clear space to call in what you desire.

Your job in this step is to pray for guidance. Then allow the universe to help guide you to whatever assignments you need. Show up for the assignments and trust that the more you clean your thoughts and energy, the more positive experiences you will attract into your life.

Principle Two: Get Clear

Clarity is king when it comes to manifesting your desires. You must have clear intentions for what you want to call in—otherwise you can manifest a lot of what you don't want. Focus on what you desire and then make a list of all that goes with it. If you're getting clear about the job you want, make a list of all the things about the job that make you happy: the office, the people, the salary, etc. Be unapologetic about what you want. This list helps you clarify your intentions and access a vibrant mental picture of what you desire.

The most important part of this step is to clarify how you want to feel. Then you can begin to access that feeling. That feeling is what makes the manifestation come into form. If you don't clearly feel what you want to experience, it will never truly manifest into form.

Principle Three: Think It, Feel It, Believe It!

Now, let's put these steps together. Take your clear intention and spend time every day sitting in the feeling of what it is that you desire. You might access the feeling through meditation, visioning exercises, when hanging out in nature or doing exercise you love. The more you feel the feeling of what you desire, the more you believe it is on the way. From a metaphysical perspective, if you believe it then it is already here.

Principle Four: Chill!

The next step is crucial to the manifestation process. In order to truly manifest your desires into form, you gotta chill out! A Course in Miracles teaches, "Those who are certain of the outcome can afford to wait and wait without anxiety." Take this message with you and allow your faithfulness to guide you into the belief that what you desire is on the way. Also trust that the universe has a much better plan than you do. Though you are clear about what you want, you cannot control the timing or the form in which it comes. Stay calm, relax, and trust that the universe has your back!

Principle Five: Know the Universe Has Your Back

When you're in the know, you're deliberate about what you want and no longer vibrate energy of fear or disbelief. You just know. As your disbelief wilts away, wanting is replaced by knowing. Getting into the know happens naturally. When you diligently practice steps one through four, you will clean house, get clear, and feel happier. This process is healing and powerful, and it leads to a deep inner knowing that you are right where you need to be. Accepting your greatness in this moment, right now, is what manifests more greatness. Being in the know helps you accept that you already are living in your desired manifestation. In time, the universe catches up with your energy and your desires come into form. This process of allowing the manifestation to follow your internal faith is true cocreation.

STAY COMMITTED TO HAPPINESS

Stay committed to this five-step process and trust that you're exactly where you need to be. Is your main desire to feel good? Trust you will be given everything you need to create that feeling. Know that feeling good is the true manifestation—and everything else is the icing on the already delicious cake!

find your direction

ROLF GATES

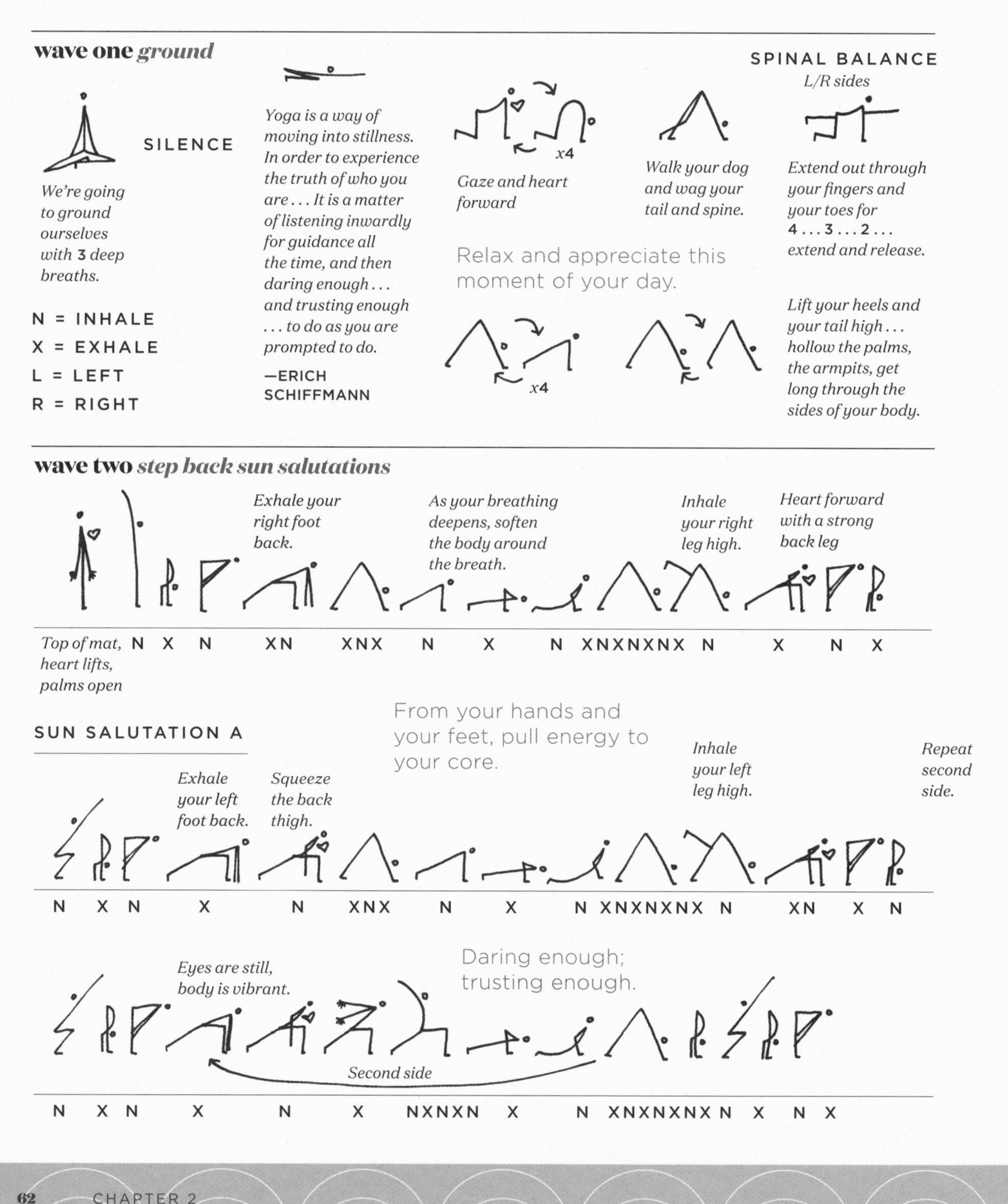

wave three *standing postures*

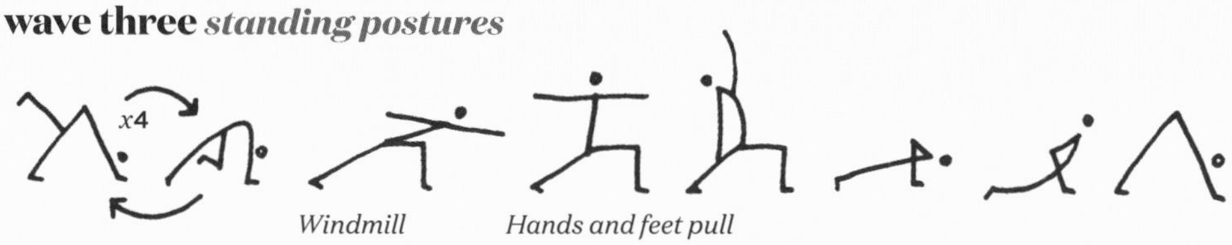

x4

Windmill up with heart down, gaze down.

Hands and feet pull energy to your center . . . from your center . . . root through your feet.

Repeat second side.

Eyes still, body vibrant, shine out.

Come into your vision, allowing the breath to move energy through the pose.

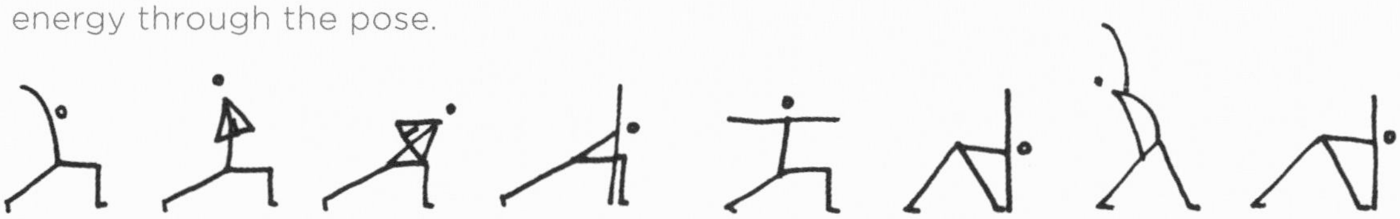

Relax and feel integrated to the point of inspiration.

Palms pressing in, feet pressing out

PARSVAKONASANA
New students, hand to the inside of the foot.

Reverse the triangle.

Awaken the heart.

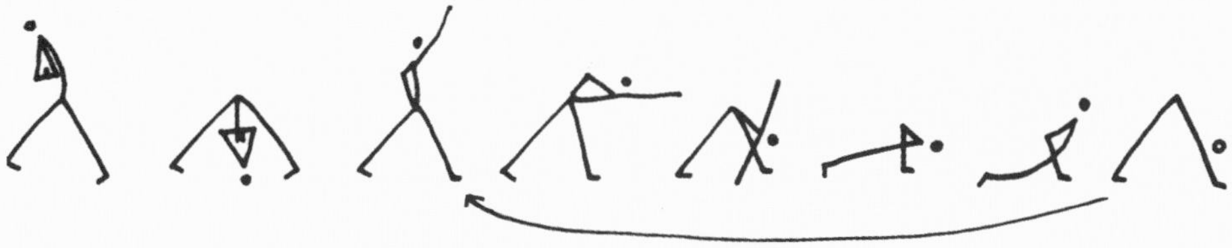

REVERSE NAMASTE
Adjust your feet, square your hips, and bring your palms together behind your back.

Take your arm high, rooting down through your back foot, reach forward and down with your hand.

PAVRITTA TRIKONASANA
Plant your hand on the floor or your block, draw your right hip back, roll your upper shoulder back.

Allow the symmetry of the pose to balance your energy.

wave four *balance*

On the in-breath, take your leg high; on the out-breath, step forward.
Back knee to the floor, palms to the top of your right knee
Palms facing each other, shoulders soft
Work the ribs down for your backbend for the count of 4.
HANUMANASANA Squeeze the thigh to protect the hamstring, shine the four corners of your front foot.
Repeat second side.
X
N
Coming up slow . . . palms to your hips
Holding energy at your center, shine out through the feet.
HORSE POSE Spin your toes out, stacking your knees over your ankles, hips low.
Gaze is steady, face is relaxed.
Toes forward, heels back
Heart slightly above the hips
Get long and melt.
SPLITS Four corners of feet grounded, core is integrated, hips are back.
Inhale lift the heart, roll the shoulders back.
GARUDASANA
wave five standing
NATARAJASANA Catch inside of your foot, take your opposite arm high.
Relax . . . integrate . . . second side.
TREE POSE
Arms wide open, heart wide open
Movements calm and precise, body language confident.
Second side, then take a full vinyasa to land on belly.
SPHINX POSE Elbows under shoulders for support, press all 10 toes into the earth.
x4
COBRA Pulsation with the hands
BOW POSE Strong with your legs, feet active, lift up . . . x2.
x2
CAMEL POSE TO DOWN DOG
Walk shoulder blades in and interlace fingers; 1 MIN Use a block to root feet down and bring hips even higher.
WHEEL POSE

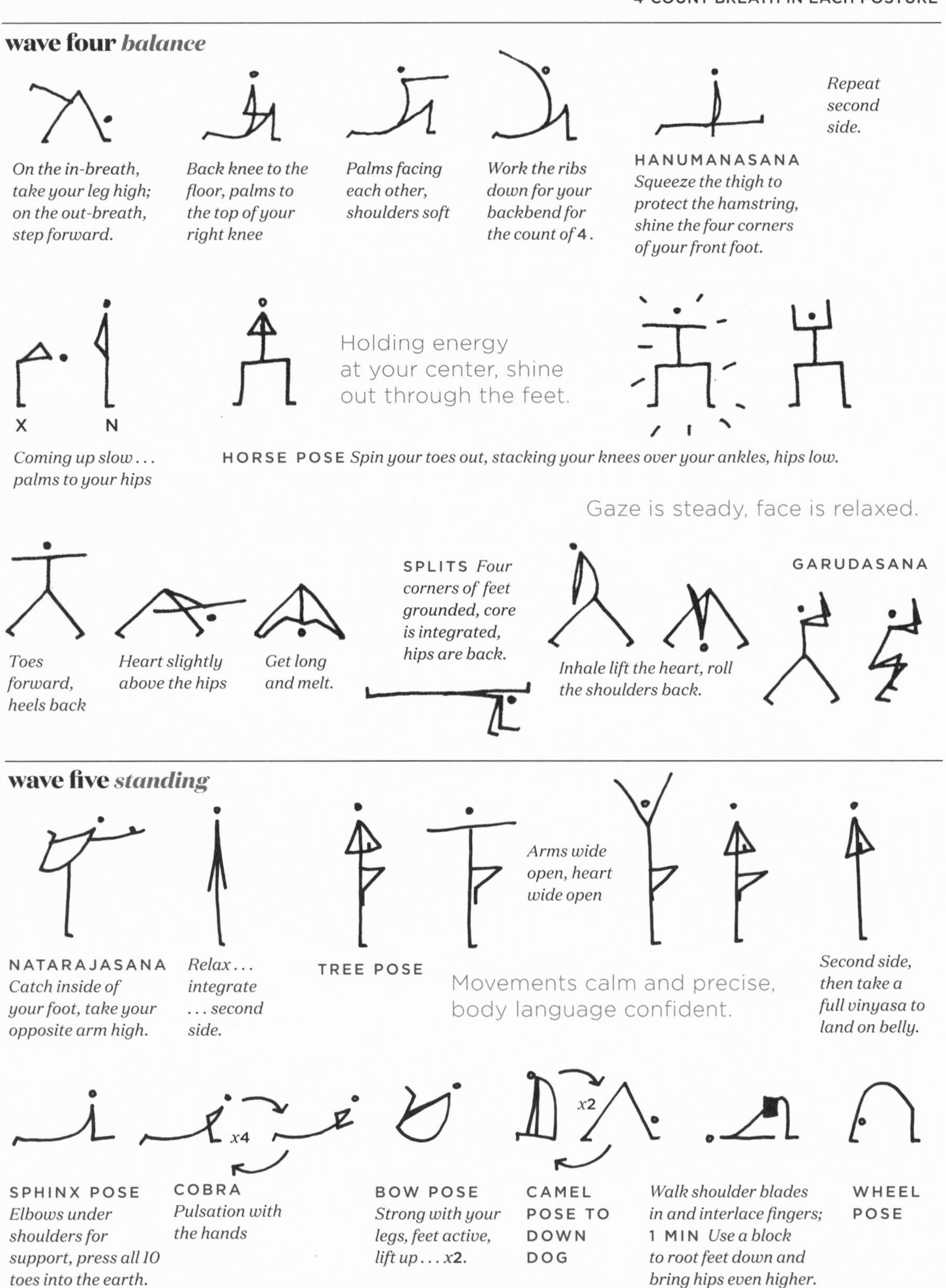

wave six *hips and finishing*

Walk your feet out toward the edge of the mat and bring your knees together, hands are on the floor by your hips, squeeze and release thighs.

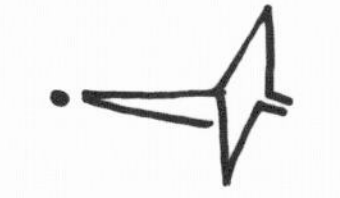

SUPTA BADDHAKONASANA *Soles of the feet together, knees apart,* 10-15 COUNTS

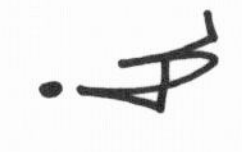

Bring your knees together . . . hug your knees to your chest, 10-15 COUNTS.

Breathing with your whole body.

Lift leg high, step through to PIGEON POSE *on your right side . . . walk your hands forward, bring your chest or forehead to the floor,* 1-3 MINUTES.

Walk your hands back to your hips . . . then bring your back leg around, AGNISTAMBASANA, FIRE LOGS. *Right leg over left, the right ankle is on top of the left thigh, right foot past the left thigh. Walk your hands forward, hold here for* 1-3 MINUTES.

Relax your body and notice how relaxation is a movement into stillness.

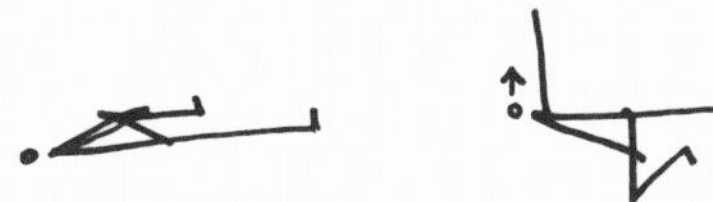

Lie back, straighten your legs, give your knee a squeeze . . . breathe into your squeeze, pause 3-5 COUNTS, *then second side.*

Take a twist, draw your knee across your body, take your arm out, chin to your shoulder, 3-5 COUNTS.

Catch your left foot with both hands, straighten your left leg.

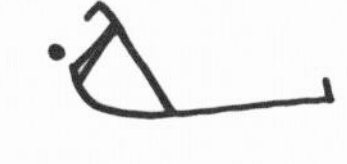

Inhale . . . as you exhale bring your forehead toward your leg for 5 . . . 4 . . . 3 . . . 2 . . . *now touch . . . come back to center and switch legs, bend your left knee, taking the twist again.*

We show up, burn brightly in the moment, live passionately, HOLD NOTHING BACK, and when the moment is over, our work is done. We step back and let go.

NAMASTE *Victory to our spirits... peace to all beings...*

Direction Playlist

complied by Kelly Casey

We've Been Inside Too Long—*Kyson*

Amateur Cartography—*Obfusc*

Awash—*Manual*

A Walk—*Tycho*

Cirrus—*Bonobo*

Sleeping Children Are Still Flying—*Blue Sky Black Death*

Kusanagi—*Odesza*

Halving the Compass—*Helios*

You are on your path, armed with a yoga practice and journaling along the way, wondering "Which way is north?" Forging your own path isn't easy. This guided meditation will help you get your bearings and forge ahead by clarifying your values and the life you wish to steer yourself toward.

Unrestricted daydreaming is a pathway into our intuitive wisdom and deepest desires.

Your Future Self

DURATION:
Thirty minutes

LOCATION:
Quiet place

MINDSET:
Contemplative

TOOLS:
Pen, timer

STEPS

1. Find a quiet place and spend a few moments connecting to your breath. Feel the inhale and exhale in turn.
2. Set the timer for fifteen minutes.
3. Read these questions. Begin to imagine yourself in five years:
   A. What do you see?
   B. What are you doing?
   C. What do you eat?
   D. Where do you live?
   E. Do you have pets?
   F. Do you have children?
   G. What does your home look like?
   H. What do you do with your time?
   I. What do you do with your money?
4. Close your eyes and answer the questions. Fill in as many details as you can by walking yourself through an ideal day in the life of your future self. Imagine that everything gives you a sense of well-being, happiness, and success.
5. Open your eyes after the timer goes off and record the answers in the space provided above.

SOME THINGS TO CONSIDER

1. Don't censor yourself; observe where the mind goes without judgment.
2. Trust what you receive, knowing your inner compass will point you in the right direction.

FIVE YEARS FROM NOW

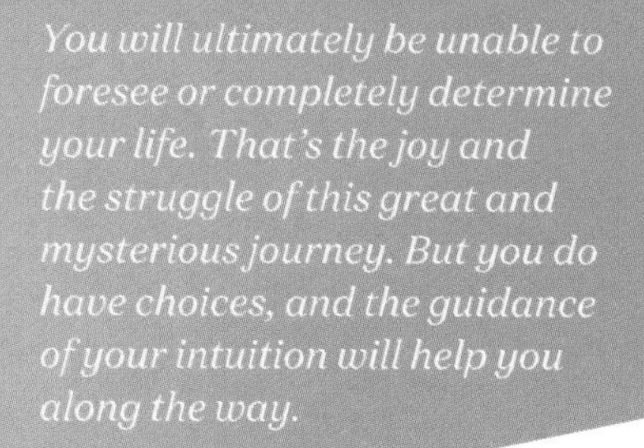

You will ultimately be unable to foresee or completely determine your life. That's the joy and the struggle of this great and mysterious journey. But you do have choices, and the guidance of your intuition will help you along the way.

Make a Vision Board

1. Get a stack of old magazines, a poster board, glue, and scissors.
2. Tear out the pages with words, images, and colors that grab your attention.
3. Cut out the shapes, objects, words, and letters.
4. Arrange them on your board and glue them down.
5. Place your vision board where you will see it and use it for inspiration or as a reminder of your path.

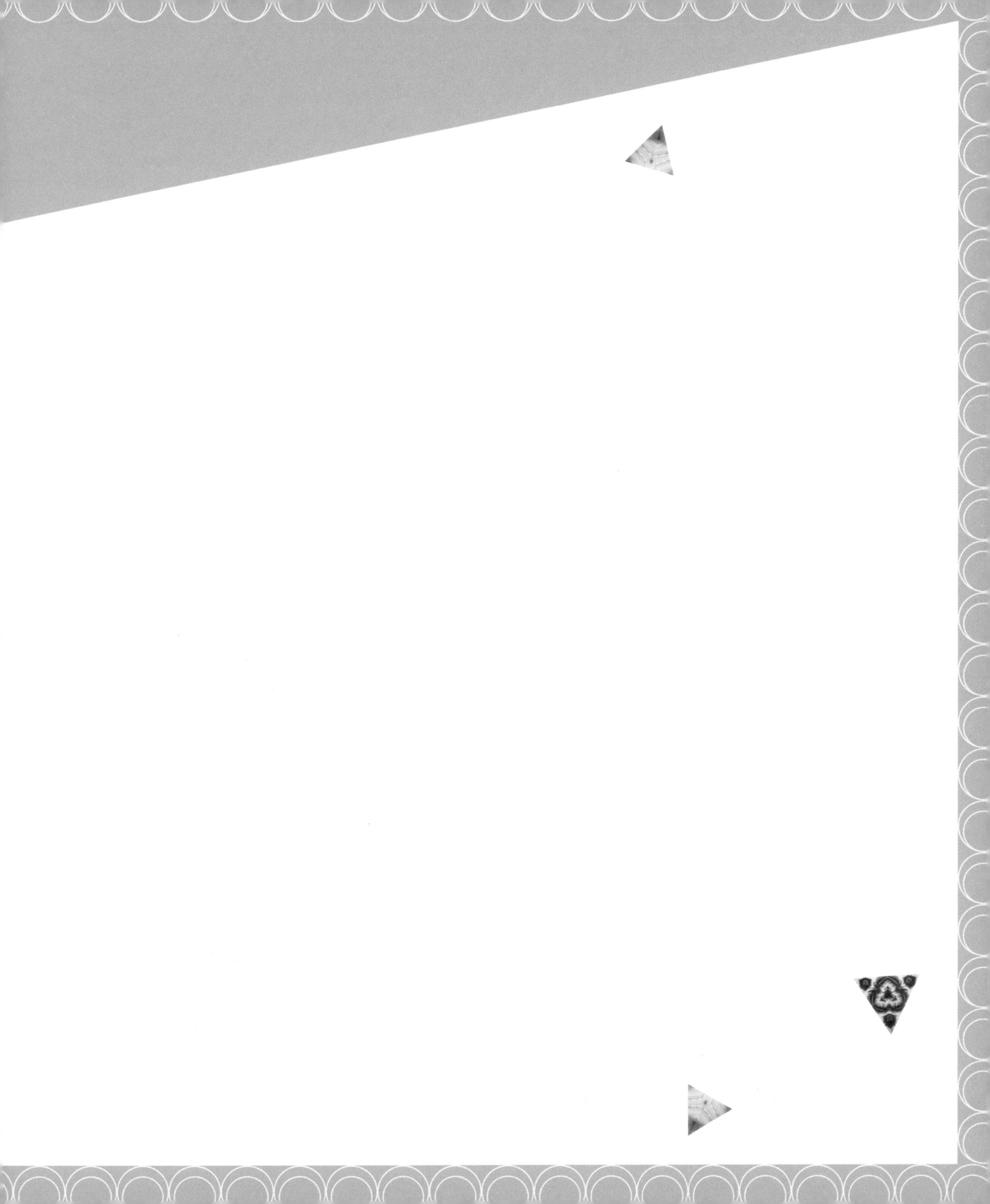

The world is the great gymnasium where we come to make ourselves strong.

—Swami Vivekananda

CHAPTER 3

find your core

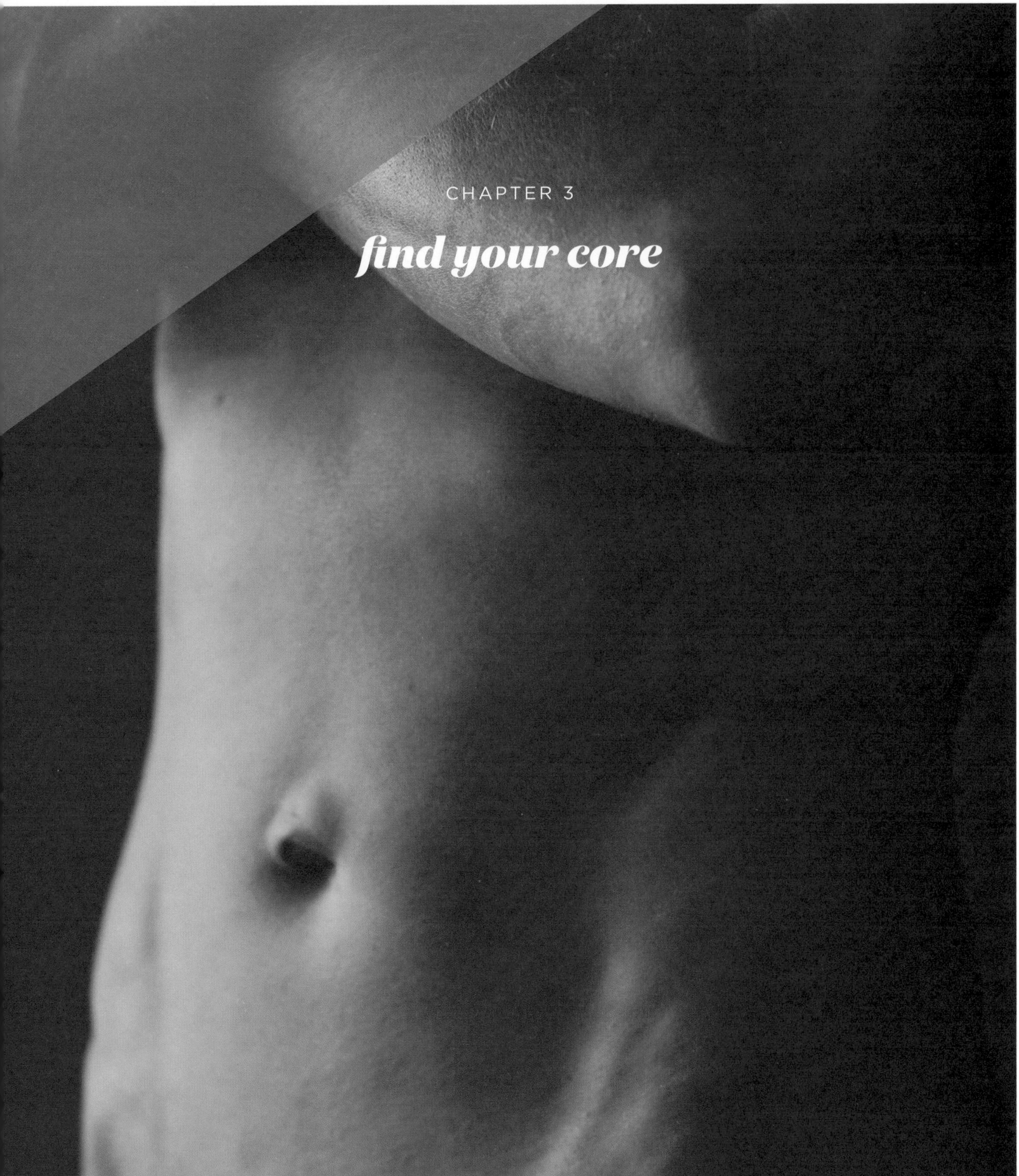

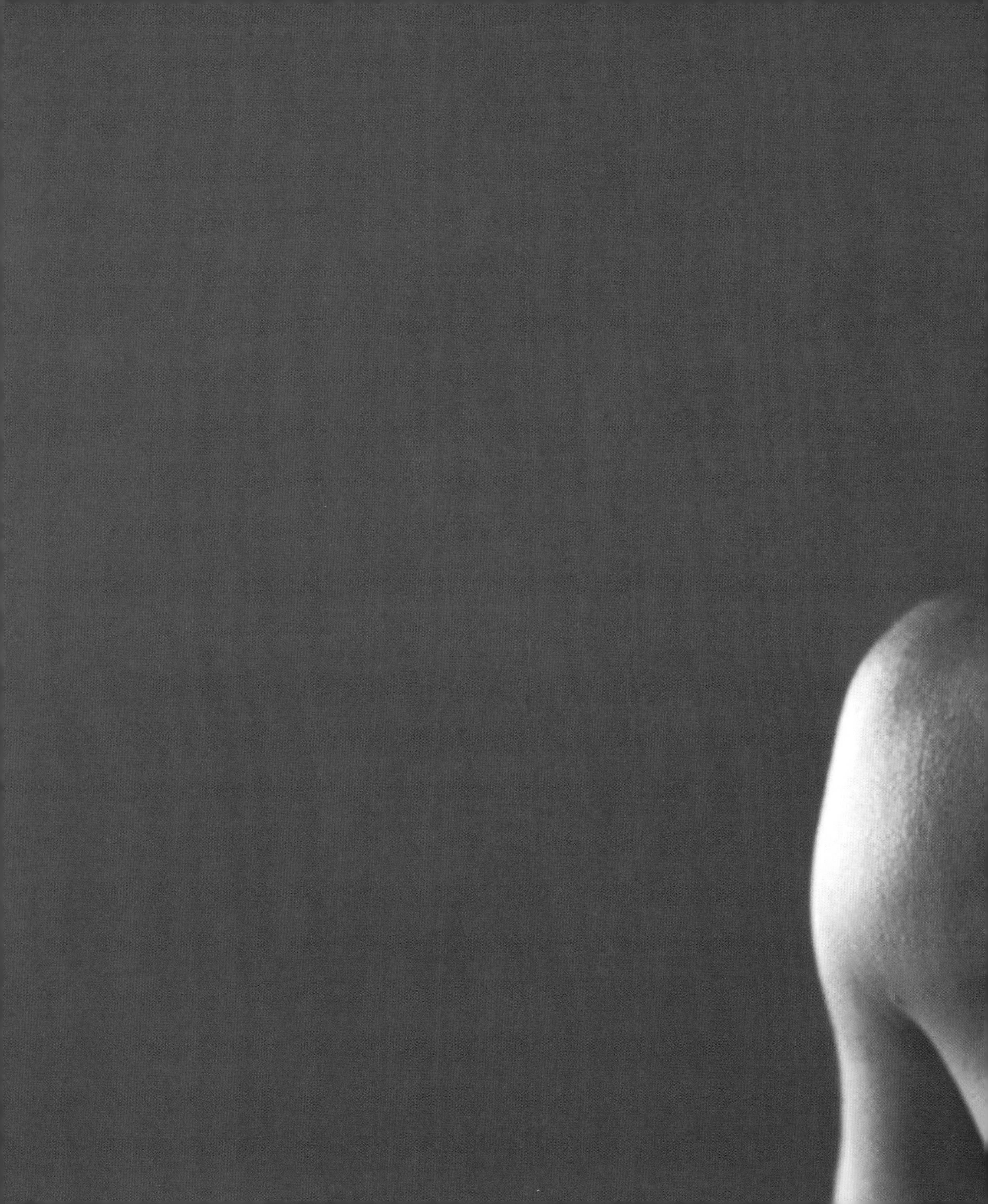

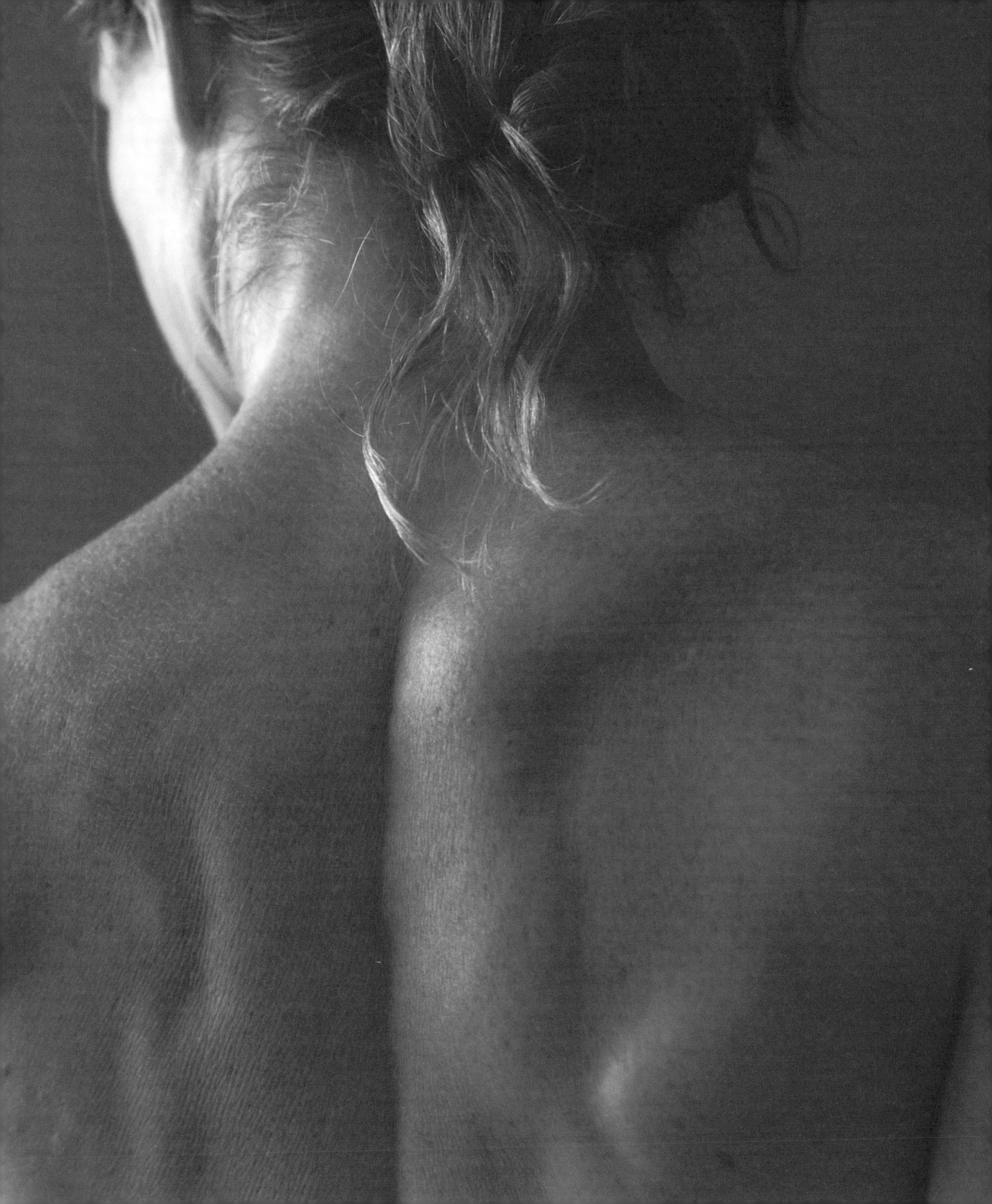

Close your eyes

The core is what is left when everything else is stripped away. When we feel naked and raw, simple and radiant. Whether in the midst of sheer brilliance or unfathomable anguish, our core connects us to something deep within the truth of who we are, the very essence of our being.

It may feel like a vulnerable place, but it is also a place of incredible strength and endurance. When the ground beneath our feet begins to quake and the world around us starts to fall, the core is there—still and untouched.

Finding it allows us to tap into our inner compass and navigate the world with earnest inquiry. In times of conflict, it teaches us how to gulp down the lump in our throat and speak our truth. In times of fear, it teaches us to untie the knot in our stomach and step forward bravely.

Tune in

Feel the gentle beat within
your chest

The soft rise and fall of
your breath

Where does it start?
What is the source?

Listen.
Ask.
Pursue.
Contemplate.
Discover.

Knowing our core is the starting
point of knowing who we are.

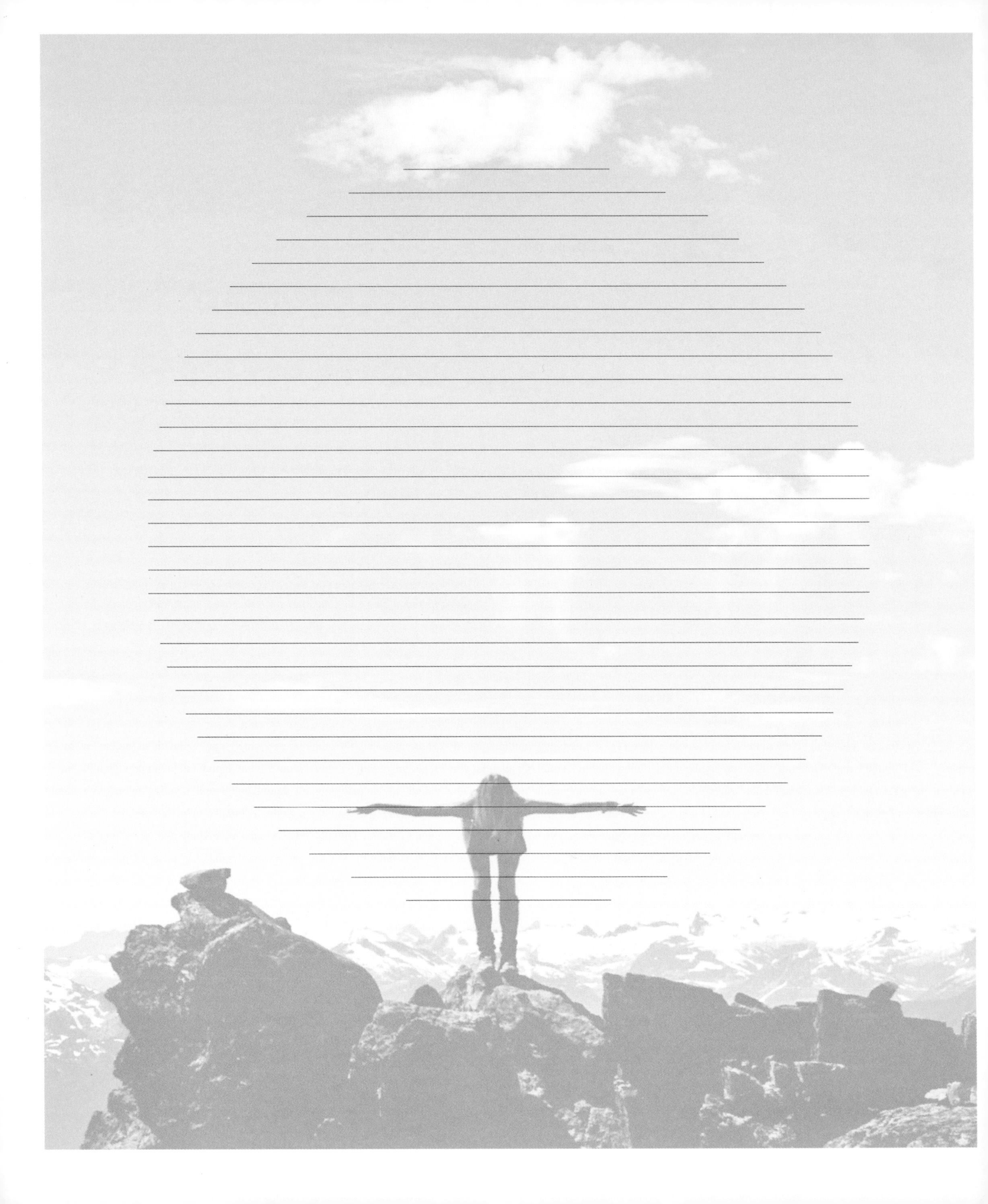

If we think of our capacity for happiness in limited ways, we form small intentions and think this is what our lives are about. When my friends and I were looking for a place to house the Insight Meditation Society, we went to look at a property for sale in Barre, Massachusetts. We noticed as we passed through the town green in the center of Barre a plaque engraved with the town motto: "TRANQUIL AND ALERT." *Because those two words are so essential to meditation practice, and the balance between the two qualities so crucial to progress on the path, we took it as an omen and bought the property.*

Some years later, we found a slim volume on the history of Barre that talks about the main building of what is now IMS. It was built as the mansion of Colonel Gaston, one-time lieutenant governor of Massachusetts. It turns out that Colonel Gaston had his own personal motto: "You should live each day so that you can look any damn man in the eye and tell him to go to hell."

I like telling those two stories in juxtaposition because I believe we each tend to have a motto, conscious or unconscious, that tells the story of who we think we are, what we are capable of, what our lives are about, and what we want to dedicate them to. Like Colonel Gaston, we may severely limit our vision.

To develop a creative sense of possibility that can guide your day-to-day intentions, I suggest:

GO DEEP. For example, you might think the thing you want more than anything is a lot of money, but no one actually wants piles of bills and coins in their homes. We want what money represents: perhaps security, leisure, freedom, choice. If we look more deeply at what money represents to us, we might realize several ways, in addition to piling up money (which might or might not work to give us the feeling we want), to experience greater security, leisure, freedom, choice.

GO WIDE. Sudha Chandran, a well-known contemporary classical Indian dancer, seemingly faced the end of her dancing career when her right leg had to be amputated. Amazingly, with her artificial leg she returned to dancing and, despite the odds, once again attained top ranking in her field. When asked how she had managed to do it, she said quite simply, "You don't need feet to dance." We are generally capable of so much more than we are conditioned to think. If you feel the constraints of tunnel vision, do a thought experiment in which you go wide.

STAY IN TOUCH. Periodically tune in to your own personal motto—what do you want most out of life, what is your vision of where the greatest happiness is to be found—and see if it is reflected anywhere in the choice you are about to make, the course of action you are about to embark on, the way you are about to treat yourself or someone else. And if it is nowhere to be found, remember that the essence of all transformation is the ability to begin again. We blow it, we can start over. We make a mistake, lose sight of that aspiration, stray from our chosen course, fall down, we can always, and must always, be able to forgive ourselves and, without rancor, begin again.

THIS IS YOUR LIFE.
DO WHAT YOU LOVE,
AND DO IT OFTEN.
IF YOU DON'T LIKE SOMETHING, CHANGE IT.
IF YOU DON'T LIKE YOUR JOB, QUIT.
IF YOU DON'T HAVE ENOUGH TIME, STOP WATCHING TV.
IF YOU ARE LOOKING FOR THE LOVE OF YOUR LIFE, STOP;
THEY WILL BE WAITING FOR YOU WHEN YOU
START DOING THINGS YOU LOVE.
STOP OVER ANALYZING,
LIFE IS SIMPLE.
ALL EMOTIONS ARE BEAUTIFUL.
WHEN YOU EAT, APPRECIATE
EVERY LAST BITE.
OPEN YOUR MIND, ARMS, AND HEART TO NEW THINGS
AND PEOPLE, WE ARE UNITED IN OUR DIFFERENCES.
ASK THE NEXT PERSON YOU SEE WHAT THEIR PASSION IS,
AND SHARE YOUR INSPIRING DREAM WITH THEM.
TRAVEL OFTEN; GETTING LOST WILL
HELP YOU FIND YOURSELF.
SOME OPPORTUNITIES ONLY COME ONCE, SEIZE THEM.
LIFE IS ABOUT THE PEOPLE YOU MEET, AND
THE THINGS YOU CREATE WITH THEM
SO GO OUT AND START CREATING.
LIFE IS SHORT.
LIVE YOUR DREAM
AND SHARE
YOUR PASSION.

MICHAEL RADPARVAR

There's something magical that happens when you allow yourself to first identify, then put into words, your true north. It may lead you to an unconventional risk or two, but you will always be happy you dared to do it.

It was spring of 2009. My brother Dave approached cofounder Fabian Pfortmüller and me, suggesting that we take some time to put into words exactly why we chose to create our company, Holstee. We were just three weeks old, had millions of things on our plate, and were in the midst of the worst recession of our generation. Still, we knew this would help us on our journey, and neither of us questioned his proposal. We agreed that whatever we wrote would be an important message to our future selves, coming from a time when our thinking was crystal clear. We used this as an opportunity to define success for ourselves, in nonfinancial terms. We talked about everything important to us: life philosophies, love, food, travel, our hopes and dreams, insights from friends and family. Everything. Then we put these ideas on paper. And for good measure, we decided to put them in a place we knew they wouldn't get lost: on the "about" page of our website. We called it our manifesto.

Over the following months and years, this manifesto took a completely unexpected journey. It grew to become one of the most actively shared images across the web and around the world, and it eventually took the form of letterpress print for better offline sharing as well. Since the day we put those words to paper, they have been reflected in Holstee's culture and products, and became more deeply ingrained into the lives of the three of us than we could ever have imagined.

We are humbled and excited that the Holstee Manifesto continues to impact so many people around the world. But to be honest, we had really just written it for ourselves. People have asked us what strategy we used to create a viral manifesto. We had no secret recipe and, most important, we didn't have any expectations. Whenever you choose to write your own authentic intentions, there is only one rule—write it for no one but yourself. And don't ask yourself what you want to do, but why.

At the end of the day, nothing resonates like the sound of honesty.

We cannot approach the idea of "core" without addressing truth. We can think of core as an aligned, centered state of ease, a way of being that is available to us all the time, both emotionally and structurally.

While truth is never a fixed constant amid any two humans, it's easy to see that secrets, hiding, and lying take their toll on our physical bodies. When we lie, keep a truth hidden, or hold secrets for ourselves or others, we move AWAY from our core, toward distracting habits and relationships. That's when the body settles into a place of constant, chronic stress, which actually initiates a neurologically degenerative process that causes misalignments in our resonance circuitry. Mental stress caused by lying frays the nerves in the brain, which, over time, can cause cellular damage to brain matter, decreases motivation and creativity, and diminishes our self-worth and our capacity to coherently relate to those closest to us. When there is a secret or something unsaid, we have to maintain a difficult divide within ourselves, between what can and cannot be said. Stress hormones flood our circuits, leaving the body in a state of agitation. On high alert for so many moments of the day, our internal organs and glands react and work far harder than normal. This manifests as exhaustion, frequent illness, or just plain sadness.

"Chronic stress can lead to a rut in which the wiring of our neural networks keeps us repeating the same dysfunctional behavior and hoping for a different outcome. As we experience depression and repetitive behaviors that stem from chronic stress, we're less capable of analytic thought. The stress hormones released into the bloodstream keep us at a lower order of brain function, unable to attain synergy."

—Villoldo and Perlmutter, POWER UP YOUR BRAIN

Basically, lying steals our resonance. And we all do it, and we all know that anxious feeling that surrounds us when we aren't honest. Whether it's a longtime habit or a relationship you know isn't serving you, realize that it's the worrying, overthinking, and lying about it that are responsible for your body's stress response. Those actions (worry, thought, lying) are all a choice. I choose to worry, I choose to overanalyze, I choose to lie, even about small matters. And I pay the price for those choices: my skin, hair, muscle tone, alertness, happiness all suffer. I lose my sense of devotion. As soon as I clear the air, create the space, have the conversation, I'm back, and feel my stride again. Truth is sometimes a difficult thing to wrangle, but when I do, I feel better.

And luckily for us, we have our yoga practice. Yoga encourages, demands, honesty. We place the physical body into alignment, and seek the optimal flow of energy in each pose. In our physical sequence for this chapter, we'll define that core in an unexpected way, and place our attention structurally on that understanding. The practice will allow us to sense what core resonance feels like, and then we can begin using that sensation to align our relationships and interactions in the direction of more truth.

And just one simple writing exercise will get you on the road to recognizing honesty—and feel way more easeful in your body and your mind. When we practice, we naturally move toward the feeling of right alignment and sense more space in the body when we're telling the truth. Both great alignment and a good hit of honesty allow our body a chance to relax on a cellular level.

WRITING EXERCISE: *Note for one day all the little lies: Make it funny—see the humor.*

1.

2.

3.

4.

5.

6.

7.

8.

9.

10.

11.

12.

EXTRA CREDIT: *Make a list of the lies you have to own/ 'fess up to.*

Curing Common Ailments with Sujok

JOSEPH GIACONA

In my experience, a successful healing modality accomplishes three things: It **detoxes, nourishes, and harmonizes.** *Of all the healing techniques that do these three, one of the most effective and simplest is Sujok© acupuncture.*

In the Korean language, SU *means hand and* JOK *means foot. Sujok therapy is hand and foot acupuncture. Acupuncture involves inserting very fine needles into the skin in order to stimulate the natural healing abilities of the body. Developed in China between two thousand and four thousand years ago, this ancient healing modality remains prevalent and extraordinarily effective in the twenty-first century.*

In Sujok acupuncture, all needles are placed in the hands or feet. The hands and feet contain hundreds of energy points that stimulate the natural healing abilities of the body. However, if you're not about to start practicing acupuncture on yourself, you can begin with acupressure, using pressure and massage to activate the areas desired.

According to Sujok, the hand is a representation of the entire body, often referred to as a microsystem. In its most basic form, the thumb corresponds to the head, the index finger and pinky correspond to the arms and the middle finger and the ring finger correspond to the legs; the back of the hand corresponds to the posterior parts of the body, such as the kidneys, and the palm corresponds to other vital organs on the front of the body, such as the large intestine.

Via a representation of the body—the hand—we can access and heal all the major organs, organ systems, cells, and even chakras of the entire body. All you need is a palpation instrument of some kind, such as a pencil eraser, a small Phillips head screwdriver, or a retractable pen.

TREATING HEADACHES

Find the point on your thumb that corresponds to the general area of your headache. For instance, let's say your headache is on the top of your head. This corresponds to the tip of your thumb. Using the pen tip, press into the top of your thumb, fishing around for a sensitive area, almost like a small ball of pain or tension. You are likely to find at least one sensitive spot. This sensitive spot shares a similitude to the area of your actual headache.

Gently massage the area for a few minutes, gradually increasing the pressure. It should be a bit uncomfortable, but not excruciating. If every point is sensitive, you are pushing too hard. Within a few minutes you may notice your headache isn't as intense and is maybe moving or dispersing.

As you do this, remember to breathe! Breathing helps increase circulation, removes waste (detoxifies), and transports nutrients to tissue. The breath is the source of life and must be cultivated through whatever form of Sujok you do.

RELIEVING NECK PAIN

Find the point on your thumb that corresponds to the general area of your neck pain.

CERVICAL 1 = *just below first knuckle in the back of the thumb*

CERVICAL 7 = *just below the second knuckle on the back of the thumb*

THORACIC 8 = *top border of the anatomical "snuff box"*

THORACIC 9 = *top of the wrist/ ulnar bone*

For neck pain originating from just below the base of the skull—in the C1 vertebra—find a tender spot slightly below the first knuckle on the back of the thumb. Gently massage the area for a few minutes, gradually increasing the pressure until some relief is experienced.

FIXING TMJ PAIN

Most people unconsciously clench their jaw—at home, at work, even while sleeping. If left untreated, jaw clenching may result in temporomandibular joint disorders, more commonly known as TMJ.

All things being connected, what happens with the jaw affects the spine and more. When the jaw is misaligned, the

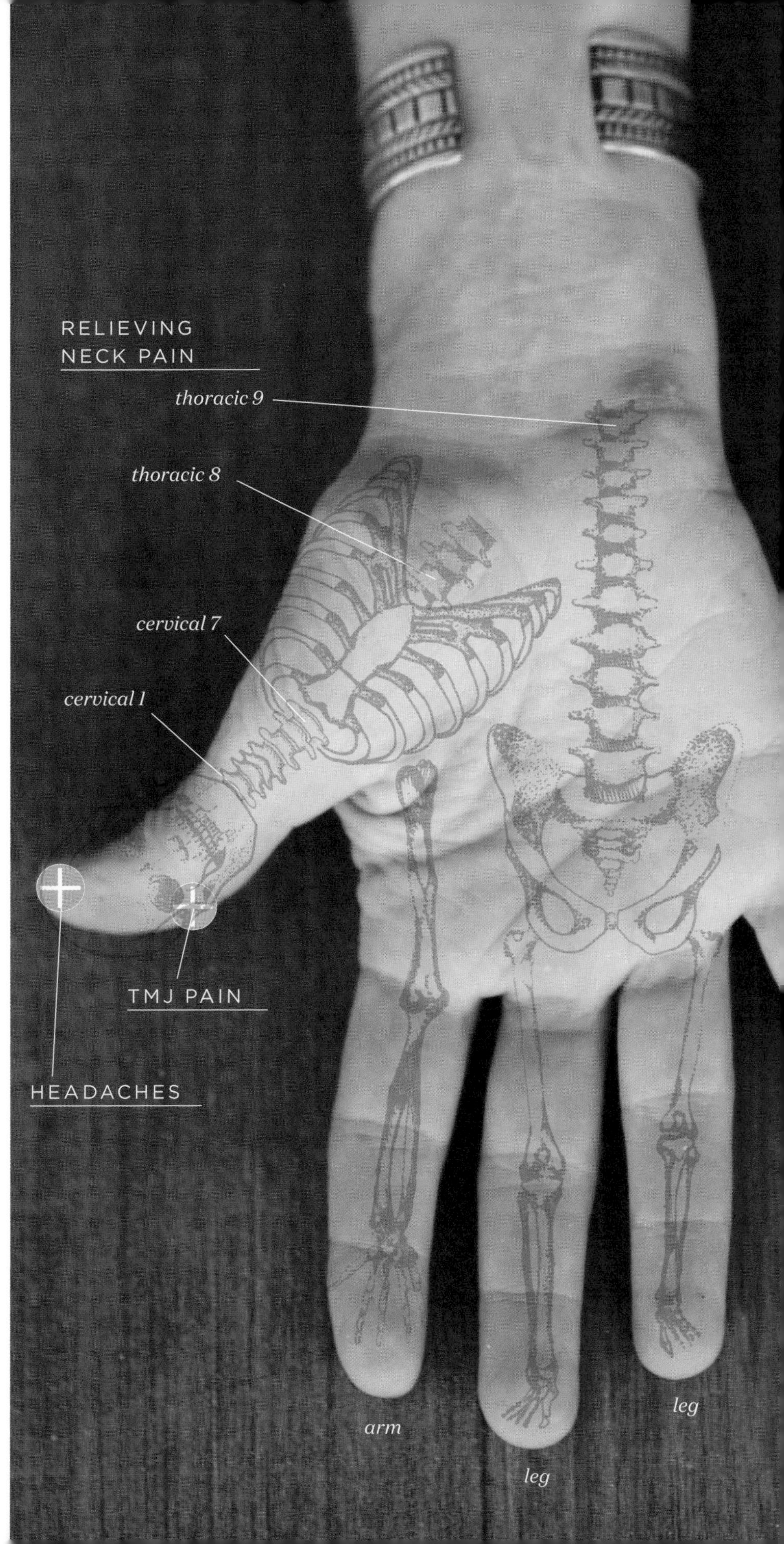

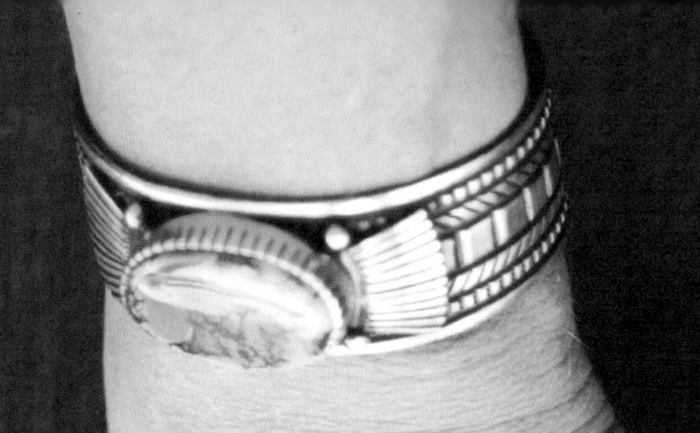
THE LIVER
HEART POINT
ADRENAL FATIGUE

entire musculature and fascial network of the skull and neck is thrown off. This imbalance spreads throughout the spine at large and farther down into the hips and pelvis, often causing knee and foot issues. In fact, many knee and foot problems originate in the jaw.

The two important Sujok acupuncture points associated with TMJ are located slightly anterior to the ears of the skull image on the thumb of the Sujok model on page 83. Follow the palpation techniques already described, massaging for tender points.

ADDRESSING ADRENAL FATIGUE

Stress, allergies, panic attacks, sleep disorders, low energy, and general weakness are all symptoms of adrenal fatigue.

The adrenal glands sit on top of the kidneys and are a major immune and endocrine organ in charge of a whole host of functions within the body. In our modern, fast-paced, high-stress lives, they are the first organ to become weak, impaired, and, quite honestly, somewhat tortured. To relieve stress, allergies, panic attacks, sleep disorders, and general weakness, stimulate the points associated with your adrenals.

HEALING THE LIVER

The liver is the main hormone organ in charge of detoxification and digestion. If you are a person who stays out late at the bar every weekend, you may notice a few sensitive spots when you palpate the liver area of your hand. To stimulate the liver, massage your hand, just down from the wrist crease on the pinky side. If you do not get a response within ten seconds, change the correspondence point.

PREVENTION AND STAYING HEALTHY

Sujok is very helpful for relieving acute symptoms. But it also functions to prevent disease, increase vitality, and increase your overall sense of well-being. The best point to stimulate for disease prevention in general is the heart point, located at the center of the fleshy mound of the palmar side of the thumb just below the thymus point. You have medicine in your hands.

Many people ask me how to get free of fear. Fear is a big part of climbing. Learning how to manage fear can change not just your experience on a climb, but your entire life. My feelings about fear have evolved a lot over time. Nowadays I think that the idea of getting rid of fear is not really what I'm after. Fear will always exist, and in fact it is an important motivator to stay safe and be on the very top of your game. It can make you sharp and make you perform your very best. So the real question is how to coexist with fear, how to manage it rather than allowing it to control you and crack your performance.

Trying an unknown climb can be scary—you've never been on that rock before, you don't know how hard it will be to climb or when the difficult sections will come at you. Since difficulty is always subjective, there's a chance you will find it much harder than others did, and the hard sections might be just the type of thing you don't happen to excel at. There's a good chance you will fall, or simply fail. So the real problem here is the unknown, which tends to be scary for humans.

Managing this type of fear is actually pretty simple: All you need to do is figure out how to reduce the number of unknowns in the picture. This can be done by information gathering and preparation, both of which will dramatically raise your confidence in climbing into the unknown.

I try to get as much information as possible about an unknown climb from other climbers and the Internet, and simply by looking up and analyzing it from the ground. Even just knowing where the hardest part of the route is can allow you to plan for that difficulty and feel that you've reduced some of the unknown.

I know that if I spend three days a week training with a finger-strength workout, then I have the extra strength to hang on a little longer on vertical terrain, and so I make that workout a priority. I also know that you get good at whatever you practice, so I make sure to consistently climb routes I don't know whenever possible, rather than always returning to my familiar favorites around home.

If you can step back from the feelings of fear and doubt, you can categorize those feelings as simple fear of the unknown, and you can list all the unknowns you have eliminated through your research and preparation. This will raise your confidence and let you feel that you do belong there and that you will do a good job and enjoy it.

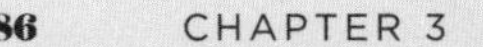

Another big part of climbing is practicing an extremely difficult climb over and over again until you can climb it with no falls. This is similar to what a dancer, musician, or gymnast does. The fear of the unknown does not figure in, since sometimes a climber will try the same route up to a hundred times before succeeding in climbing it perfectly.

An entirely different, maybe even more complicated, fear comes into play here: the fear of failure. Every time you try the climb and fall off just at the very end, you become more invested in the route and you become more susceptible to pressure. Every time you almost succeed, but not quite, you have to decide to try again rather than abandon this climb and doing something easier, more fun, more achievable. Each attempt increases the feeling of investment, of time and effort that could be "wasted" if you give up on it or never manage to finish it. It's very difficult not to become focused on the outcome—climbing the route with no falls—and it's easy to stop enjoying the process of trying to do so.

Every dedicated climber who has tried a climbing "project" is familiar with this mental journey, and I think it's a really valuable life lesson and perhaps the single best reason for doing this type of climbing.

The hardest thing about a climbing project is the need to try as hard as you can, yet simultaneously remain unattached to the outcome. If you don't care a lot, you won't have the desire needed to push past your limits. But caring too much can cause mental conflict: stress, anxiety, and pressure. I've learned that when I try a route like this, I need to remove that feeling of mental pressure right before I start climbing. Rather than stepping off the ground thinking, "I really wish I could complete this route cleanly today. If I have to try it one more time I might go nuts," I remind myself that it really doesn't matter at all if I do the climb now or later. If I fall off, I'll just try again. I'll do it eventually, whether today or another day. It does not matter at all. Taking this attitude immediately reduces the stress level and the mental pressure, which makes me enjoy the climbing and often allows me to be in the right mind state to actually do it.

Having done a lot of big climbing projects in my life, it didn't take long to realize that there's actually a surprising feeling of letdown after you succeed and finish the route. Of course it feels great in the first minutes, and sometimes even days, after you finish it. You feel excitement, pride, satisfaction, and often relief that you finally made it after so much effort and time. After all, that's what you wanted more than anything, to be at the top of the route, successful at last. But soon that wears off, and you realize that you miss the experience of working on the project and are actually dissatisfied until you find a new climb to work on. Funny enough, it's the process of working on a climb that is so much more enjoyable than finishing it—finishing feels good, but it also means that the process is over.

This is a reminder that life is a journey, not a destination, and every second should be cherished.

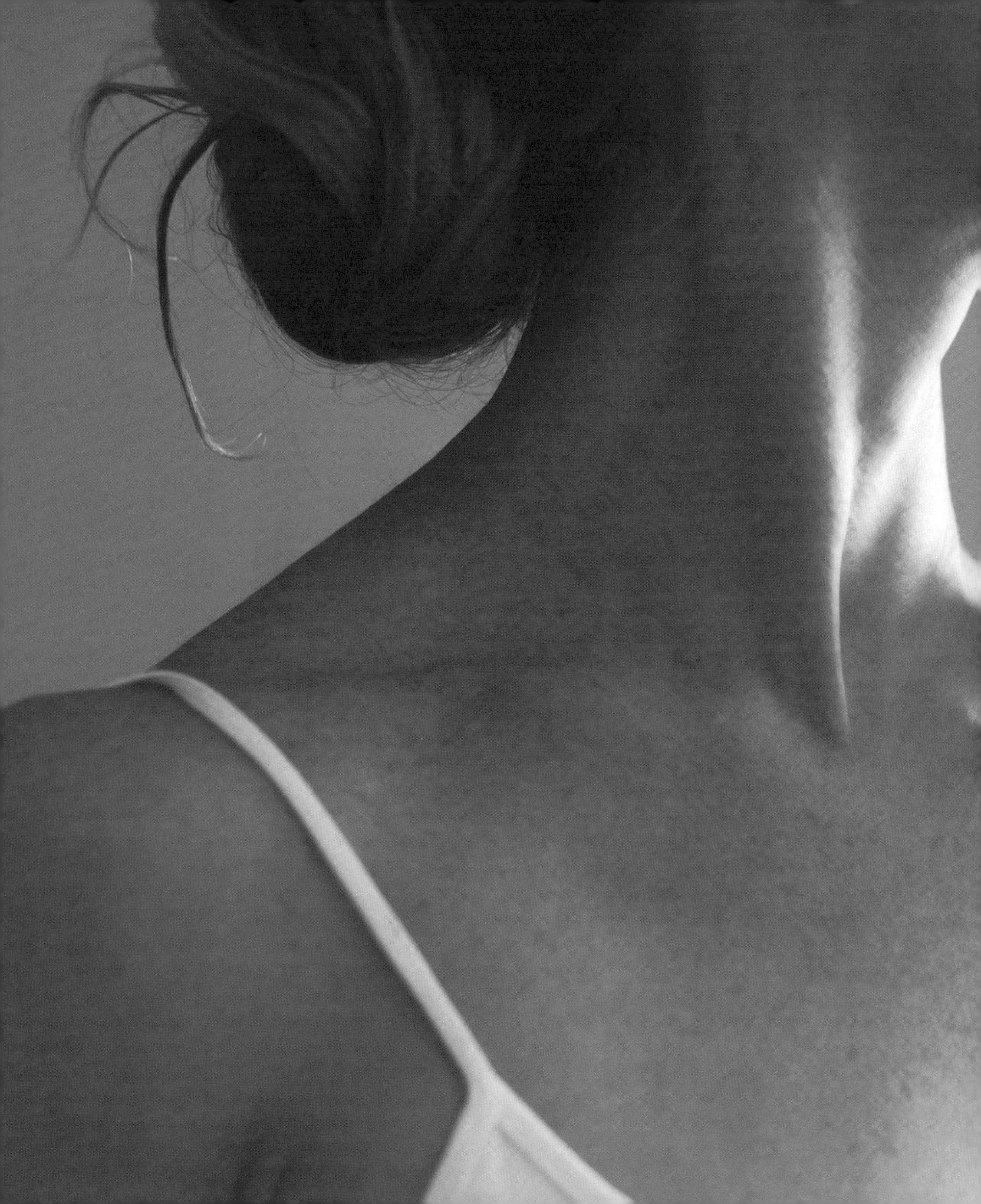

occiput *base of skull*

biceps brachii *biceps*

cervical spine *neck*

triceps brachii *triceps*

upper trapezius *upper traps*

scapulae *shoulder blade*

pectoralis major *pecs*

thoracic spine *middle/upper back*

serratus anterior *serratus*

sacral spine *lower back*

iliac crest *hip points*

sacrum

piriformis

iliospoas *psoas*

coccyx *tailbone*

pubis *pubic bone*

ischium *sit bones*

hamstring

quadriceps *quads*

femur *thigh bone*

tibia *shin bone*

gastrocnemius *calf*

THE TAO OF CHAKRAS

THOMAS DROGE

In the spiritual traditions of India, the body is viewed in both its physical and its energetic form. This energetic form is known as the "subtle body." Within the subtle body we find chakras. These are meeting points of the energetic pathways of the body known as the nadiis. Prana (our life force) uses these pathways to travel throughout the body.

The seven main chakras span the area from the base of the tailbone at the pelvic floor to the top of the head. Each corresponds to a different physical and spiritual developmental state, with a unique connection to particular organs, emotional and spiritual issues, physical ailments, colors, and sounds.

Chakras can be accessed by asana, meditation, breathing, environment, and touch. As we look at each individual chakra, you will see how we can activate and transform our issues at the physical or psychological level through the spiritual asana practice of opening and activating our chakras. These vortices of energy are doors of perception that can literally transport our consciousness into multiple dimensions.

So let's begin at the root chakra and work our way from the earth to the heavens.

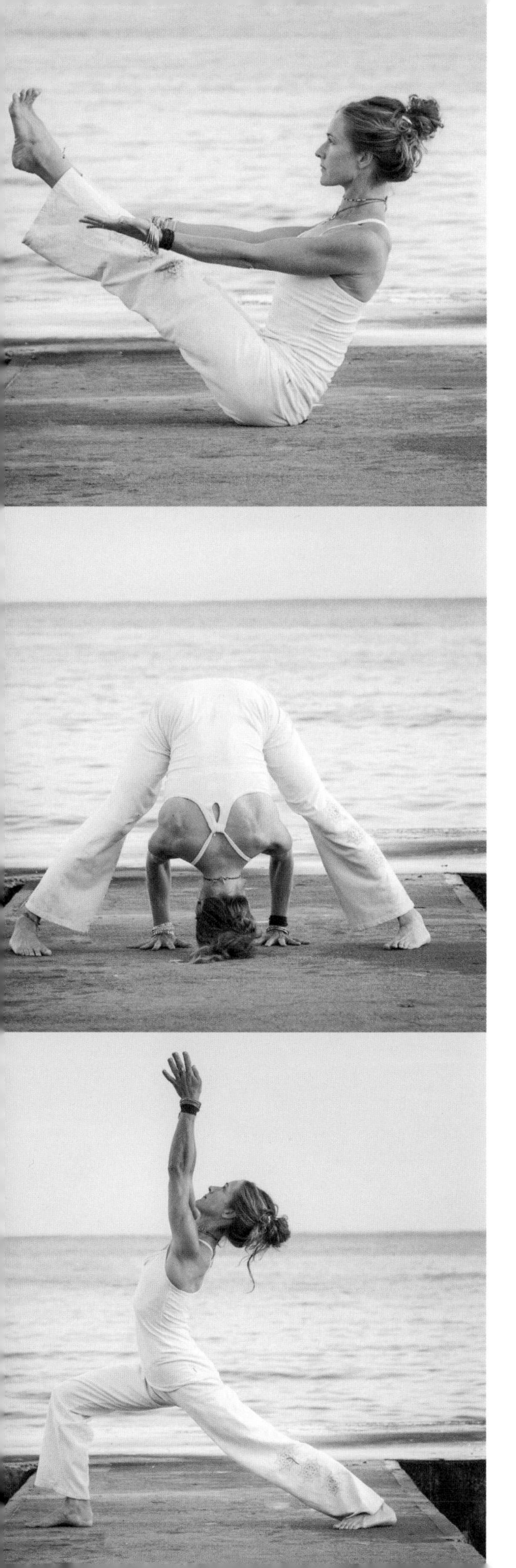
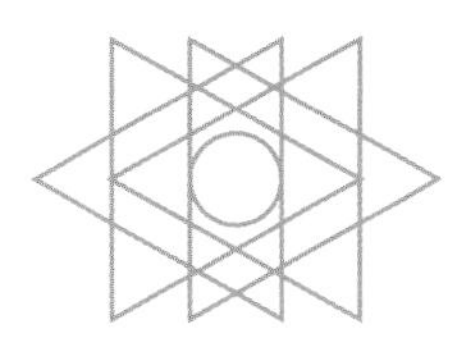
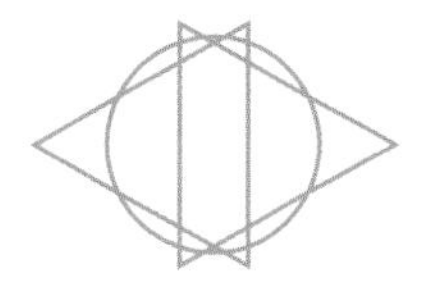
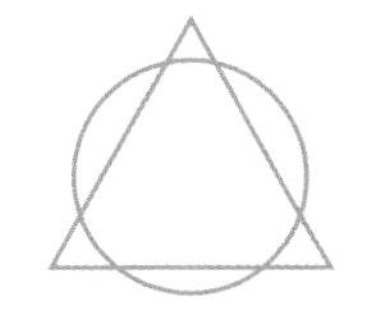
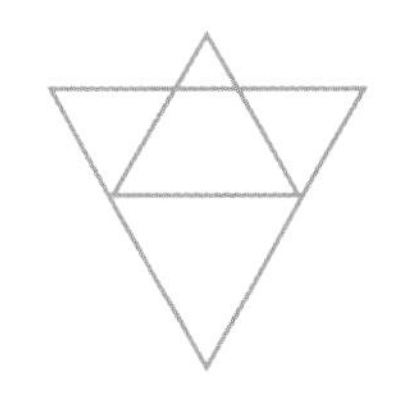
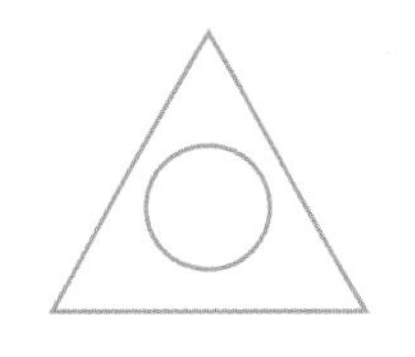
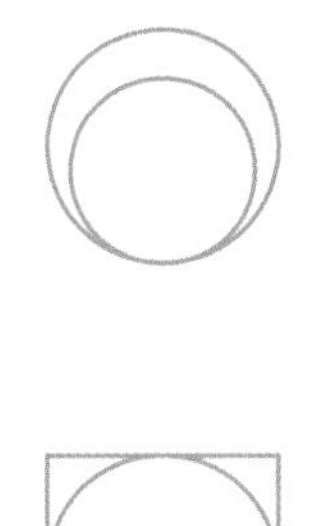
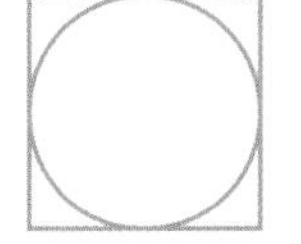
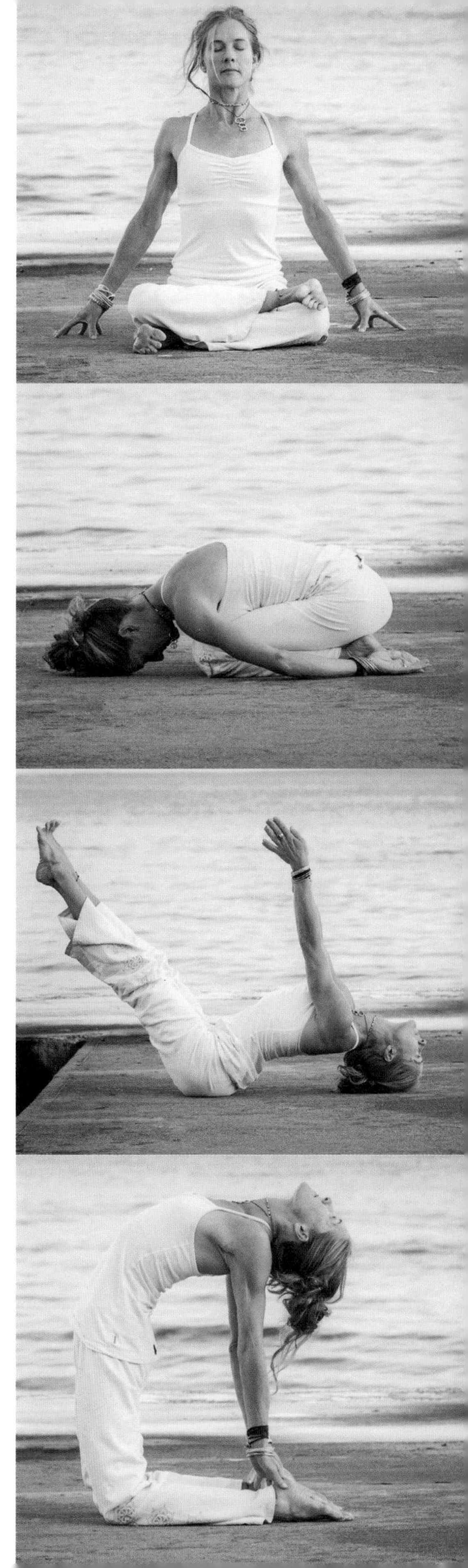

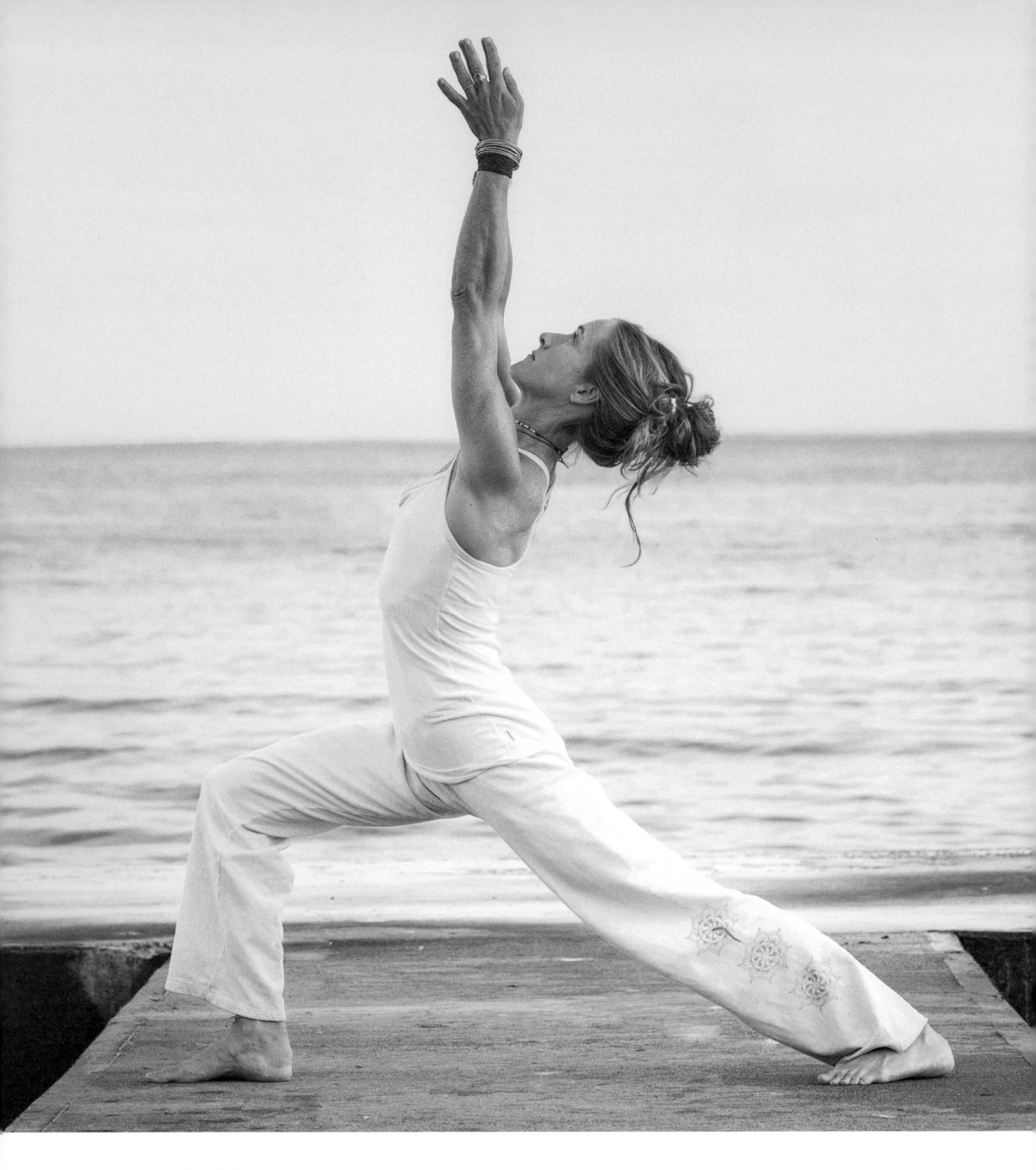

THE FIRST CHAKRA

Muladhara: Mula (root) adhara (support)

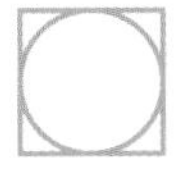

Located at the tip of the coccyx and the pelvic floor, this chakra is associated with physical identity, survival, stability, and instinctual nature. Psychologically it relates to fear, ungroundedness, and anger. Physically it corresponds to tiredness, poor sleep, lower-back pain, immune disorders, and obesity.

To strengthen muladhara, we build strength, physically grounding the body with the stability of the earth so we can be rooted, self-aware, courageous, and fearless.

ASANAS: *Mountain pose, warrior pose, standing forward bend.* **COLOR:** *red;* **ELEMENT:** *earth;* **SENSE:** *smell*

THE SECOND CHAKRA

Svadhisthana: Seat of Vital Force

Located between the sacrum and pubic bone, including the genitals, svadhisthana corresponds with the center of gravity of the body. This chakra relates to the cultivation of the emotional and sensual self. It is the home of the reproductive organs, the kidneys, the hips, and the sacrum. Fluidity, sensual pleasure, and dance, as well as physical and emotional expression, are all rooted in this second chakra. It is psychologically connected to power and control issues, morality, obsession, guilt, blame, and addiction. The power released in the physical world with this chakra is not to be trifled with. This chakra often relates to emotional identity, desire, procreation, self-love (especially physical), and relationships. It relates to health issues associated with libido, sciatica, lower-back pain, vertigo, menstrual issues, and hormonal imbalances.

When balanced, svadhisthana produces a balanced, vital, sexually uninhibited, prosperous, satisfied way of being.

ASANAS: *Hip openers, wide-stance forward bend, wide-stance seated position, and seated bound angle position.* **COLOR:** *orange;* **ELEMENT:** *water;* **SENSE:** *taste*

THE THIRD CHAKRA

Manipura: City of Jewels

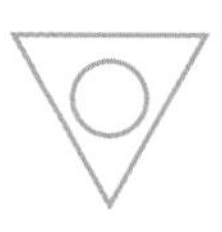

Located at the solar plexus, manipura is a central point of transformation in the body. In these alchemical practices, when we really want to change, we engender fire (manipura's element) and burn away our former selves to allow for a new self to emerge. Jewels also function as prisms, bending light to change the look of reality, thereby reminding us that reality is shaped by perception.

Some of the organs associated with manipura include the stomach, liver, gallbladder, midspine, and small intestines. This chakra can help you deal with psychological issues like low self-esteem, timidity, depression, fear of rejection, perfectionism, anger, indecisiveness, and rage.

When manipura is balanced, one feels confident, clear, decisive, productive, and focused, and one's digestion is excellent.

ASANAS: *Half twist, boat pose, backbends, reverse warrior, and, of course, "breath of fire" are all excellent for this chakra.* COLOR: *yellow;* ELEMENT: *fire;* SENSE: *sight*

THE FOURTH CHAKRA

Anahata

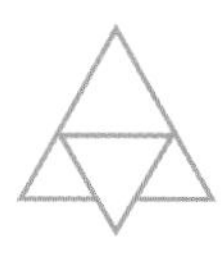

Anahata literally means "unbeaten." It is the heart chakra and the center point in the chakra system, standing between the three lower earthly chakras and the three celestial chakras above. Through the heart chakra we harmonize heaven and earth, finding the dynamic balance between spiritual practice and living in the earthly realm. It is my belief that this chakra holds the power to transcend pain and suffering. At the core of this chakra is love, and love IS the unifying healing force that links us all together. One of the best ways to strengthen the heart chakra is to offer it openly to the world.

ASANAS: *Eagle pose, cow pose, backbends, and chest opening poses.* COLOR: *green;* ELEMENT: *air;* SENSE: *touch*

THE FIFTH CHAKRA

Visuddha: Purification

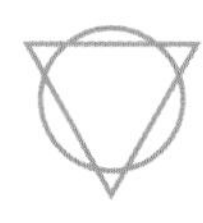

Unlike the lower chakras, visuddha is focused on the spiritual and metaphysical path. Located at the throat, this chakra connects the spiritual and physical plane through the vibration of sound. The reading of poems and prayers and chanting are all excellent ways to express the positive nature of this chakra. The throat, thyroid, and parathyroid glands are always associated with visuddha, and they are often healed through communication and creativity.

ASANAS: *Fish pose, lion, and supported shoulder stand.* COLOR: *blue;* ELEMENT: *sound;* SENSE: *hearing*

THE SIXTH CHAKRA

Ajna: Third Eye

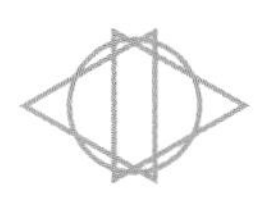

Located between the two eyebrows, ajna is related to inner vision. This chakra sits in the acupuncture point often translated as "calm spirit," and provides us with the unique gift of being able to link our sight with our crown chakra to access the greater collective consciousness. This is the chakra we use to scan our body and energetic field for disturbances. This chakra requires rooting in the earth element through the breath in order not to overactivate it. Dysfunction of this chakra can lead to headaches, nightmares, eyestrain, and learning disabilities. When balanced, this chakra produces a deep, clear calm and is capable of creating reality from thought.

ASANAS: *Breath work, meditation, child's pose, yoga nidra.* COLOR: *indigo;* ELEMENT: *light;* SENSE: *ESP*

THE SEVENTH CHAKRA

Sahasrara: One-Thousand-Petaled Lotus

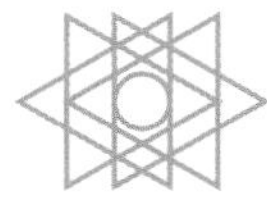

The lotus represents the infinite creation and destruction of all things. Located at the crown of the head, sahasrara allows you to directly receive celestial information and to connect with deities and other energy forces available to you. This chakra when open can collapse time and space and allow the future and past to be available to you simultaneously. Often misinterpreted as seeing the future, a deep connection with sahasrara allows you to see everything in the now.

ASANAS: *Tree, eagle, and seated meditation.* COLOR: *white (sahasrara carries all the colors in its spectrum);* ELEMENT: *thought;* SENSE: *unity and interdependence of all things*

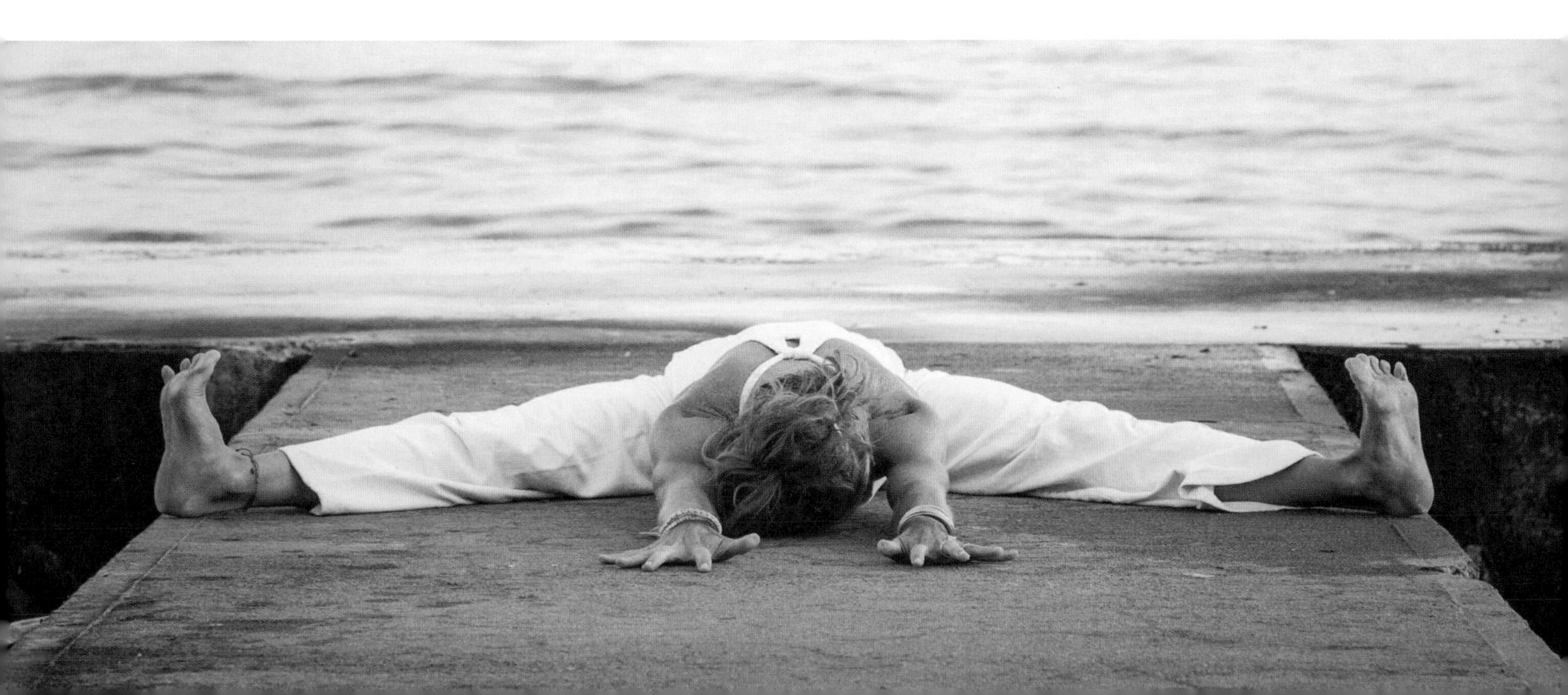

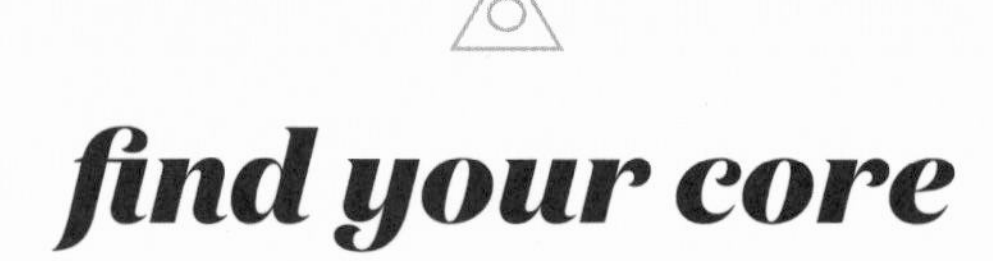

find your core

ELENA BROWER AND
JONINA TURZI

Imagine the body is an apple. The core of the apple is the spine. In this short sequence, you'll practice stabilizing from your core in simple postures at first. Increasingly larger dynamic movements become possible "on axis" as you move consciously. While practicing these poses, notice how your pelvis is actually two separate segments, right and left. Feel those two bones lead the actions of the poses you take. As an advanced practice, allow the breath to move first, then follow with the bones.

wave one *initiation*

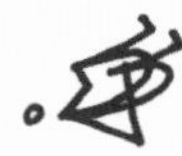

FETAL FOLD

Spread your sit bones away from one another and lift them up off the floor.

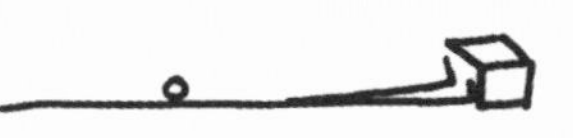

ELONGATION STRETCH

Stretch your arms and legs long, perhaps feet against a wall or yoga blocks. Lengthen your pubic bones and sit bones toward the feet.

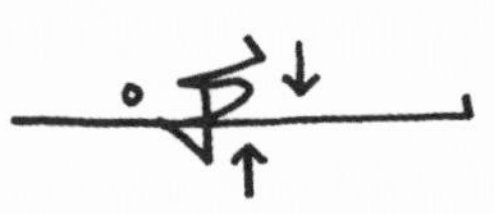

SUPINE LEG LIFTS

Keep your left leg and arm anchored in the elongation stretch, lift your right knee into your hand. Use your right sit bone to initiate the lift of your whole right leg. Breathe and feel a healthy segmentation within your pelvis; feel both sides working gently in opposition, creating strength along your spinal axis.

wave two *acceptance*

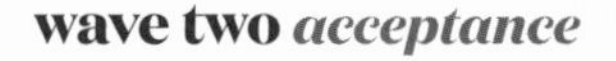

ROCKING BOAT

From any variation of boat pose, shift your weight side to side, lifting the opposite hip/sit bone up off the floor. Keep your spine as long as possible.

"Physical integrity and personal integrity are inherently connected."

—JONINA TURZI

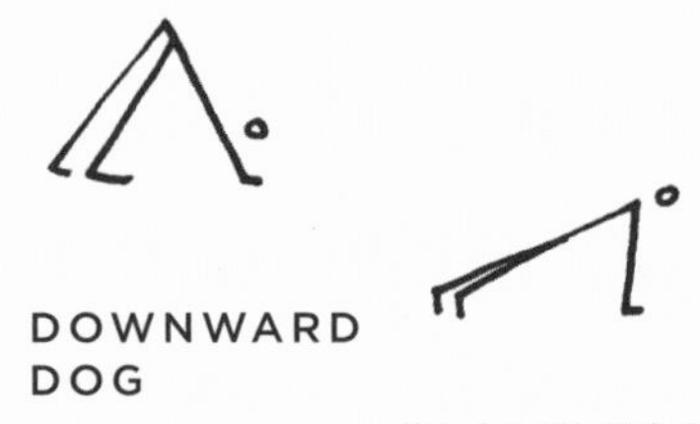

DOWNWARD DOG

PLANK POSE

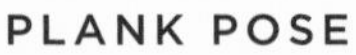

Core Playlist

compiled by Kelly Casey

- **10 Laws**—*East Forest*
- **Bron-Yr-Aur**—*Led Zeppelin*
- **Theme from Prince Avalanche**—*Explosions In The Sky*
- **Heartbeats**—*José González*
- **Wonderwall**—*Ryan Adams*
- **Soak It Up**—*Houses*
- **Vapour**—*Vancouver Sleep Clinic*
- **Big Light**—*Houses*
- **Parade of Wind**—*Slow Dancing Society*
- **Grandmothersphere**—*East Forest*

wave three *expansion*

ASHTANGASANA

Knees, chest, and chin elongate to the floor.

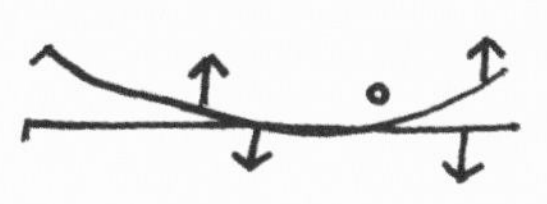

PRONE LEG LIFTS

Root your left pelvis onto the floor. Lift your entire right pelvis and extend the right leg a few inches off the floor. Be certain your right pelvis has cleared the floor (can feel with hands under your hips). Slowly lower and anchor the right pelvis to lift the left leg and repeat.

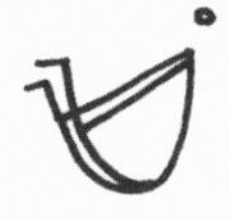

ROCKING BOW POSE

Hold your feet, extend both hips to lift knees and shoulders evenly off the floor. Again rock your weight laterally and lift one pelvis at a time; if possible, turn fully onto one side of your body for a few breaths.

wave four *concentration*

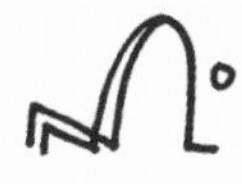

CAT POSE

From table, root the pelvic bones toward the knees and lift your abdominal organs for a rounded lower back stretch.

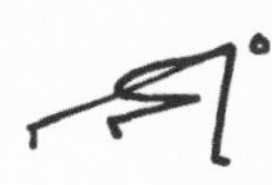

Can do this entire movement from plank to step a foot forward as an advanced alternative.

HOVER CRAWL

Bring your right knee to hover just inside your right wrist. Shift the right pelvic bones forward and up toward the right shoulder. Gently place the knee down, crawl your hands forward, and switch to the left leg's hovering lift.

STANDING FORWARD FOLD

Stack hips over the heels (weight shifted forward) as you fold. Move your chest and chin toward your feet as deeply as your pelvic bones can initiate.

wave four *conscious evolution*

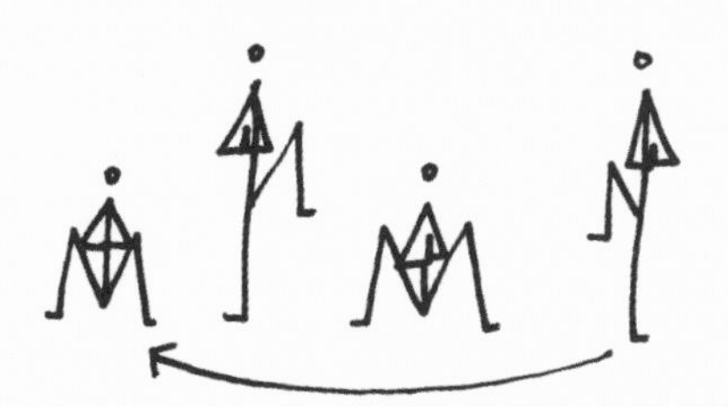

STANDING SQUATS TO LEG LIFTS

From squat, transfer weight onto the right leg to lift the entire left pelvis and leg. Push to stand, keep the left hip lifted. At the top of this move, the right hip will be down and back and the left hip will be up and forward. Sit down through squat to switch sides, repeat.

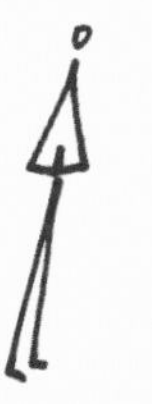

MOUNTAIN POSE

As we step off the mat, from/within/ atop the mountain.

MARA MUNRO

The core is far more than your abs. It is the mental and emotional stamina that keeps you connected and moving forward. Core values shape your life and the stories you tell yourself about who you are, what you can and cannot do. These stories can set you free—and they can also imprison you.

What stories do you tell yourself? What outdated narratives are not serving you? What new stories would you like to tell? It's time to flip the script.

Flip the Script

DURATION:
One week

LOCATION:
Anywhere

MINDSET:
Observant

TOOLS:
Pen

PART ONE:

1. Make a note of every time you say or think, "I can't."
2. Record the context of each moment:
   A. Where were you?
   B. Who did you say it to?
   C. What was the situation that you were trying to create, or to avoid?

I CAN'T
A.
B.
C.

I CAN'T
A.
B.
C.

I CAN'T
A.
B.
C.

I CAN'T
A.
B.
C.

I CAN'T
A.
B.
C.

I CAN'T
A.
B.
C.

I CAN'T
A.
B.
C.

PART TWO:

1. Recognize when this occurs.
2. Ask yourself:
   A. What is the real story?
   B. What is the source of this story?
   C. What if it wasn't true?
   D. How would the opposite change your life?

PART THREE:

1. Flip the script! When you say/think the following:

I COULD NEVER ____________________

BECAUSE ____________________

IF THIS WASN'T TRUE, I WOULD ____________________

Change it to:

I CAN ____________________

BECAUSE ____________________

THIS IS TRUE, SO I WILL ____________________

AND EXPERIMENT WITH MOVING FORWARD IN THIS NEW STORY.

2. Observe and record the differences:

   A. What happened after you began with "I can"?

   B. How was it different?

   C. How did it make you feel?

You are now coming into your power to create your life by choosing what to believe about yourself. Every time you rewrite an outdated story, you free a part of yourself and move closer to your true north.

We delight in the beauty of the butterfly, but rarely admit the changes it has gone through to achieve that beauty.

—Maya Angelou

INSPIRE

It is only with the heart that one can see rightly; what is essential is invisible to the eye.

—Antoine de Saint-Exupery

CHAPTER 4

find your heart

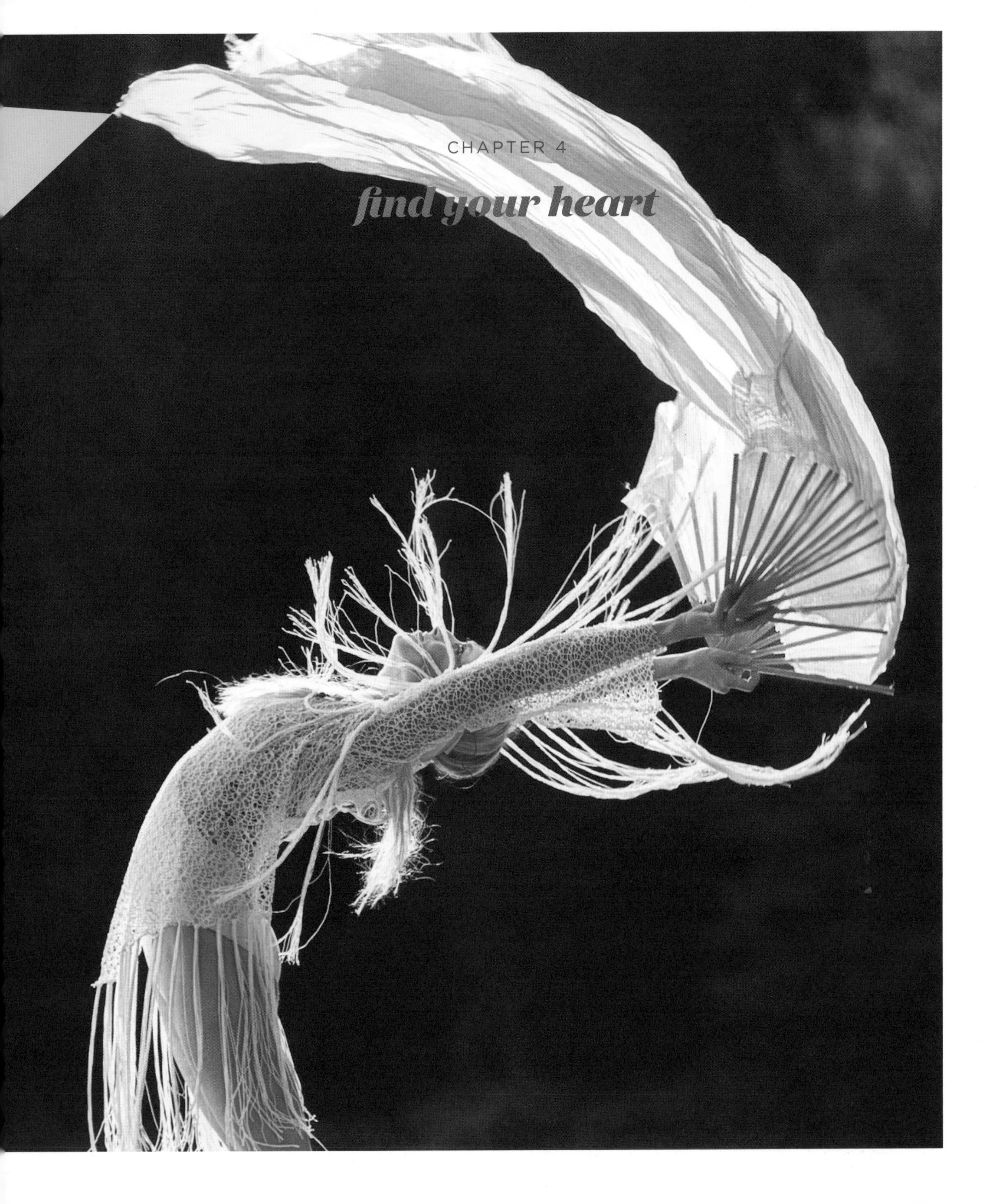

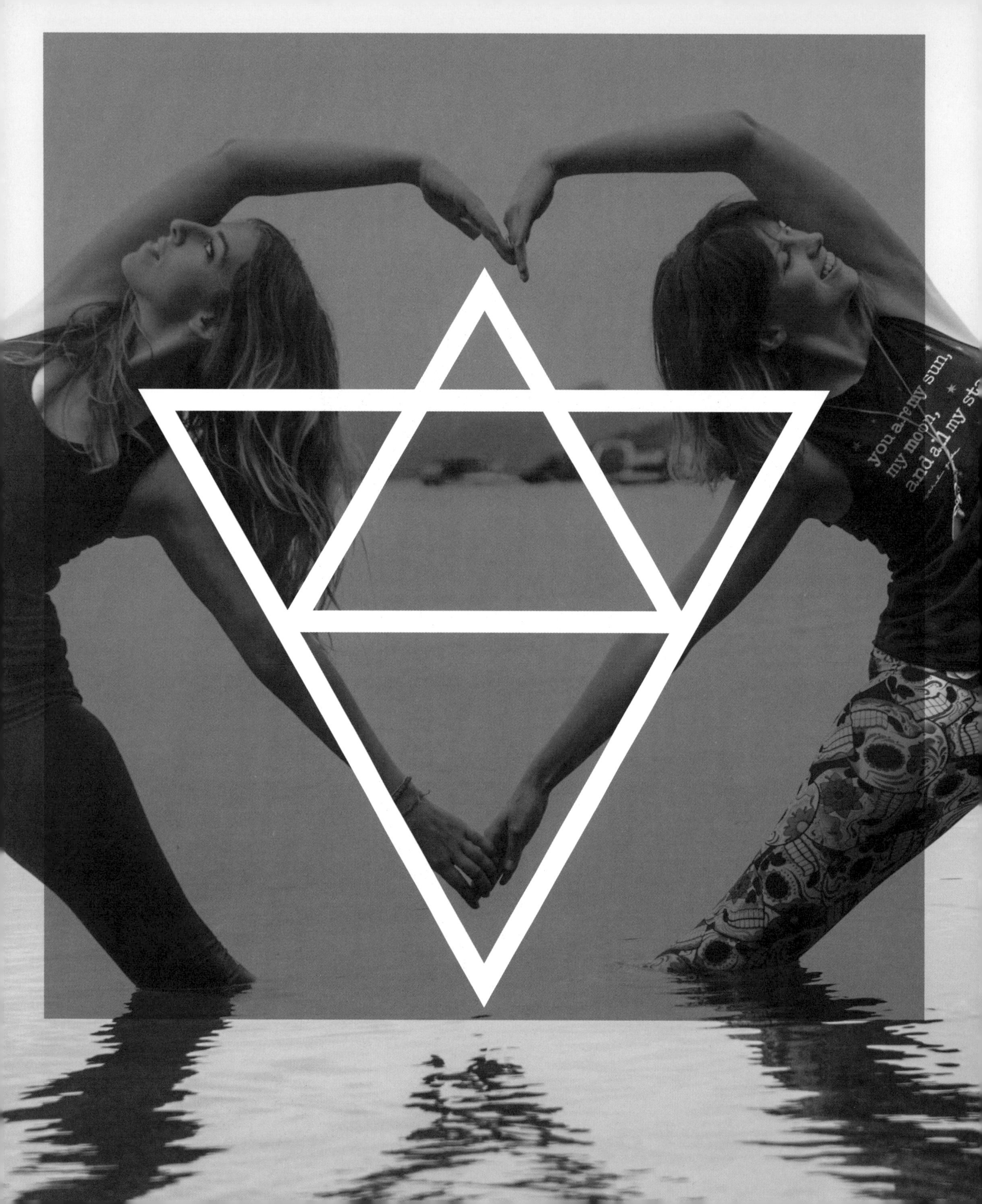
my sun,
my moon,

We cannot talk about Wanderlust without journeying into the most wild and powerful terrain: the heart.

The heart is a movable object, enigmatic.

is an engine, propelling us,
valves and all.

it opens like a door and closes like a flower.

can bruise and mend.

has voice, telling us what's true.

We cannot talk about yoga without the heart. In poses, we think about which way it turns: toward the sky in upward dog, tucked inward in a forward fold. We practice: speaking from it, acting from it, and bowing it, in devotion, to whatever we praise.

In ancient Egypt, the heart was the only organ left inside the body during mummification. They thought of the heart as the center of being, the seat of intellect and feeling. Science may have disproved this, but we know better.

Grief is nondiscriminatory, often inconvenient, can hit us like a brick, render our lives utterly and infinitely transformed, and open us to levels of vulnerability, tenderness, and even gratitude. It is so raw, so inexpressible, that it can only truly be considered—unapologetically, perfectly, blindingly—as purely human and ultimately unavoidable if we live long enough to endure both the pain and the joy that is this life.

My father died in 2010 after a long, brutal struggle with cancer that left his body ravaged, his soul exposed, and us, his tiny family, bewildered in the strange toss-up between acceptance and disbelief. He held me once, not too long before that was physically impossible, and told me I would never again feel so ripped open. "Remember this feeling," he told me, as I studied the new tumor on his shoulder that I could swear wasn't there just hours before. "Your grief will either consume you or set you free. It won't feel this way right now because you're in it," he said, "but you will come through, you will heal, you will grow, and you will be grateful." I told him to go fuck himself and we laughed hard, until we cried, at the horror of it all and the beauty that we knew we would both one day come to understand. Me, as I struggled to let him go. Him, as he accepted he had no choice but to.

I won't pretend to understand your heartbreak, your loss, or the power of your grief. I will never say, "I know just how you feel." I don't. I only know how my grief felt and I honor that place in you that tastes some version of that sadness. I do know that if you have the strength to sit side by side with it, breathe into it, open yourself up to the wave after wave after wave of impossible and sometimes conflicting emotions that arise—healing is possible.

One of my father's last requests of me was that I was to eulogize him at his funeral. I stood there, my father's wasted body in the coffin behind me, and looked around the room into the eyes of the different expressions of grief staring back at me. I saw devastation in my grandmother. I saw relief in my mother. I saw anger in my brother. I saw numbness in many. I took a breath and said, "I always knew this moment would happen, that I would stand before you all and say good-bye to my father, and I knew it would be hard. But I underestimated the intensity of this moment. It is beyond hard. The pain I feel is worse than I imagined, and my grief feels palpable. But to grieve this hard can only mean that in this lifetime I got to love that big . . . and for that I am grateful."

May your journey through your own grief awaken you to levels of knowing, empathy, and peace that free your own soul, open you to love big, and allow you to embrace the beauty, the sweetness, and the unbearable, but glorious, impermanence of it all.

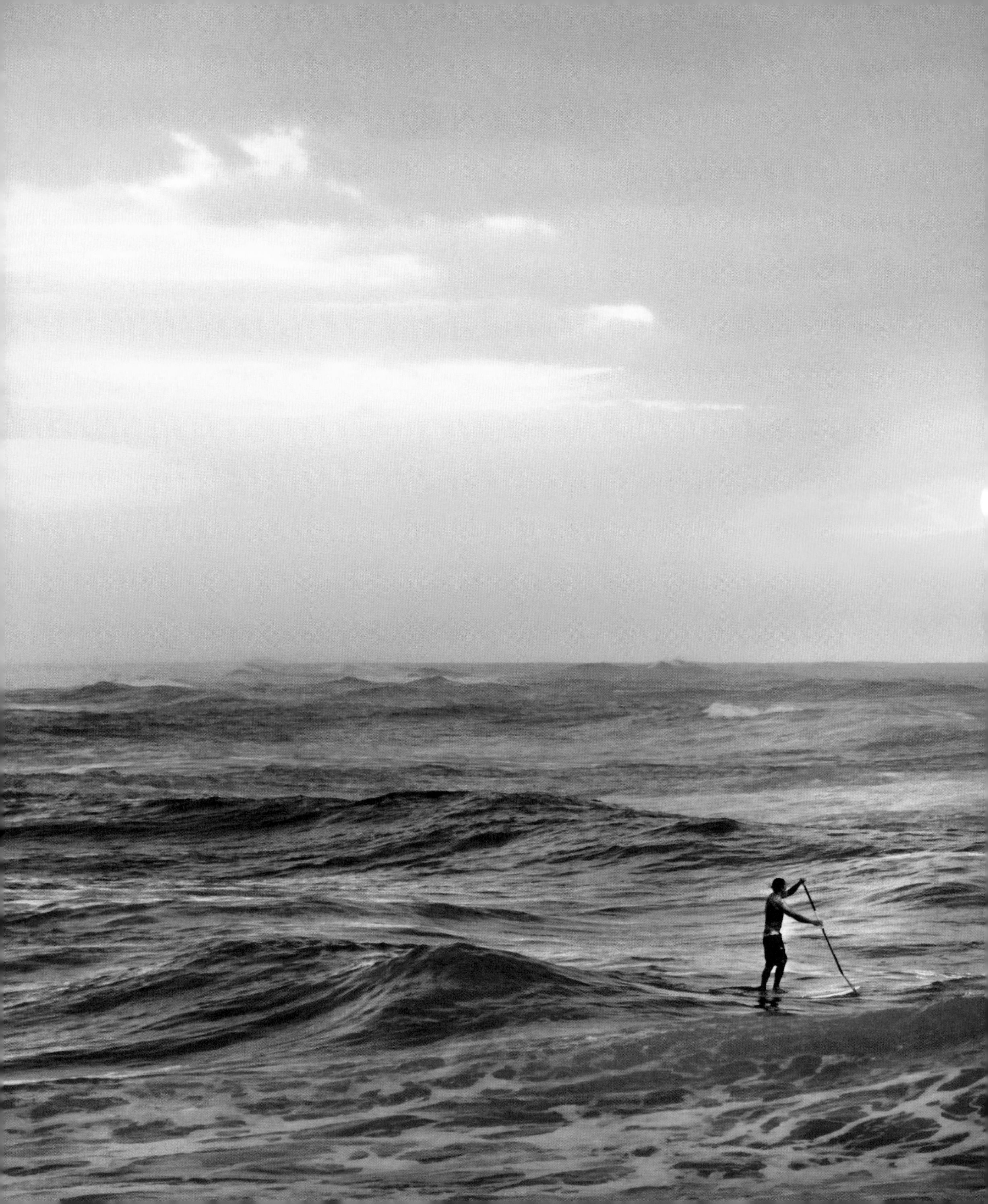

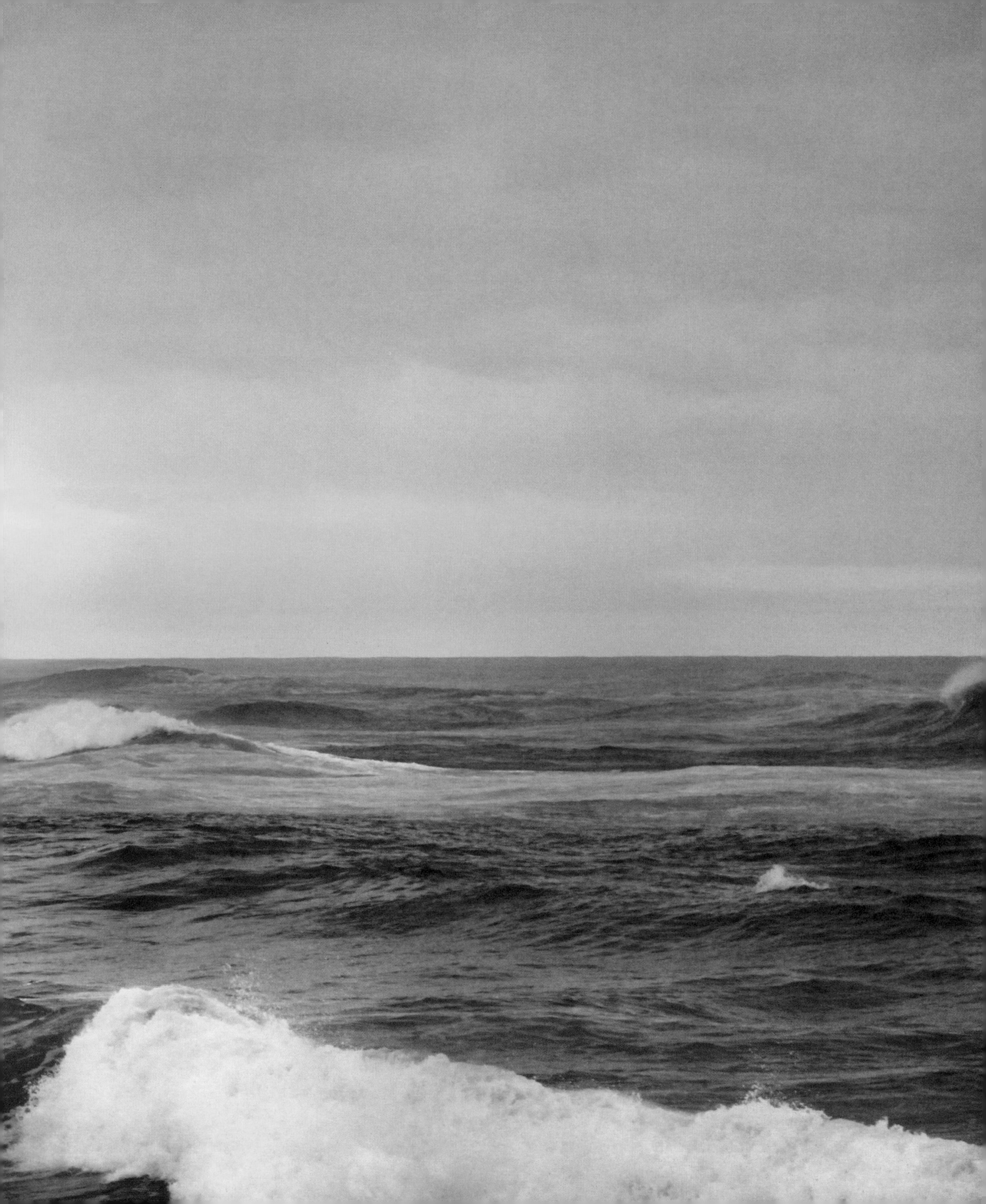

One weekend I was driving home with a group of students. We had finished a training in Indianapolis and were heading back to Chicago. Tornadoes had touched down on our route, abandoned trucks were overturned on the side of the road, and the sky was a creepy mix of purple and black. Despite the buffeting of the wind and our concern for the fate of the truckers, the ride was filled with the usual joy and laughter that arise when yoga people get together. At some point, my friend who had lost her husband began talking about her love for him, and her appreciation for having had him in her life. She described a moment toward the end when her husband was frail from his illness and disoriented from the medications he had been given for the pain. He looked at her and his eyes were clear and he said to her, "If I could have scripted my life, I would not change a thing." The silence that followed was filled with an understanding: If that was all our friend would ever know of love in this lifetime, it would be enough.

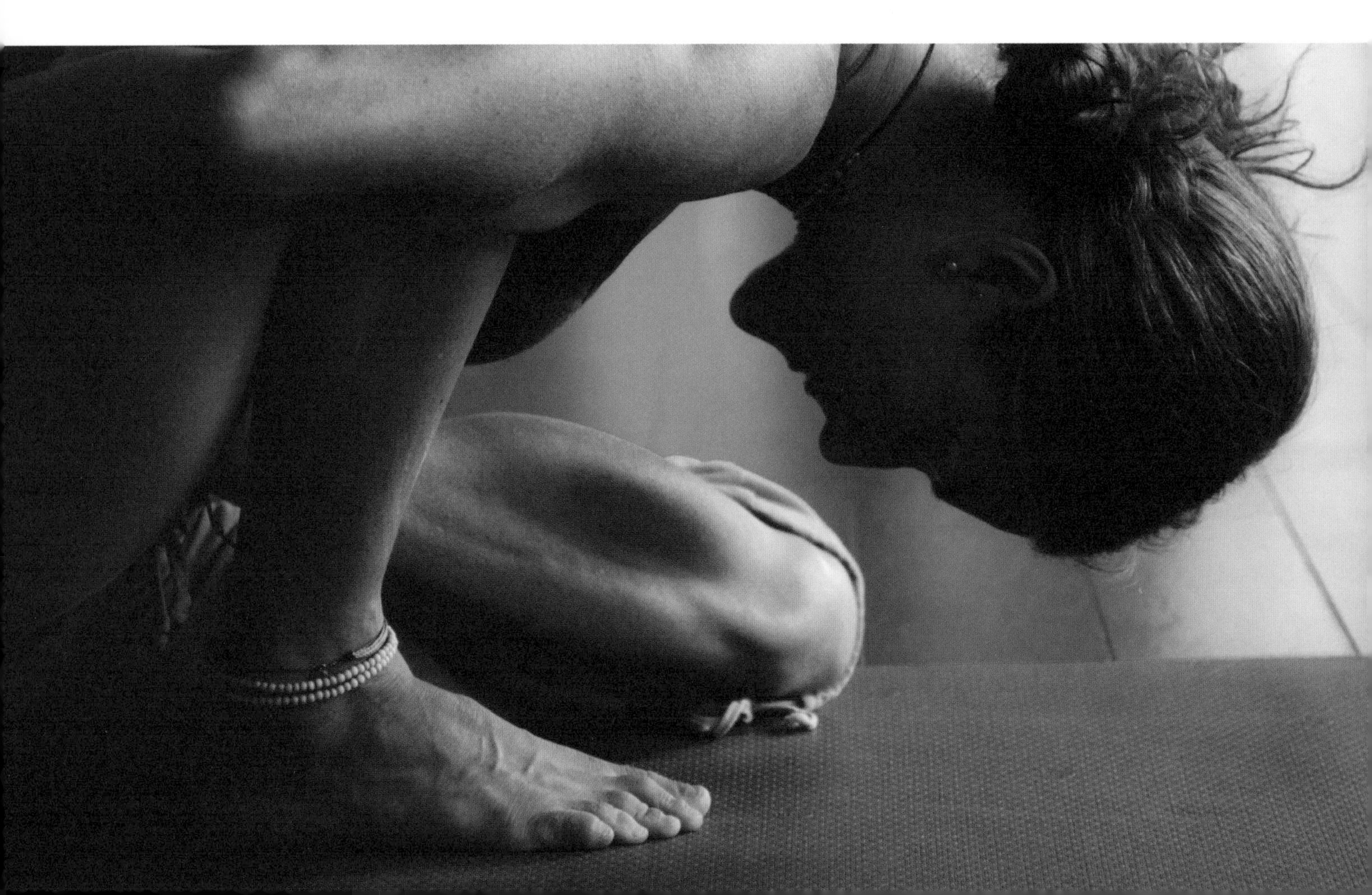

I had struggled all year with what has seemed to be too much pain, too much loss. So much so that I have not been able to speak of it, let alone understand what I thought of it.

My mother was a teacher, my father was a minister, and being a yoga teacher allows me to be a little of both. This year I taught at a memorial service for my friend's eighteen-year-old son, a memorial service for a new father, and a fund-raiser for a twenty-year-old who had just passed. It was a lot to hold, and I noticed I often relied upon being needed to avoid taking in the depths of pain.

In the silence, in the car, in the windy darkness, I understood. The overwhelming pain of loss brings with it a teaching. To have known those we have loved and to have been loved by them is enough. Loss teaches the meaning of the Hebrew word DAYENU, from a song at Passover. If these are all the blessings we will receive, if loving this person I so dearly miss is all I will know of love in this lifetime, it would be enough.

Flying back to California the next day, I finally let myself feel my grief and pain over the massive loss I had witnessed that year. I cried for close to an hour; fortunately the person next to me was asleep. As I cried, I felt all that has been enough in my lifetime. I was adopted, but my parents were at pains to tell me how much the nuns who cared for me as a baby loved me, that I was special to them and loved by them—it would be enough. I grew up in a family of people who wore their hearts on their sleeves—it would be enough. I prayed one morning and my desire to drink was lifted from me and has never come back—it would be enough. I knew my older sister Wendy for twenty-six years and loved her with all of my heart—it would be enough. I went to work one day and met a young woman who would become my wife—it would be enough. I watched my daughter Jasmine come into the world—it would be enough. I held my son Dylan in my arms as his eyes opened and saw light for the first time—it would be enough. Before my friend Jude passed away, he shared with me his love of nature and art; to this day, I cannot see a beautiful landscape without thinking of how much he would have loved it—it would be enough. I have felt the grace generated by groups of people in twelve-step meetings, yoga classes, and meditation retreats—it would be enough. If I am willing to feel the pain of loss I am able to feel the depth of my love and gratitude—it is enough.

Loss also brings with it questions: What now? How do I live on? What life would do justice to the blessing of having known someone so precious? If I know that I have been given more than enough already, if my life does not need more, what am I living for?

Our loved ones leave us a teaching. In the silence of their passing there is a whisper. It says:

"Love the way you loved me, laugh the way we laughed together, be kind the way we were kind to one another, see me in everyone you meet; that would be enough."

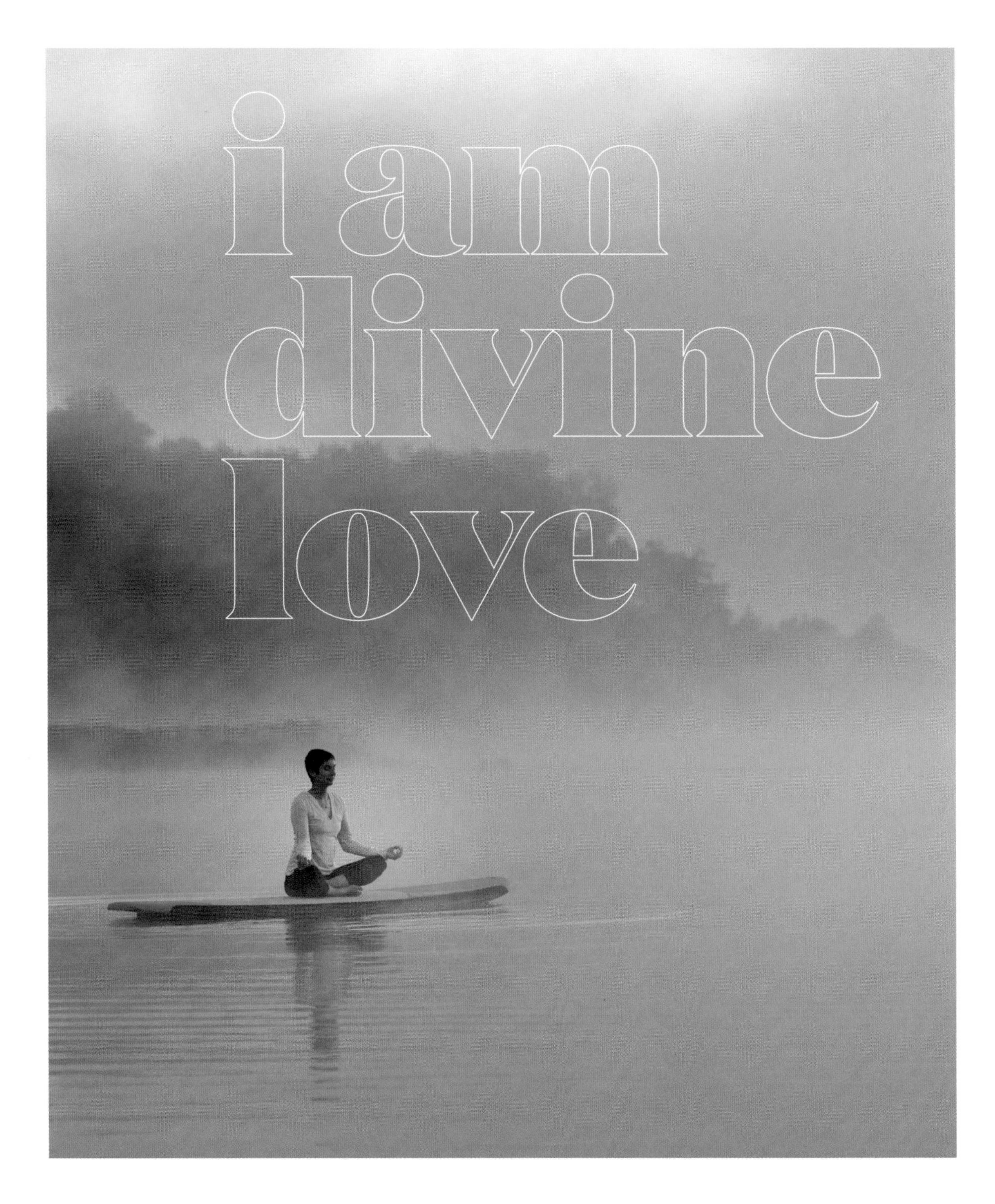
i am
divine
love

MEGGAN WATTERSON

Your task is not to seek love, but merely to seek and find all the barriers within yourself that you have built against it. Love is the bridge between you and everything.

—Rumi

After six months of couples' therapy, my husband decided the summer before our son turned one that we needed to separate. I was at a low I had never reached before. I felt unlovable. And yet, ironically, this heartbreak proved to be a turning point in humbly understanding true love.

Through loss I became conscious of my addiction to the idea that love would arrive from outside of myself. I thought I had to earn it somehow. I had to get one more degree, have one more relationship, cut one more notch in that proverbial belt, and then I'd be ready. Deserving.

I came to realize that any and all outside sources of love were too inconsistent to rely on as a mainspring. I needed me.

But how do we love ourselves?

I started leaving love notes for my soul. With red lipstick, I wrote on the mirror in the center of my wall altar and on the long mirror where I check out my full-length look before going out at night.

Miracles came gradually. Day by day the awe of my own love returned to me. I finally, completely, turned within and found the love I'd been looking for my entire life. It came little by little but the utter transformation was nothing short of a slap on the forehead.

Now I experience myself as love in action.

For me this is the most radical thing I can embody. This is the most profound activism I can participate in, more than any protest I could attend or op-ed I could write: the act of loving myself, fiercely. Because in my experience, everything becomes possible when a person dares to meet with the soul of love inside them.

Now a fire alarm sounds whenever a negative thought about myself enters my mind. I blow it a kiss and let it leave as quickly as it can hightail it out of me. This is the path and practice of self-love.

To me love, true love, means no longer waiting.

This soul-voice meditation can help you discern if there are any places within that still hold a sense of being unworthy of love.

Even the darkest moments in your life have profound teachings to give you, not just more "baggage." Both the happy and the hard moments so far have been opportunities to acquire more of the precise attributes to flex and exercise your capacity to love.

Try the exercise on the following page. It can be practiced daily.

SIT VERY STILL. Let the stories of your life, which often feel like agitated water at the surface, settle so you can see clear down to the bottom of what matters most. Find those stories that have left the loudest, darkest, and deepest imprint on your soul—the stories that allow you to believe you're not worthy of love.

QUESTION THOSE STORIES. Ask your soul to show you what still needs to be healed within you. Resist nothing; invite all of those hard-to-reach memories to come back. Trust that you are ready to see and receive them in a new way. You are strong enough. Maybe you see a memory of a bully from high school, or of a moment when you experienced a humbling or humiliating experience that still lives in you somewhere. Maybe you were not there for someone in a time of need and hold regret and guilt. Maybe you have believed all this time someone else's truth about you: for example, that you are not good enough or worthy, or that you are much too much for anyone to handle. One by one, allow these memories to return to consciousness. Invite them in like dinner guests. Be grateful they have shown up.

LOVE THEM. I know I'm asking you to do something really hard. I know from experience. I do this practice daily. Initially, it felt like moving through stone. But over the years, it has become far more light-filled.

If you are having a hard time bringing love to a memory or a moment, if some limiting belief is just too convincing for you to find a way to shower it with love, then work in a more general way. Focus on conjuring a feeling of unconditional love within. If you're a writing type like me, write out all the excuses and stories you have held tight that have blocked you from love. Let them exist now in your journal rather than within. Let the journal hold them. You don't need to anymore.

Ask yourself if there is anything left you can still learn from these still-loud moments. And ask if there is anything left for you to forgive. What are you keeping, holding silent inside you? What stories are still held tightly sealed inside your heart?

Open them all up. Let your love reach where it never has before. And then, see if you can sit in silence. This is the very peace that allows you to hear a voice of compassion that wants to lead you, real and trustworthy as the earth beneath you.

FOLLOW YOUR WANDERING HEART: INCREDIBLE ADVENTURES FOR THOSE WITH INCURABLE WANDERLUST

Il Palio festival—Siena, Italy (July 2 and August 16 each year)

WHERE TO STAY: The Airbnb room I found was within a hundred steps of the piazza and was run by a lovely woman who runs an antiques shop around the corner. Stay within the community.

WHERE TO EAT: San Giuseppe for great, classic Italian dishes

WHAT TO DO (TOP ACTIVITY): The medieval pomp and circumstance around the two bareback horseback races gives you a sense you have popped into a century half a millennium ago.

SOMETHING RANDOM ABOUT THE PLACE: Definitely get a ticket to one of the neighborhood dinners the night before the races so you'll get an authentic flavor of how Siena hasn't changed much in five hundred years.

Burgos, Spain

WHERE TO STAY: AC Hotel Burgos

WHERE TO EAT: Cerveceria Morito is so good I ate there three nights in a row.

WHAT TO DO (TOP ACTIVITY): The Museum of Human Evolution gives you a twenty-first-century feeling of what a museum can be. While you're at it, stroll around the car-free downtown and check out the Gothic cathedral.

SOMETHING RANDOM ABOUT THE PLACE: You have to go in early June to experience El Colacho in the village of Castrillo de Murcia, the famed baby jumping festival.

Harbin, China

WHERE TO STAY: Shangri-La Hotel

WHERE TO EAT: Across the square from the stunning Russian St. Sophia's church is the Dingxin hot pot restaurant where you cook your own meats, seafood, and vegetables at your table.

WHAT TO DO (TOP ACTIVITY): Harbin Ice and Snow Sculpture Festival is in January and February and is one of the most visually stunning festivals I've ever experienced. Check out Ice and Snow World, Zhaolin Park, and the Snow Sculpture Art Expo on Sun Island.

SOMETHING RANDOM ABOUT THE PLACE: If you're in this intersection of Siberia and Manchuria during the Ice and Snow Festival, check out the crazy folks who do a daily swim in the swimming pool next to the river in thirteen-degree-below-zero temperatures.

Telluride, Colorado

WHERE TO STAY: Hotel Telluride

WHERE TO EAT: 221 South Oak, classic cooking in a charming home

WHAT TO DO (TOP ACTIVITY): Telluride is a great place to go to a festival due to the womblike nature of the physical setting. The Blues Festival is legendary, but I've gone to the Telluride Film Festival two of the last three years over Labor Day weekend, and, in my humble opinion as a film buff, this is the best film festival in the world.

SOMETHING RANDOM ABOUT THE PLACE: Dunton Hot Springs is almost an hour away by a gorgeous drive, and there are steaming hot springs in this small, funky, luxury resort.

Fes, Morocco

WHERE TO STAY: The classic Riad Fes

WHERE TO EAT: Dar Roumana

WHAT TO DO (TOP ACTIVITY): Go in early June for the Fes Festival of World Sacred Music where you'll listen to everything from Mongolian throat singing to southern US gospel to Balinese gamelan orchestras.

SOMETHING RANDOM ABOUT THE PLACE: Get lost in the medina winding your way around the ancient alleys.

Cappadocia, Turkey

WHERE TO STAY: Argos in Cappadocia Hotel, a cave hotel

WHERE TO EAT: Seki, the restaurant at Argos in Cappadocia, has stunning views of the geologically odd-looking valley below.

WHAT TO DO (TOP ACTIVITY): The best hot-air ballooning in the world given the rock formations

SOMETHING RANDOM ABOUT THE PLACE: Highly recommend you go in the off-season and experience the Whirling Dervish Festival in Konya, Turkey, a few hours away. This ten-day festival from December 7 through 17 honors the first whirling dervish, the poet and philosopher Rumi, and there's even a Rumi museum in this town of nearly one million people.

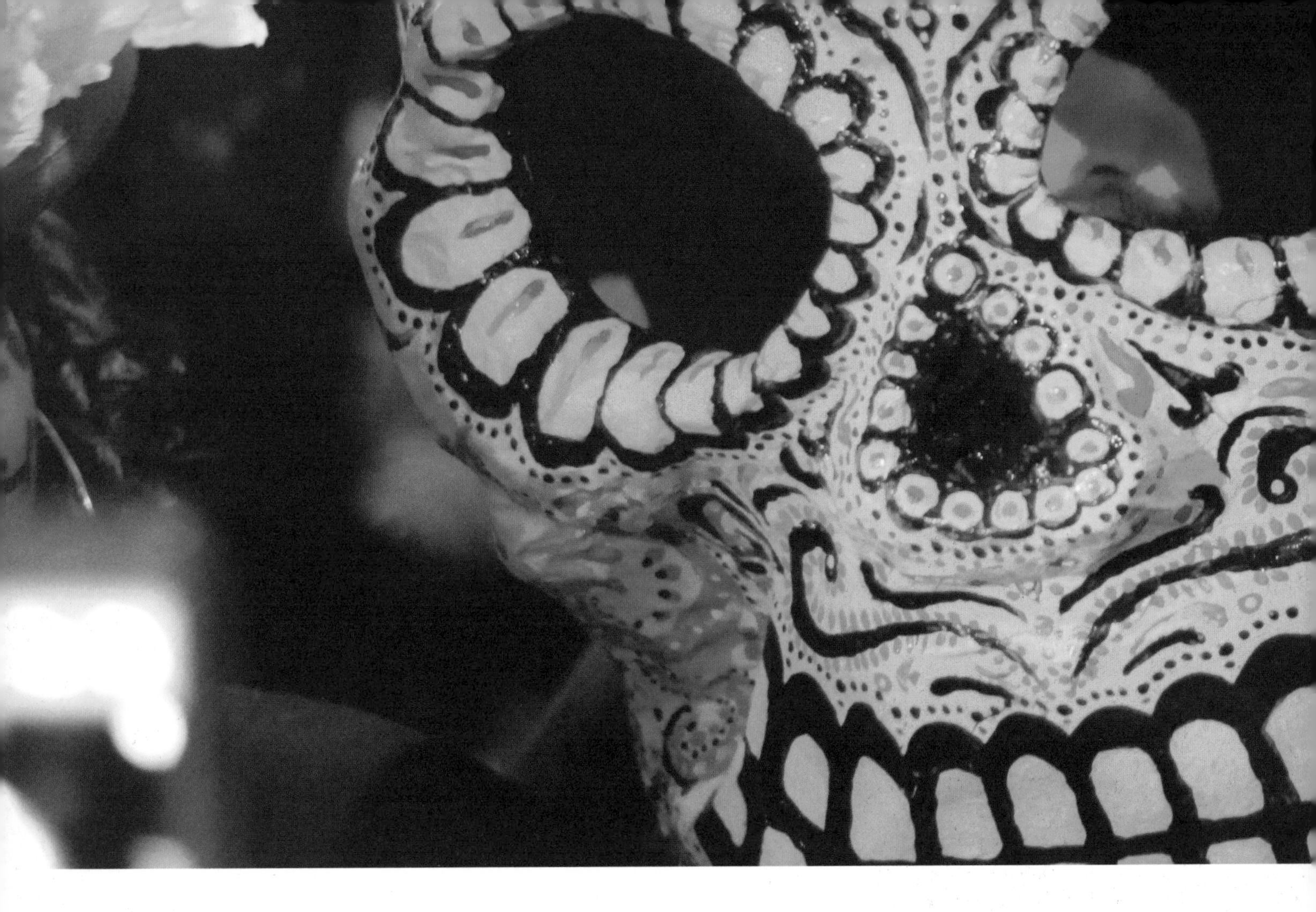

Oaxaca, Mexico

WHERE TO STAY: Casa Oaxaca

WHERE TO EAT: Mexita; try the crunchy grasshoppers if they have them on the menu.

WHAT TO DO (TOP ACTIVITY): Dia de los Muertos (October 31 to November 2), with an artistic celebration of the dead

SOMETHING RANDOM ABOUT THE PLACE: Tour a graveyard at night; some of them have enormous altars full of candles.

Ubud, Bali

WHERE TO STAY: Ibah in Campuhan, next to Ubud. Go for a hike on Campuhan Ridge.

WHERE TO EAT: With a French gastronomic spin on Indonesian cuisine, Mozaic is not your normal Balinese restaurant.

WHAT TO DO (TOP ACTIVITY): Bali is one endless festival, but Galungan is one of the more interesting festivals to experience. Also, find a guide on the street and ask if there's a cremation ceremony happening anytime soon, as that'll be an experience you'll remember the rest of your life.

SOMETHING RANDOM ABOUT THE PLACE: While traffic is both ever-present and dangerous, on the outskirts of Ubud you can find some lovely country roads that will lead you to waterfalls, temples, and some of the most stunning rice paddy fields you've ever seen. Get lost in paradise.

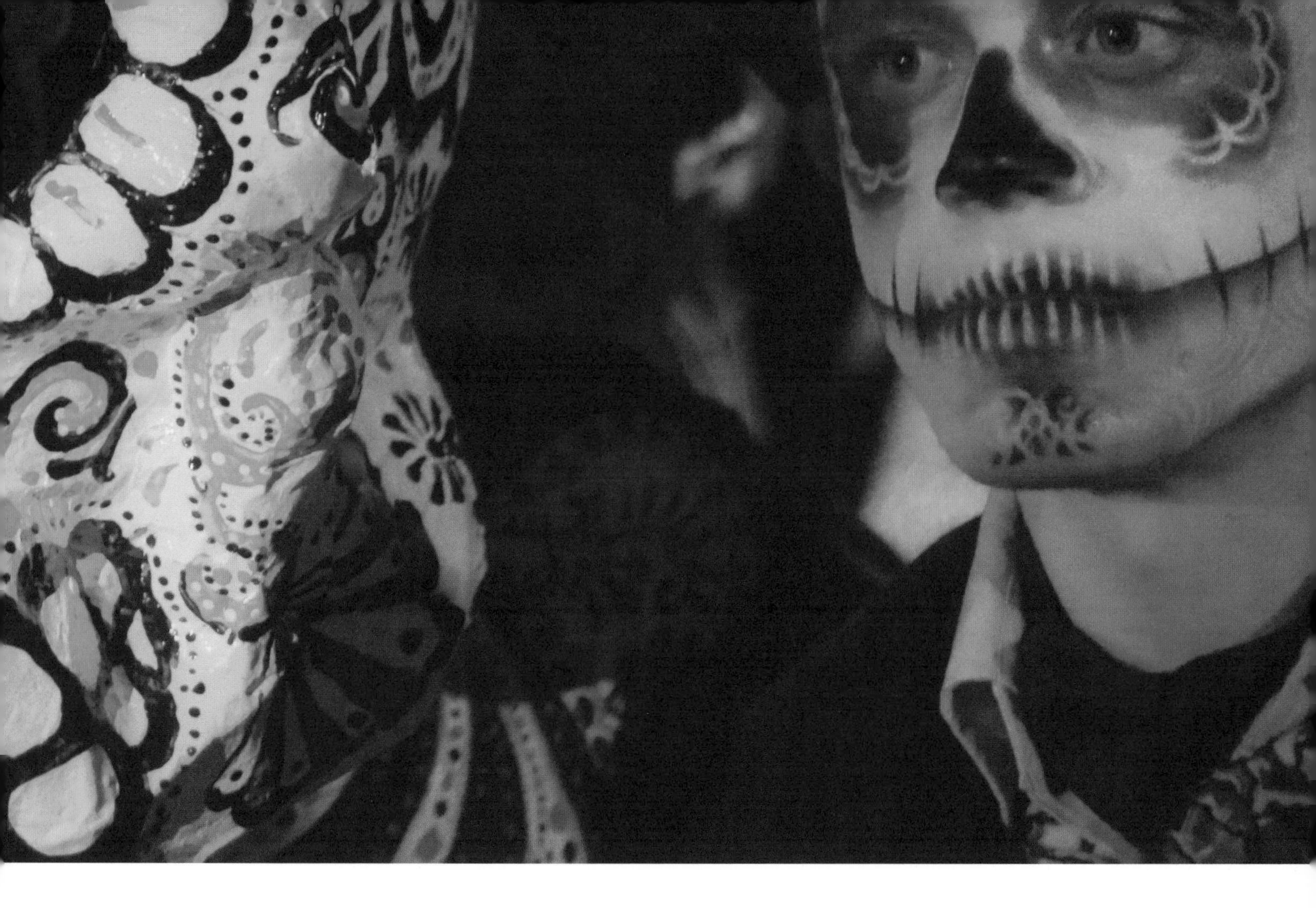

Cusco, Peru

WHERE TO STAY: Hotel Monasterio

WHERE TO EAT: Cicciolina in an old colonial house with "farm to table" tapas from the nearby Sacred Valley

WHAT TO DO (TOP ACTIVITY): Go during the Inti Raymi festival in June, a spectacular reenactment of the Sun God festivals of centuries ago.

SOMETHING RANDOM ABOUT THE PLACE: If you're in the area, you must travel to Machu Picchu for one of the more transformational moments of your life.

San Francisco, California

WHERE TO STAY: Hotel Vitale, a hotel I, admittedly, built on the waterfront across the street from the historic Ferry Building

WHERE TO EAT: Gitane, a Basque restaurant on charming Claude Lane

WHAT TO DO (TOP ACTIVITY): There are many great festivals in San Francisco, from Outside Lands to Hardly Strictly Bluegrass to San Francisco LGBT Pride to the Bay to Breakers running race.

SOMETHING RANDOM ABOUT THE PLACE: I used to live on the Filbert Steps and Napier Lane on the east side of Telegraph Hill. This set of steps that takes you from Coit Tower down to Levi's Plaza is one of the more quaint and atmospheric places in San Francisco.

Mantras are tools for inner connection and conscious living. One of the most recognizable is the single-syllable mantra of OM. Mantras are highly vibrational sounds that the seers of the ancient yogic tradition heard while absorbed in the unified state. They can bring us back to center while aligning us with something elevated, all at once.

THE PRIVILEGE

The amazing thing is that we get the privilege to access what the yogis learned from their immersion in yogic practice. We access this by chanting from the notes they left behind in the form of mantras. In today's traditional yogic schools, this essential knowledge about the self gets imparted to students through a kind of reverse process. Students follow the trail of the mantras that the yogis of old left, and by saying the sounds, they reach the same unified experience.

A teacher will say, "Repeat this mantra, but stay conscious. When you do this, you will experience a lot of vibration. Stay with this feeling. You will be drawn from the feeling that there is only worldly life. Stay awake and follow the sound to the serene experience of energized inner peace beyond your thinking mind. Stay conscious in this discovery and feel what you are."

Thirty-Day Practice

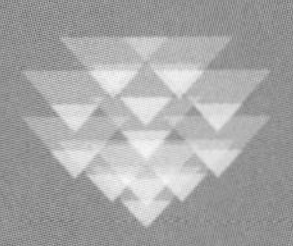

LUMINOUS SOUL SHIVA MANTRA PRACTICE:

Shiva Mantra

om namah shivaya

Reverence to Lord Shiva, god of completion, tranquility, and transformation.

EACH MORNING:

Repeat this mantra with awareness 108 times.

Sit quietly.

For ten minutes, be present with space.

Allow the quiet to fill you with yogic energy and strength.

Before you end your practice, bring your palms together in front of your heart and bow your head reverently.

Begin your day with gratitude.

Notice throughout your day, week, and month what effect this mantra practice has on you and your life.

MANORAMA'S PRACTICE TIPS:

Set aside twenty minutes each morning for this practice.

Pronounce the mantra slowly and with attention.

Once you've started, don't interrupt the practice.

Know that practice isn't always comfortable or easy. Increase your capacity by working with your threshold.

track your daily progress

1	2	3	4	5	6	7	8	9	10	11	12	13	14	15
16	17	18	19	20	21	22	23	24	25	26	27	28	29	30

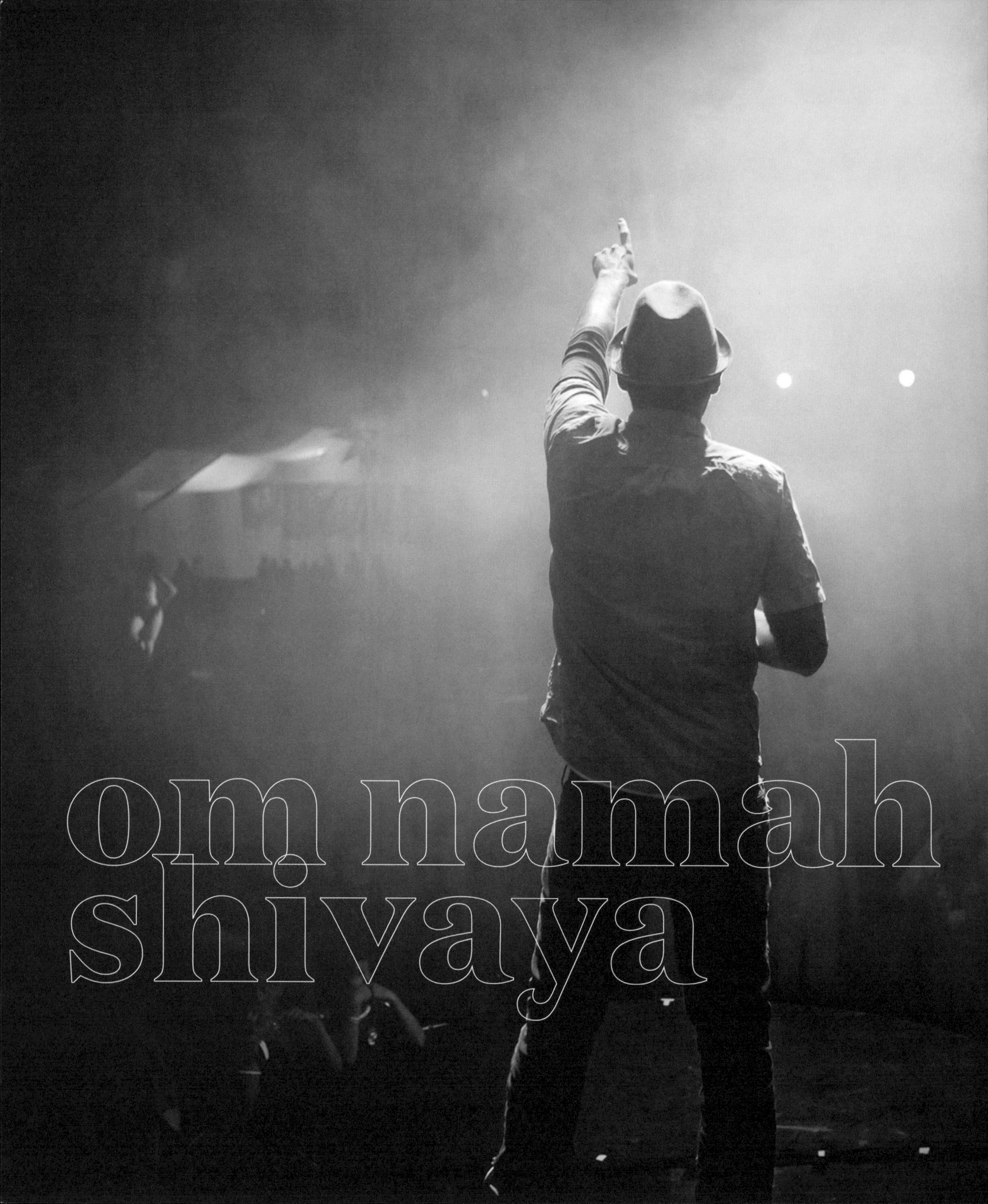
om namah
shivaya

HOW DO YOU WORK WITH A MANTRA?

Traditionally, a teacher will select a specific mantra for you based on what he or she feels you need to work on. Optionally, you can work with a mantra by noticing which mantras you feel drawn to. Sometimes a mantra will sound pleasing or feel healing for you. Follow that inner feeling and work with it. It's important when you decide to work with the selected mantra that you do it regularly for at least one year. Chant the mantra 108 times daily. Over and over and over, repeat the sounds and work to stay conscious. When you fall unconscious, lift up and feel conscious again until at some point in the repetitive process you become aware that your thinking mind calms and is no longer acting in its usual guiding role. Notice this will happen when you feel steady in awareness.

With repeated mantric practice, the thinking mind calms and you access the pure energy that underlies the mind. Pure energy is a yogic term that means the powerful vibration that exists beyond thought. The more you practice a mantra, the more you create a relationship with this essential energy that is within you. There is a difference between knowing you are beyond the body and mind and feeling that you are beyond the body and mind. Mantras are tools for experiencing what you are beyond the body and thinking mind. With the awareness of your inner misperception of who you are comes the space to feel who you really are. You enter the center of the sound and at this point have the capacity to listen with the no-mind state. This is called nirvana through mantra.

Mantras can also be said in English.

If *om namah shivaya* seems daunting to you or you prefer to work with a mantra in English, here are some Luminous Soul tools you can focus on as English mantras:

Work to develop greater patience.

Grow your capacity by listening more.

Notice energy in you and around you.

Read these phrases throughout your week and they will act like modern-day English mantras, infusing your day and life with practice that builds the strength to feel who you truly are.

All yogic practices teach you to align with your inner strength. In mantra, the strength you want to access is the feeling that exists on a no-mind level. In order to experience this, you will need to cultivate patience, the ability to listen, and the courage to feel what you are as energy.

In the mantra *om namah shivaya,* Shiva is the strength of patience, steadiness, and energized tranquility. So instead of saying the mantra in Sanskrit, you have the option to connect with these teachings by working with what he signifies in English.

Whether you say mantras in Sanskrit or English, the key is to practice regularly. When you consistently practice, you make yourself a channel for understanding. Continuously focusing on a mantra draws its hidden meaning to you. By chanting mantras, you make yourself ready to receive your own spiritual essence. Mantras help you grow in inner peace and in a strong connection with the divine that you are.

BHAKTI YOGA + CHANT: SING, OFFER, REPEAT

KRISHNA DAS

It's good to do practices. It's good to do asana and meditation and chanting. But it is also important to think about and understand what we are trying to accomplish with these practices. Many of us are trying to find something, and are trying to slow down.

The pace of Western life is so insane. We forget what it is like to really go slow. We return home after work and turn on the television or music or get busy reading the paper or talk on the phone. We don't really slow down until we try to sleep at night and then we watch all those ninety channels as we fall asleep.

Chanting, the repetition of the names of God, can unpeel layers of ourselves and encourage a real, true slowing down.

Chanting is not about getting something. It's not about becoming the best yoga practitioner in your part of town, on your block. It's about trying to find out who you really are and find some sweetness in life, a sweetness that lasts and doesn't depend on how the outside world is treating you at that particular moment.

We often chant Sanskrit terms that mean things like divine presence, God, the soul, the oversoul, but the real meaning of these names is not something we can think about. It is something we have to and will experience directly from within. It's something we feel. That's the whole difference. Everything comes from inside. It's subtle. Through the repetition of these names, it is said that gradually, but inevitably, the presence that is hidden within us, our own divine presence, and the atman, the soul, God, whatever you want to call it, is uncovered. And that means it's already in there. We are not getting anything from the outside. We're not making anything. We're not creating anything. We don't have to emotionally manipulate ourselves to get high. We are not pushing away any bad feelings to grab ahold of good ones. We are peeling away to an essence. What's underneath—good and bad, holding on and clinging, pushing away, attachment and aversion, fame and shame, name and gain—is who we are. That's what these practices actually uncover. Simply uncover it.

Remember, all these practices are really offerings that we make to the Heart of All. You are offering your labors up to others, to the universe, to God, in joy.

After all, how are we to find peace if we can't be at ease with ourselves?

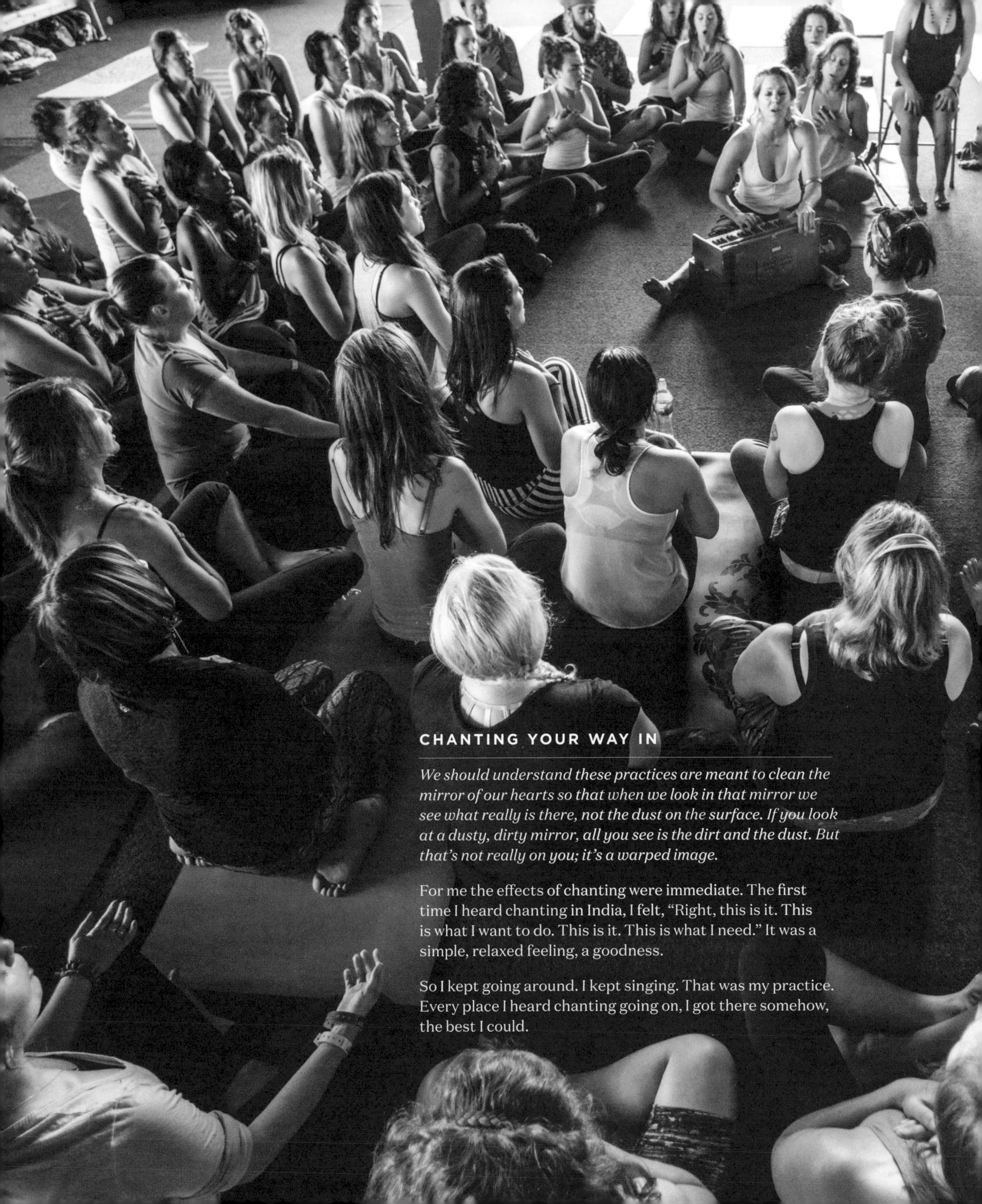

CHANTING YOUR WAY IN

We should understand these practices are meant to clean the mirror of our hearts so that when we look in that mirror we see what really is there, not the dust on the surface. If you look at a dusty, dirty mirror, all you see is the dirt and the dust. But that's not really on you; it's a warped image.

For me the effects of chanting were immediate. The first time I heard chanting in India, I felt, "Right, this is it. This is what I want to do. This is it. This is what I need." It was a simple, relaxed feeling, a goodness.

So I kept going around. I kept singing. That was my practice. Every place I heard chanting going on, I got there somehow, the best I could.

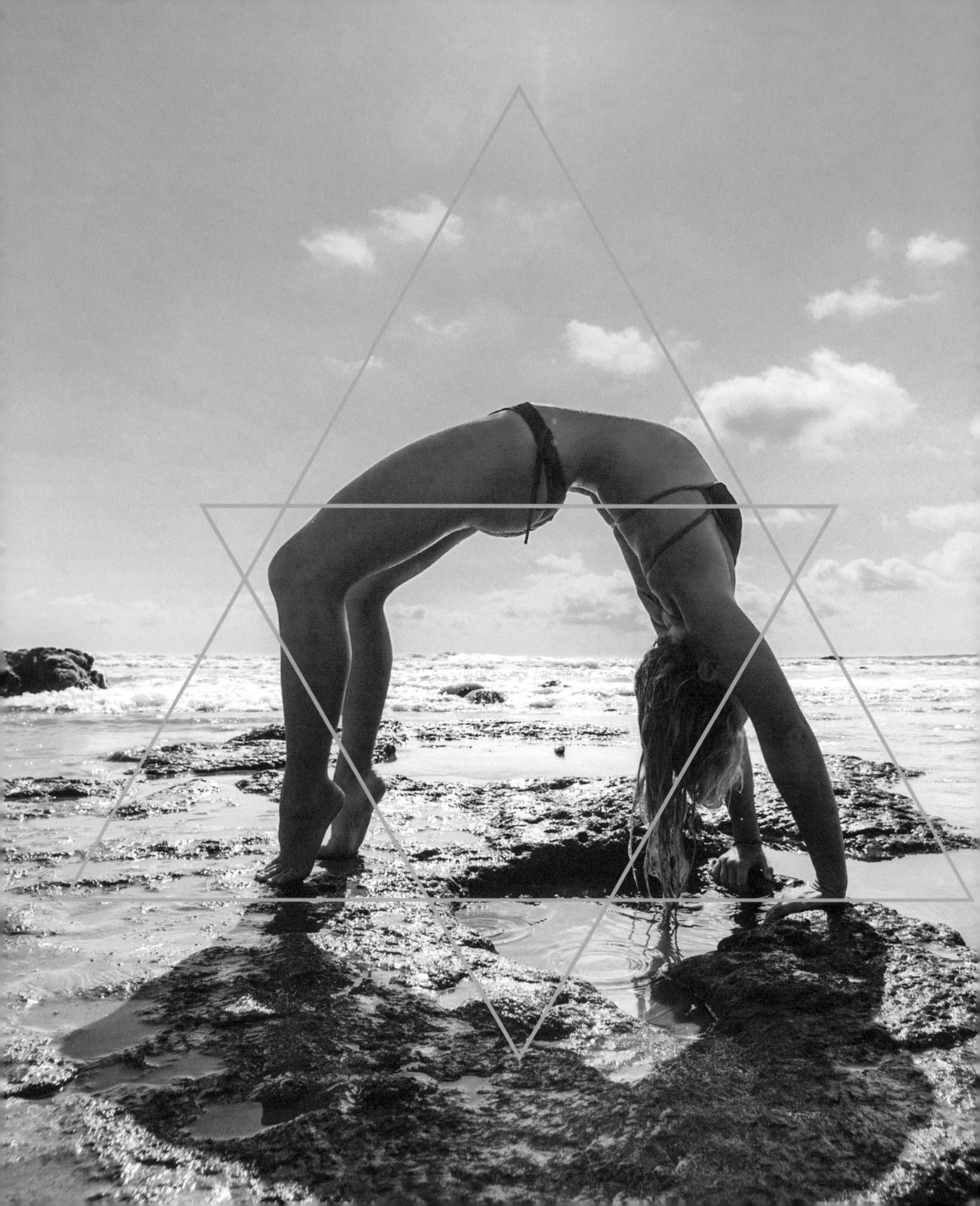

BLOSSOMING OF THE LOTUS OF THE HEART

ANAND MEHROTRA

Within the city of Brahman, which is the body, there is the heart. Within, there is a space. This space has a shape of a lotus and within it dwells That, which is to be sought after, inquired about, and realized. As large as the Universe outside, there is the Universe within the lotus of the heart. Within it are sky and Earth, the sun, the moon, all the planets, and all the stars. What is in the macrocosm is in this microcosm. Though the body is bound by time, the lotus of the heart is timeless. At the death of the body, it does not die. The true self dwelling therein is untouched by any deed, any story, any judgment, and resides in all her glory.

—Chandogaya Upanishad, seventh–sixth centuries BCE

The lotus of the heart, also known as anahata chakra, is the seat of our true self. It is the seat of our intuitive and spiritual intelligence. Connecting to this is fundamental to living an awakened life. Only when we can connect to the lotus of the heart and let it blossom can we experience life in all of its beauty and love. Without the blossoming of the lotus of the heart, we are constantly driven by an underlying current of threat and fear and we end up living a life driven by the ego, a life that is unfulfilled. In order to allow the blossoming of the lotus of the heart, the Vedic and Tantric wisdom teachings refer repeatedly to these fundamental teachings.

The Three Fundamental Teachings of the Lotus of the Heart

In order to allow the blossoming of the lotus, these three fundamentals wisdom teachings of the heart have to be cultivated and understood. As you make contact with this wisdom, keep them in the forefront of your consciousness. Meditate upon them, and let them enter into the movement of your life.

AHAM BRAHMASMI:

I Am Totality—Identifying the True Self

The fundamental thing that keeps the heart from blossoming is the misidentification of self. While we are identified with our small, time-bound self, our ego, we cannot enter the heart center fully. This is from where our issues of self-hatred arise. Until we are connecting to the true self, we will always feel inadequate, not enough, and will be pushed constantly to try and fix ourselves. It is fundamental to our evolution that we start making contact with our timeless self, our higher self. As we connect with the higher self, we begin to realize we are not our stories; we are not people's stories of us. This experience in yoga is what is described as detachment, Vairagayam, nonidentification. Your life becomes an expression of who you are, and not a search for who you are. You have a deep shift from a position of effect to a position of cause. This awareness strengthens the heart center and allows the blossoming of the lotus of the heart. You begin to realize that even though you exist in time, you belong to eternity. Essentially, you were never born and you shall never die. This teaching is not an intellectual idea, but rather the deepest truth of who we are. So in your meditation, in your life, develop a daily practice where you really connect. Allow yourself the gift of really experiencing your own timeless nature.

1

I am totality

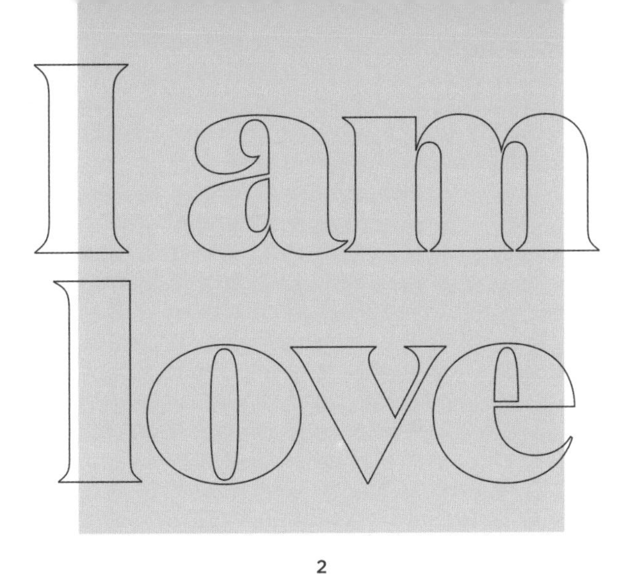

2

AHAM PREMA:

I Am Love—Allowing Love

The heart cannot fully blossom while we are looking for love. Love is not something we can find outside of ourselves. That love that you seek outside is a mere shadow of the love within your heart center. Instead of looking for love, we need to allow love. Because the truth is that we come from love, we exist through love, and unto love we shall return. No matter where you are reading these words, if you pause in this very moment and just allow yourself to realize the immense love that is supporting you constantly despite all the stories of the mind, in this very moment you are alive and aware. If this is not love, what is? When you realize this, there is an awakening to radical trust and radical gratitude in you. As you experience these two qualities of love, you develop a strong spine, which allows the heart to keep opening. Trust is not about trusting someone or trusting in something, but it is rather realizing the sacred love, the divine love, that has carried you to this moment. This field that we exist in is essentially love. It is constantly supporting us without asking anything in return. This is existential love. Only when we can begin to experience life through this awareness does our primary experience of life become existential love, and not existential burden. Only then our neediness dissolves and our compassion and magnetism increase.

3

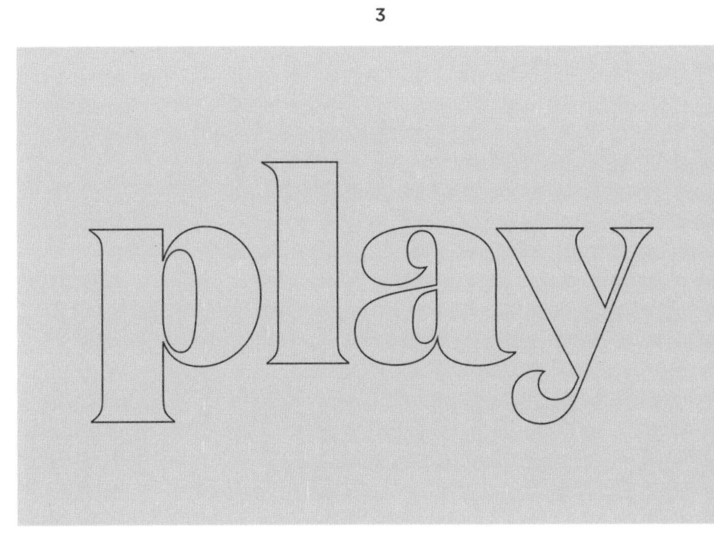

LEELA:

Realizing the Impermanence—Realizing the Play

As you make contact with this teaching of the heart, you stop holding on. There is a spontaneous letting go. Since we have chosen to enter this level of existence with its impermanence, we will all experience pain on some level. But when we have made contact with this teaching, the pain will only deepen our compassion and not turn into resentment or grief. As we realize the transitory nature of all things in time, we have a radical shift in value, and to what we give our time and attention. Whatever you give attention to will grow. The invitation of this teaching is to stop taking life so seriously and so personally. To have a sense of play with life. That is why in the yogic tradition, this world is often referred to as leela, the field of play. We have nothing to lose, but only to experience. As we deepen this understanding, we are filed with innocent, spontaneous joy, and we don't waste our life looking for safety, but rather we choose freedom.

A Meditation

1

Sit in meditation posture. If possible, cover yourself with a woolen or silk shawl. Focus your attention at your heart center and visualize a sacred lotus within it. As you inhale through the nose, mentally speak "aham" (I am), and as you exhale through the mouth, mentally speak "brahamasmi" (totality). Whatever arises within you, include everything in the space at the heart center. As you merge deeper and deeper into that space, feel time fading into nothingness. All stories, all masks, fear, and neediness coming to an end. Dissolving. Spontaneously, without any mind effort. Continue the practice for at least eleven minutes.

2

Sit in meditation posture. Bring your left hand to your heart center and right palm facing up with elbow bent. Begin to move your body very slowly and gently back and forth. Keep your lips parted softly. Inhale through the mouth and exhale through the nose. Invite the feeling of radical gratitude into the heart space. Feeling the deep love of existence that has been with you all this journey. Even at times when you denied it, pushed it back, it always was there for you. Replace any thought with the mantra "aham prema" (I am love). Practice at least seven minutes.

3

Lie down flat on your back. Let the body be fully still. Focus deeply at your heart space and feel the universe within the sacred lotus of the heart. Feel the lotus expanding and including the whole cosmos within it. See the animals, plants, trees, mountains, sun, moon, planets, stars . . . within you. Keep breathing in and out as slowly as possible. Realize how you are all and all is you.

The continuity of practice and awareness is liberation itself. May you all experience the blossoming of the lotus of your own heart.

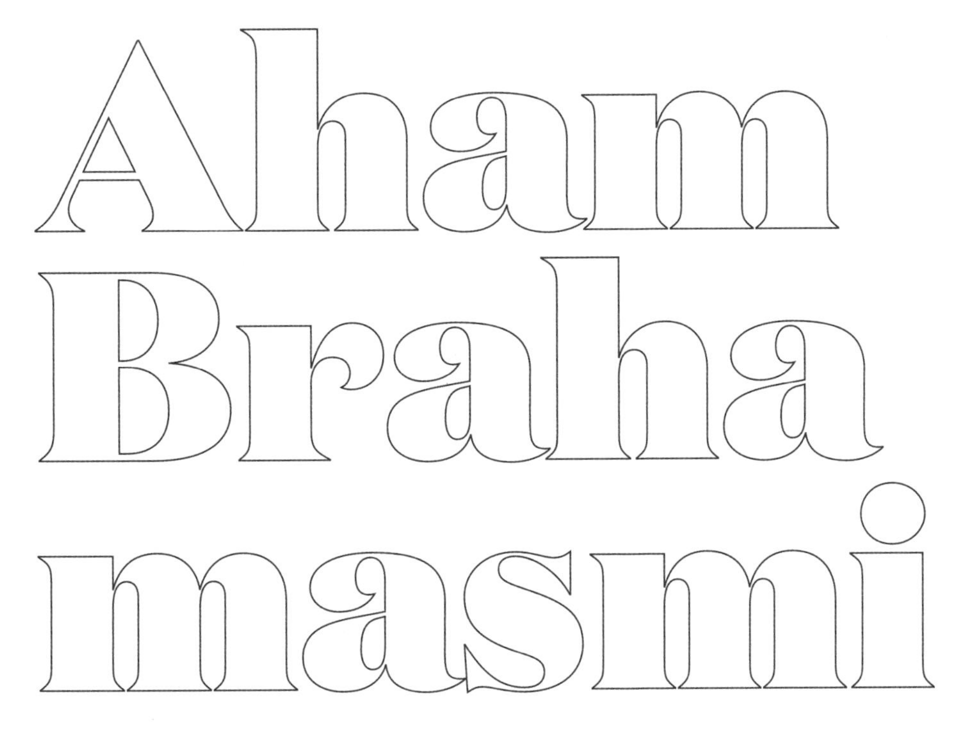

I Am Totality.

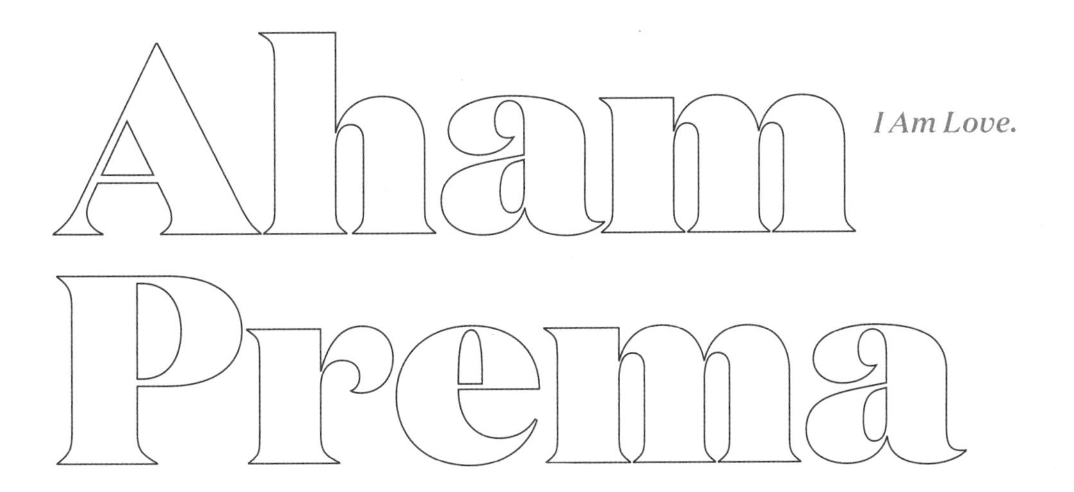

I Am Love.

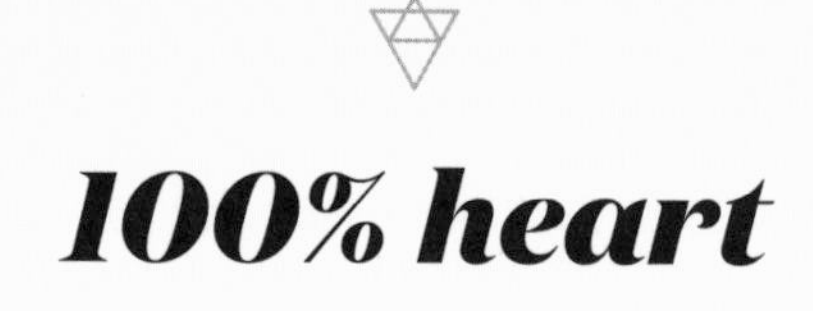

100% heart

JANET STONE

An asana practice that helps you find the strength to let yourself feel vulnerable.

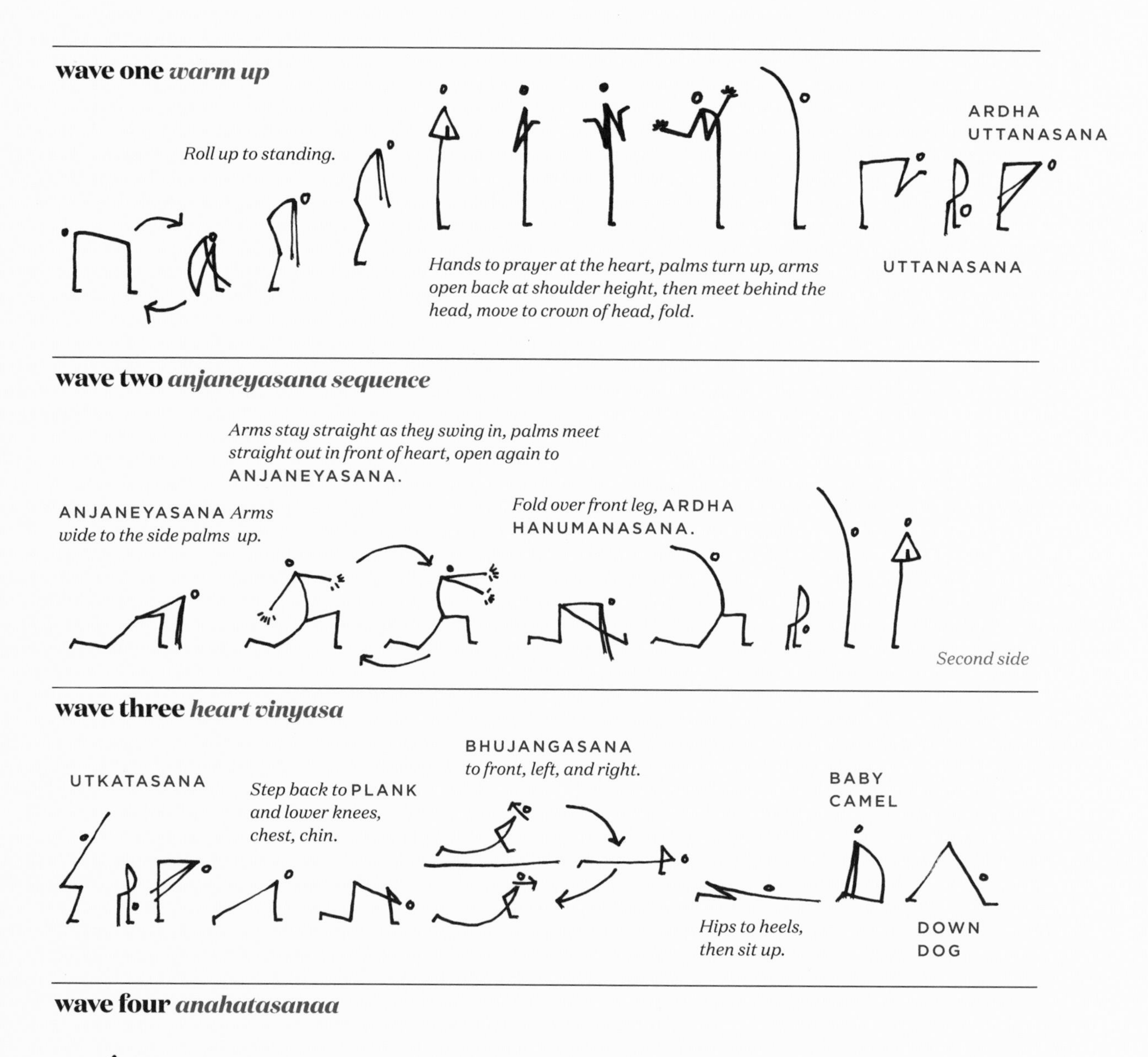

wave one *warm up*

Roll up to standing.

Hands to prayer at the heart, palms turn up, arms open back at shoulder height, then meet behind the head, move to crown of head, fold.

ARDHA UTTANASANA

UTTANASANA

wave two *anjaneyasana sequence*

ANJANEYASANA *Arms wide to the side palms up.*

Arms stay straight as they swing in, palms meet straight out in front of heart, open again to ANJANEYASANA.

Fold over front leg, ARDHA HANUMANASANA.

Second side

wave three *heart vinyasa*

UTKATASANA

Step back to PLANK *and lower knees, chest, chin.*

BHUJANGASANA *to front, left, and right.*

Hips to heels, then sit up.

BABY CAMEL

DOWN DOG

wave four *anahatasanaa*

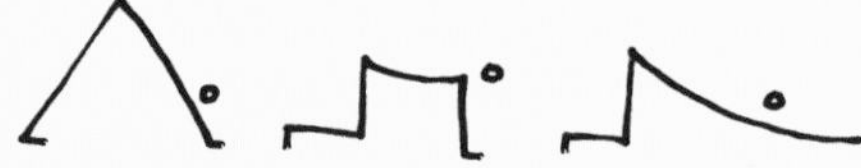

Heart Playlist

compiled by Kelly Casey

- **Ag Penthouse**—*Triola*
- **Bowspirit**—*Balmorhea*
- **Flying**—*Garth Stevenson*
- **Light**—*Dr. Toast*
- **X-33**—*Lights Out Asia*
- **Rapture at Sea**—*Eastern Sun*
- **Shanti (Peace Out)**—*MC Yogi*

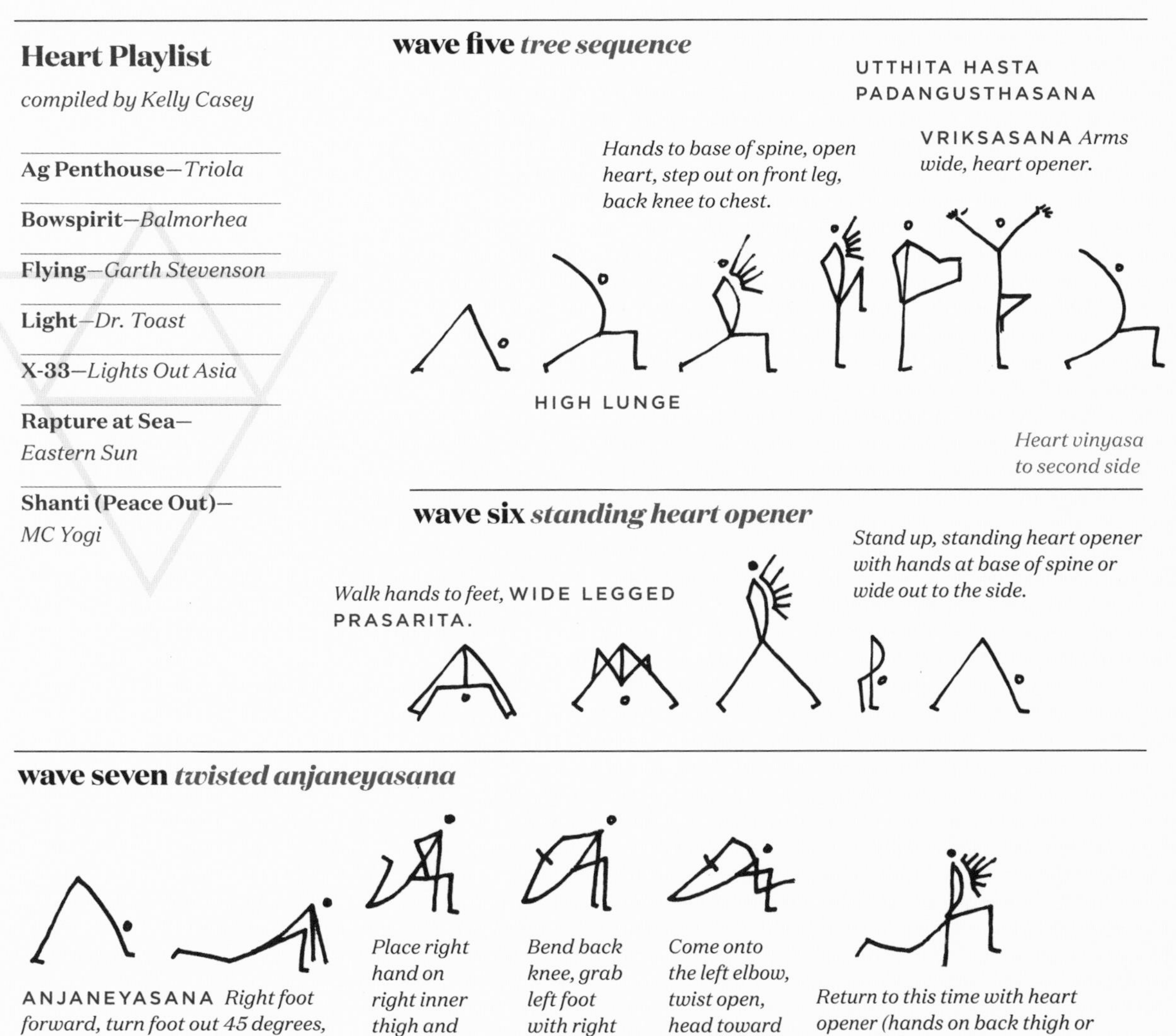

wave five *tree sequence*

Hands to base of spine, open heart, step out on front leg, back knee to chest.

UTTHITA HASTA PADANGUSTHASANA

VRIKSASANA *Arms wide, heart opener.*

HIGH LUNGE

Heart vinyasa to second side

wave six *standing heart opener*

Walk hands to feet, WIDE LEGGED PRASARITA.

Stand up, standing heart opener with hands at base of spine or wide out to the side.

wave seven *twisted anjaneyasana*

ANJANEYASANA *Right foot forward, turn foot out 45 degrees, roll to outer edge of foot.*

Place right hand on right inner thigh and twist.

Bend back knee, grab left foot with right hand.

Come onto the left elbow, twist open, head toward base of spine.

Return to this time with heart opener (hands on back thigh or touching the earth).

Heart vinyasa to second side

wave eight *closing poses*

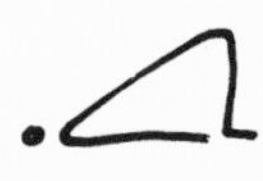

BRIDGE

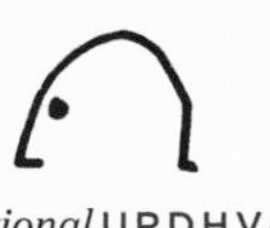

optional URDHVA DHANURASANA

SPINAL TWIST *(Supta Matsyendrasana)*

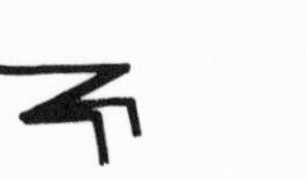

MATSYASANA

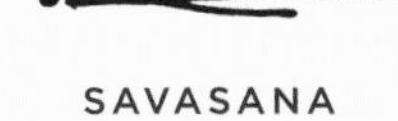

SAVASANA

As you awaken your innate capacity for compassion, your challenge is to stay in the heart center and continue north. You may find that perhaps the greatest challenge of all is to love yourself and your life, with equanimity and gratitude for all your challenges and struggles.

Every day that we pursue our heart's desire is a gift.

Ten Things

DURATION:	LOCATION:	MINDSET:	TOOL:
Twenty minutes	*Your bedroom*	*Grateful*	*Pen*

Jot down a list for one of the following:

TEN THINGS YOU LOVE ABOUT YOURSELF	TEN THINGS YOU LOVE ABOUT YOUR FRIENDS	TEN THINGS YOU LOVE ABOUT YOUR LIFE
1.	1.	1.
2.	2.	2.
3.	3.	3.
4.	4.	4.
5.	5.	5.
6.	6.	6.
7.	7.	7.
8.	8.	8.
9.	9.	9.
10.	10.	10.

TEN THINGS YOU LOVE ABOUT YOUR HOME

1.
2.
3.
4.
5.
6.
7.
8.
9.
10.

TEN THINGS YOU LOVE ABOUT YOUR FAMILY

1.
2.
3.
4.
5.
6.
7.
8.
9.
10.

TEN THINGS YOU LOVE ABOUT YOUR JOB

1.
2.
3.
4.
5.
6.
7.
8.
9.
10.

TEN THINGS YOU LOVE TO DO BY YOURSELF

1.
2.
3.
4.
5.

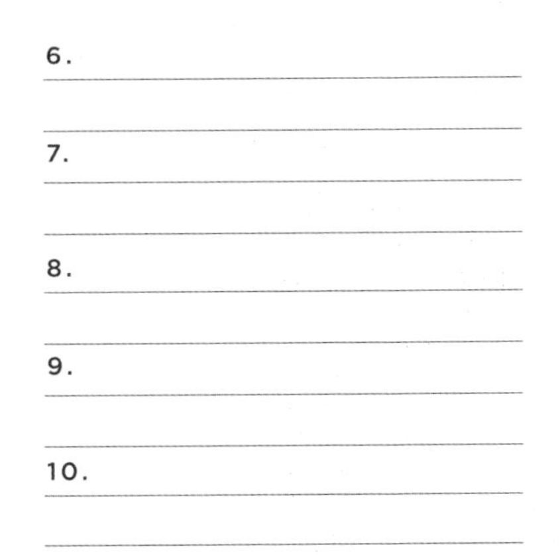

Your lists may repeat, become prayers, or help you feel better when you are angry, frustrated, or depressed. Let your lists support you and help you find gratitude through life's struggles and successes.

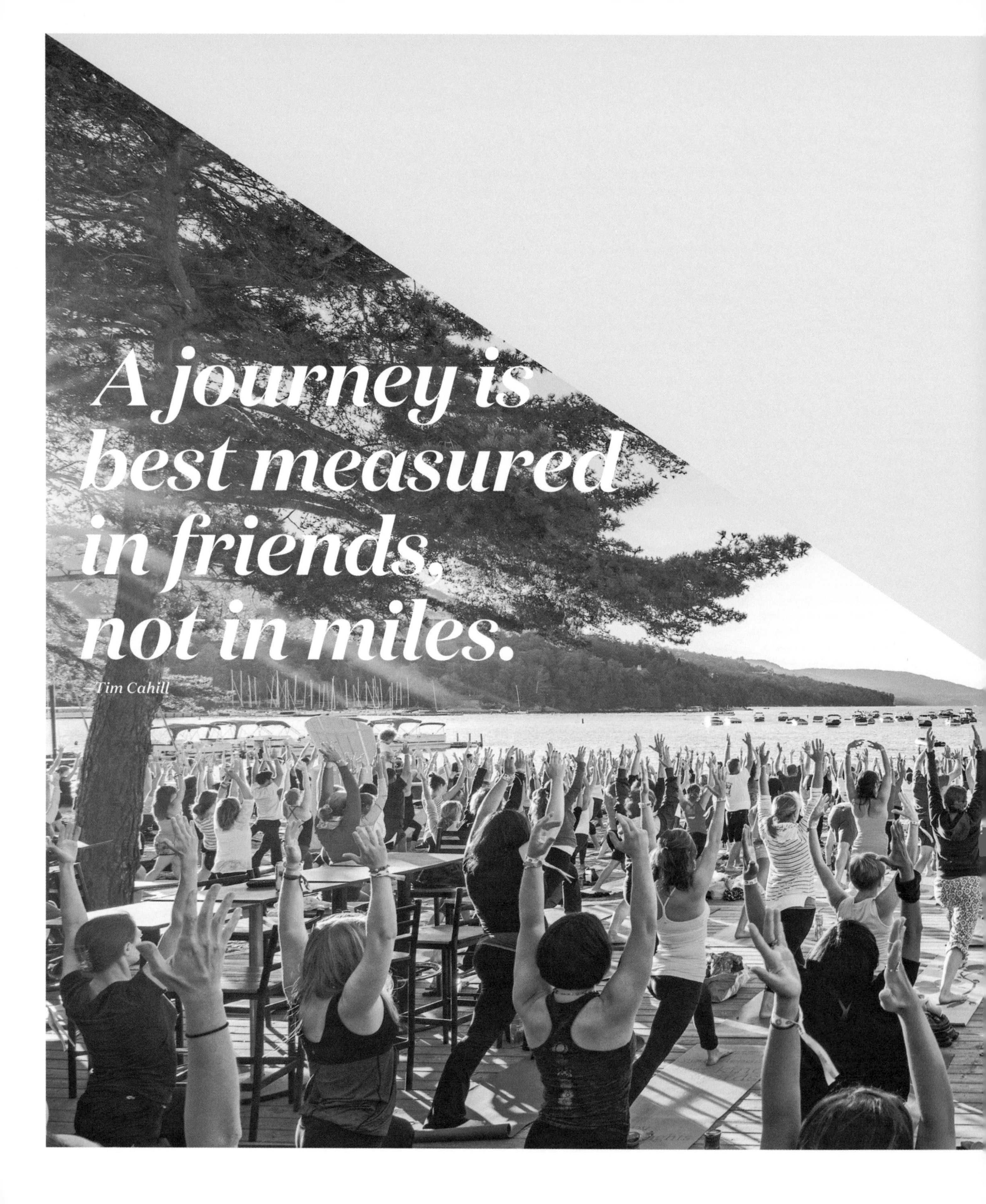
A journey is best measured in friends, not in miles.
—Tim Cahill

CHAPTER 5

find your community

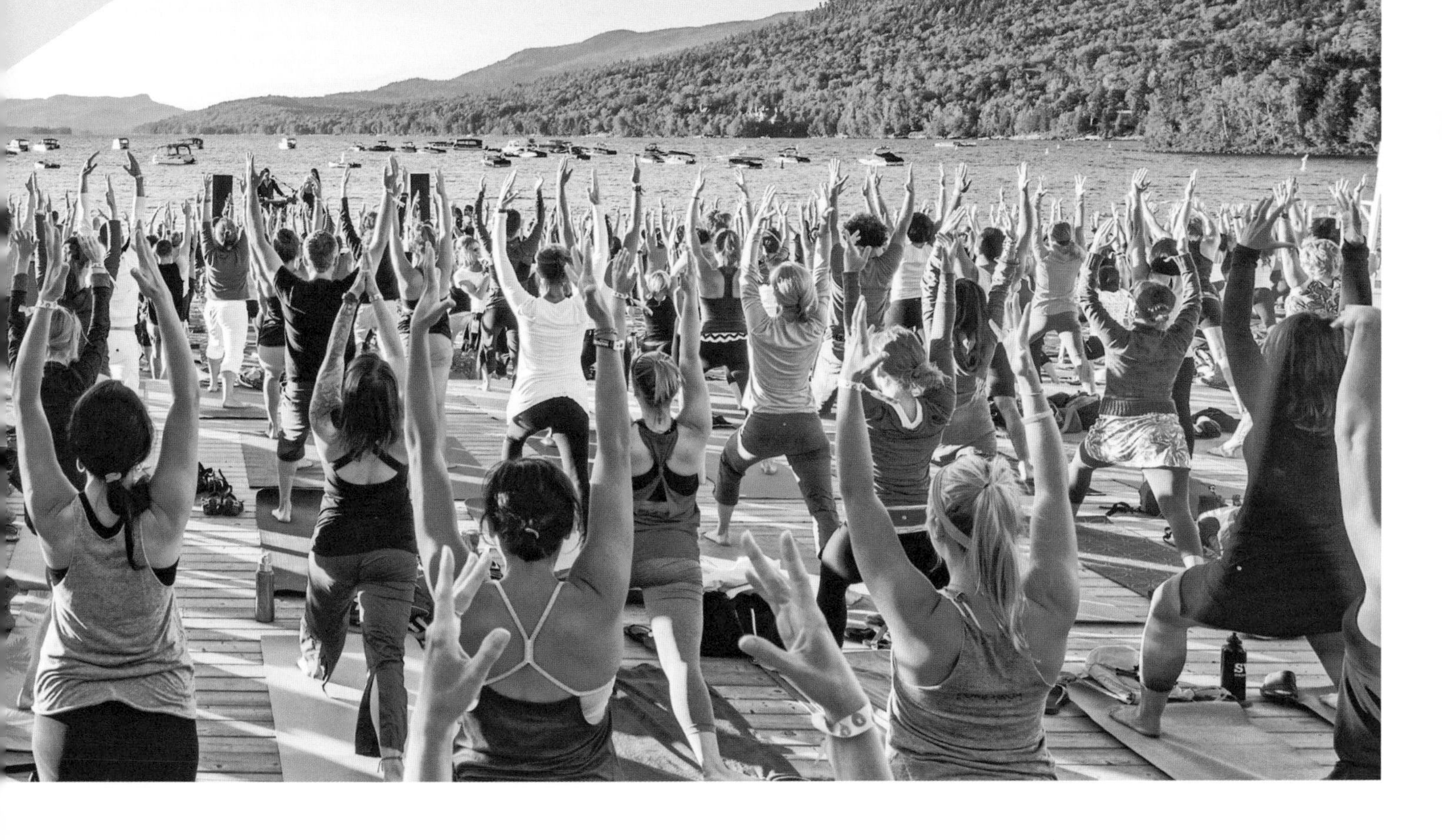

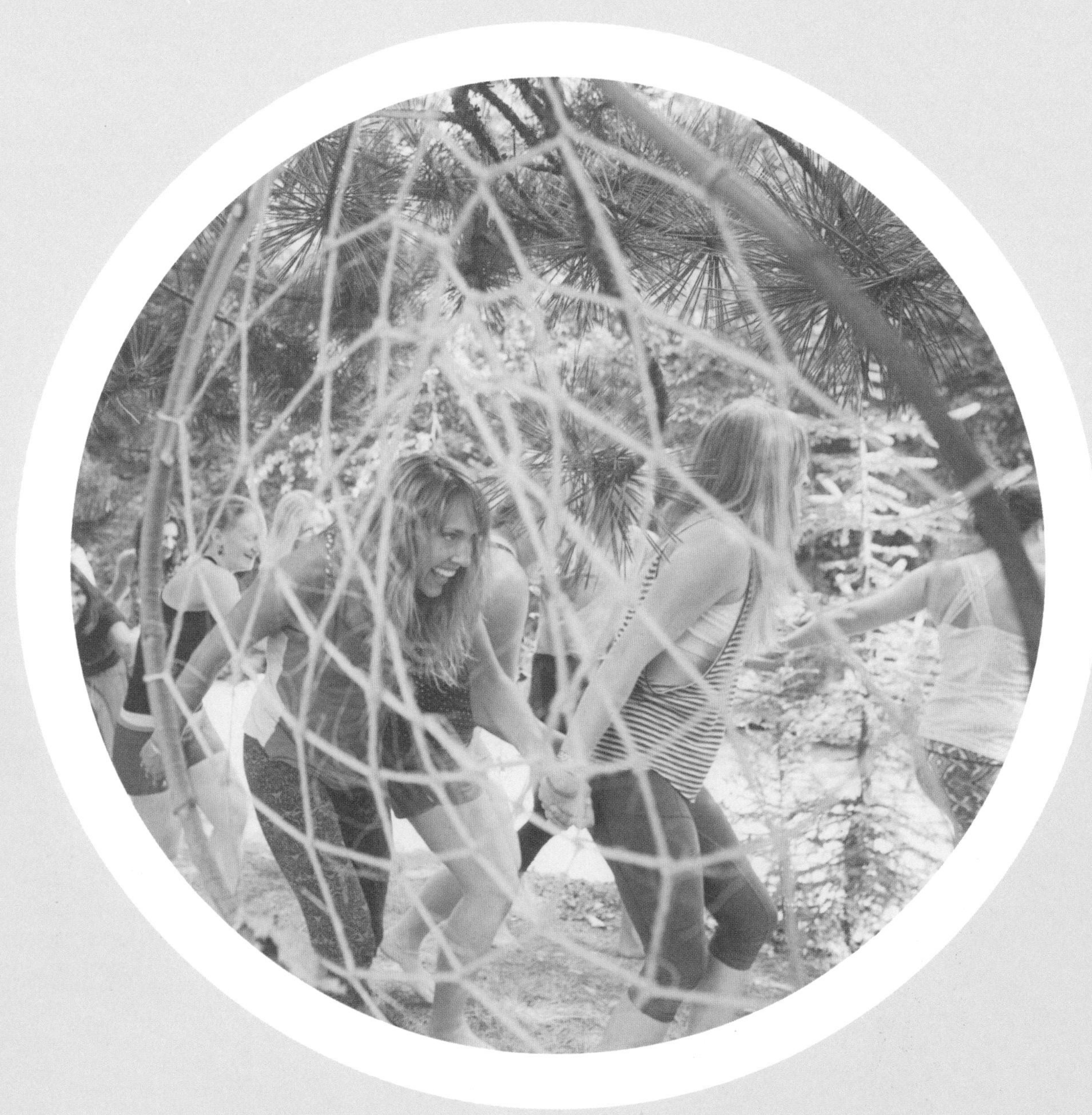

There are many different types of communities—from Buddhist sanghas to birdwatching societies, from book groups to urban gardeners. In its essence, a community is a group of people who come together around shared beliefs and behavior. In yoga, we often hear the Sanskrit word *kula,* which means intentional community. The basis of any kula is the feeling that life is best when shared.

The notion of community has been somewhat co-opted and twisted by the digital age. E-mail, texts, and social media are great organizing tools. But our modern, hyperconnected world often creates more isolation than connectedness. As we accumulate digital friends and followers, we are increasingly thirsting for real human interaction. This is one of the reasons events like Wanderlust, Burning Man, and food festivals have become so popular. People are seeking to disconnect from their "virtual" lives and reconnect with their actual community, where they can have real-time experiences and express ideas and feelings with more than 140 characters.

We started Wanderlust because we thought it would be incredible to create a large-scale communal experience of mindful living. We envisioned an event where yoga, music, personal development, organics, sustainability, ethical consumption, and the arts all came together under one big tent to remind people how powerful the medicine of connection can be. One of the most satisfying things about the success of Wanderlust is in witnessing the lasting connections made at the festival—the friendships and partnerships sparked, businesses hatched, and babies made on various mountaintops over the years.

Music, food, shared spiritual practices, athletics, and giving back (also known as the concept of *seva*—service—in yoga), these are among the strongest community builders. From singing around a campfire to Coachella, music, throughout its existence, has played a central role in bringing people together. Food plays a similar role. In the home, meals have always been the time and place where family and friends gather. From heated political discussions to romantic trysts, the dinner table is the venue for old-fashioned analog discourse. On a larger scale, farmers' markets and food festivals like Outstanding in the Field bring people together around abundance and nourishment.

Yoga, traditionally an intimate teacher/student relationship, has increasingly become a communal experience as well as a personal practice. Studios are community centers as much as they are a place to study. Like churches, yoga studios have become congregating places for those with shared values. Also like churches, studios often organize ways for people to join together and give back. If you've ever been to a soup kitchen or built a neighborhood garden, you know the palpable feeling of community that pulses through people united, working together for a common cause.

The same is true for a zendo, martial arts studio, or any spiritual or contemplative community—or even a soccer league. Though the ostensible "point" of sports is competition, athletics actually bring people together—whether you're on a team or in the stands. Marathoners and soccer players, skiers, and tennis players of all nationalities share a common bond.

Food, music, yoga, seva—whatever it is that brings people together—living in harmony with others, feeling part of something bigger than yourself, is powerful and inspiring. While posting on FB and watching the likes accumulate can give you a fleeting sense of connectedness, it will never compare to sharing a great concert or a good sweat.

Part of finding happiness is discovering, cultivating, and building one's true kula. We all long for a sense of belonging and connectedness. Often in marathons, there is one runner who sprints out to an early lead, pushing the pace. He rarely wins. Instead, the top runners group together. For years, Kenyans and Ethiopians have dominated the sport, giving credence to the old African proverb **"If you want to go fast, go alone. If you want to go far, go together."**

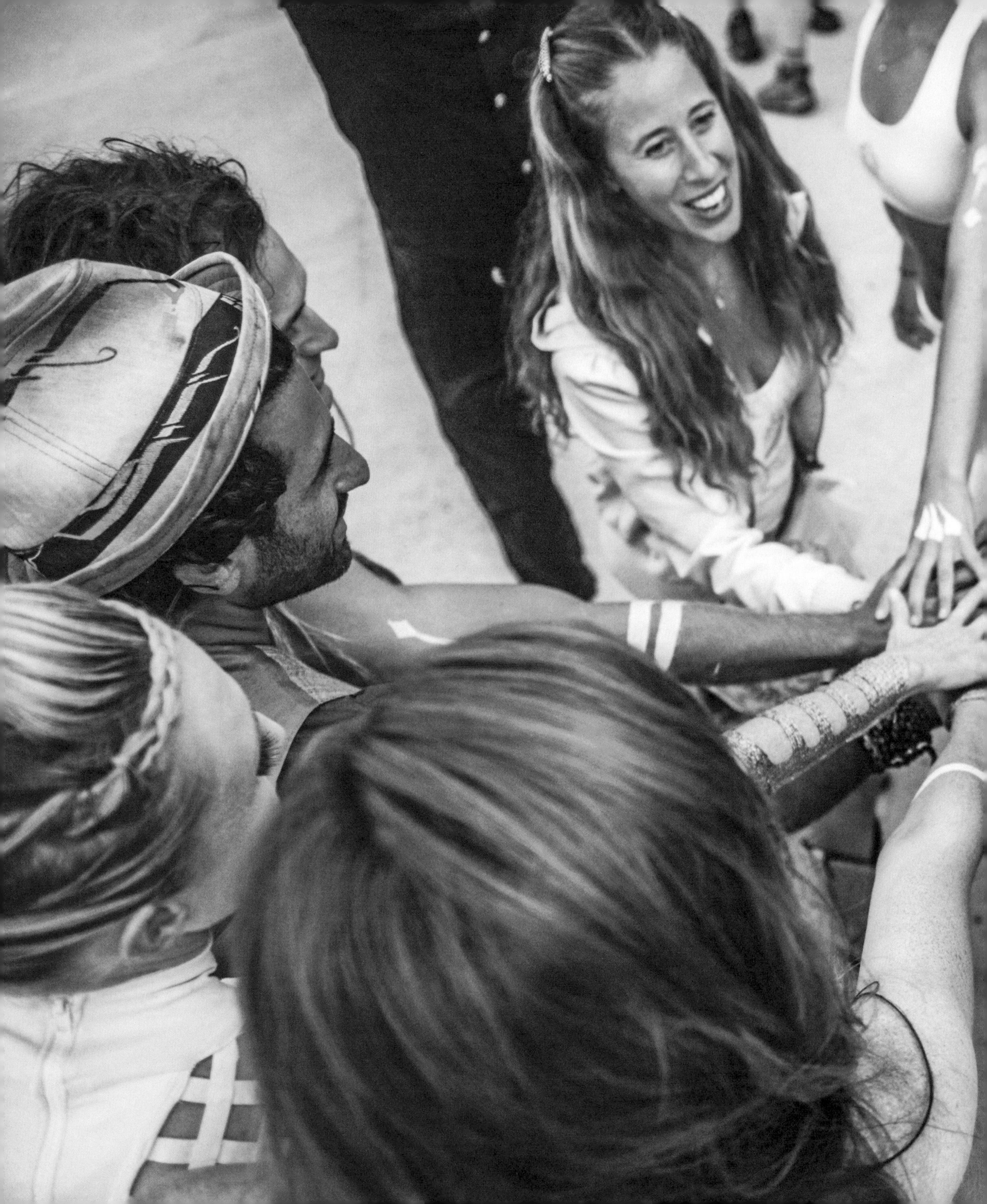

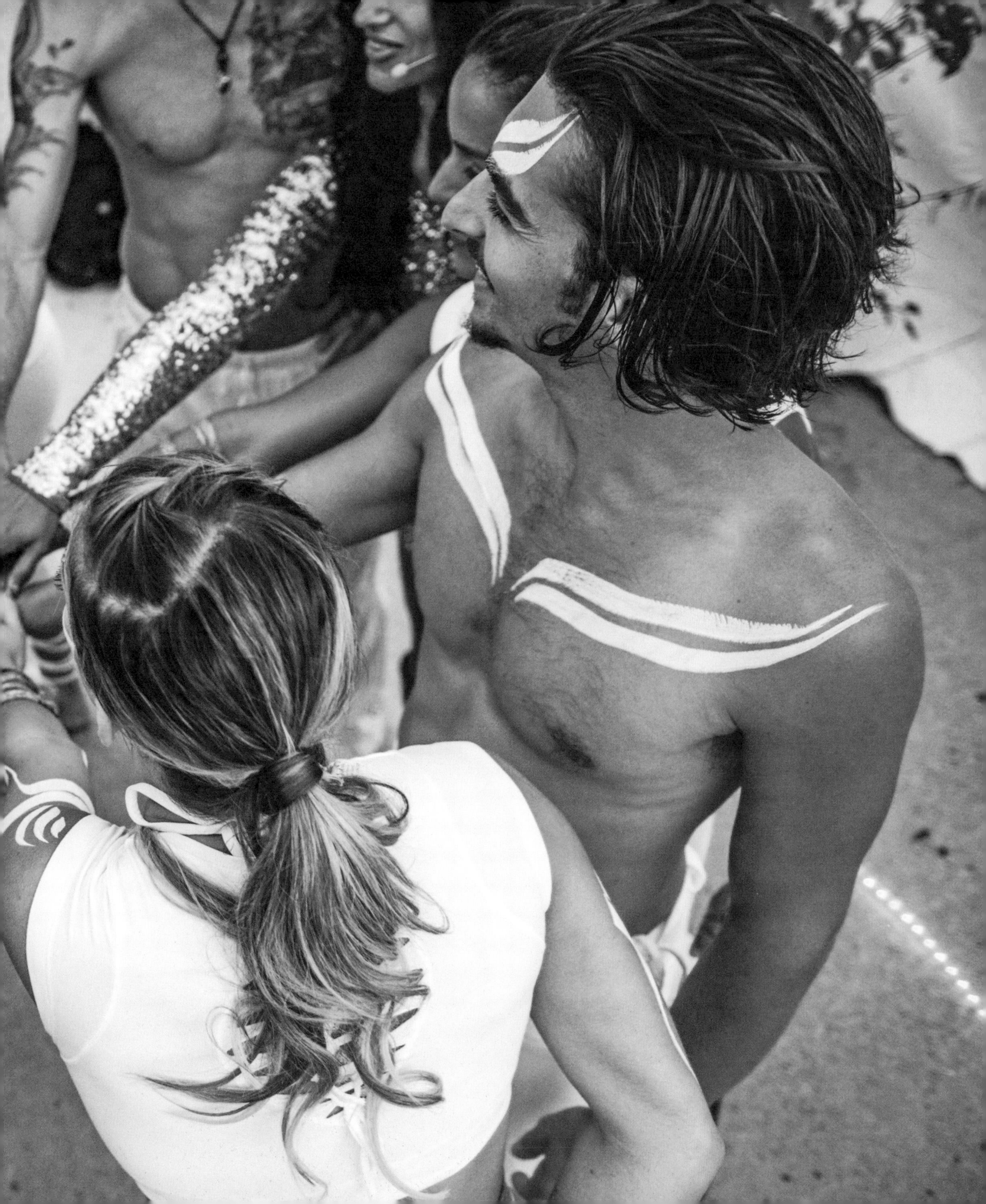

be bold

reach out beyond distraction and the trance of consumption

step out of your comfort zone

celebrate the life force in each other

invoke the sacred

ask deep questions

magnetize playmates

risk being silly, boring, or even dangerous

create opportunities to work and play together

move beyond self-interest, fear, judgment

ask how you might serve

step into play, prayer, and support

mark the passages of your lives

build, create, or save something

ask for help and ideas

cocreate

make rituals that matter and help with real problems

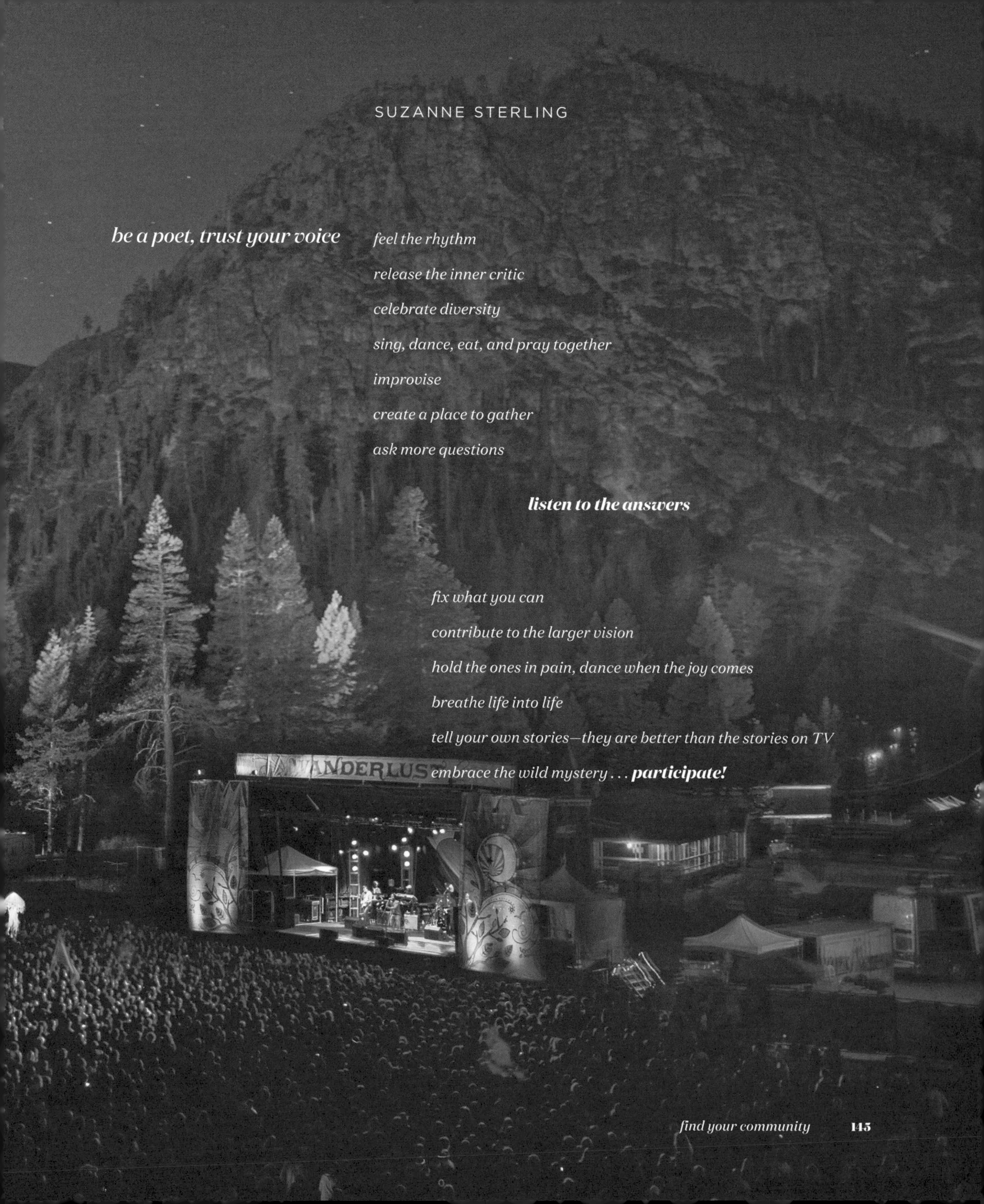

SUZANNE STERLING

be a poet, trust your voice

feel the rhythm

release the inner critic

celebrate diversity

sing, dance, eat, and pray together

improvise

create a place to gather

ask more questions

listen to the answers

fix what you can

contribute to the larger vision

hold the ones in pain, dance when the joy comes

breathe life into life

tell your own stories—they are better than the stories on TV

embrace the wild mystery . . . ***participate!***

ACT FROM THE HEART

Responsible living certainly includes being neighborly. That means we don't sweep our trash onto the neighbor's place. We don't pollute their water. We don't foul their air. Instead, we desire their happiness, health, and success. It means we don't contrive ways to exploit them by impoverishing them in order to enrich ourselves.

These are such fundamental rules of harmonious living that to clarify them seems childish. Yet in many of our systems, the way we interact with each other is far from neighborly. For example, a Concentrated Animal Feeding Operation (CAFO) stinks up the neighborhood, often for miles around. A neighborly farmer, rather than conceiving a plan to externalize problems, creates a food production model that is aesthetically and aromatically sensually romantic.

Naysayers will scoff at this notion, arguing that the CAFO is actually better because it produces the cheapest food in the highest quantity. But it's only cheap if the cost of offending neighbors isn't factored in. And who wants quantity if it poisons water and encourages pathogens?

The old Chinese adage "If every man would sweep in front of his own house the whole world would be clean" applies to neighborliness. How can we live in a community of nations if we can't figure out how to be neighborly to the fellow next door? If the sensibilities, freedoms, or rights of the neighbor next door can be assaulted in the name of business, growth, or production, then what about the country next door?

In conjunction with this neighborliness is openness, primarily because it's the foundation of accountability. Opaqueness and secrecy protect chicanery and villainy in all its forms. Living in community demands transparency.

On our farm, we maintain a 24/7/365 open-door policy to anyone from anywhere to see anything at anytime, unannounced. Rather than asking for more government regulations for food, farming, or employment standards, we encourage customers and others to visit, to see what we're doing firsthand. To be sure, this opens us up to unjustified criticism from folks who may not realize what they're seeing, but what's the alternative? No Trespassing signs?

I saw a wonderful sign on the entrance of a farm in Australia. Although it looked like a No Trespassing sign, it actually said, "Trespassers will be impressed." Now that's a community-oriented, neighbor-friendly way of doing business. A welcome mat instead of a security outpost. Parking signs instead of razor wire. Michael Pollan noted in his

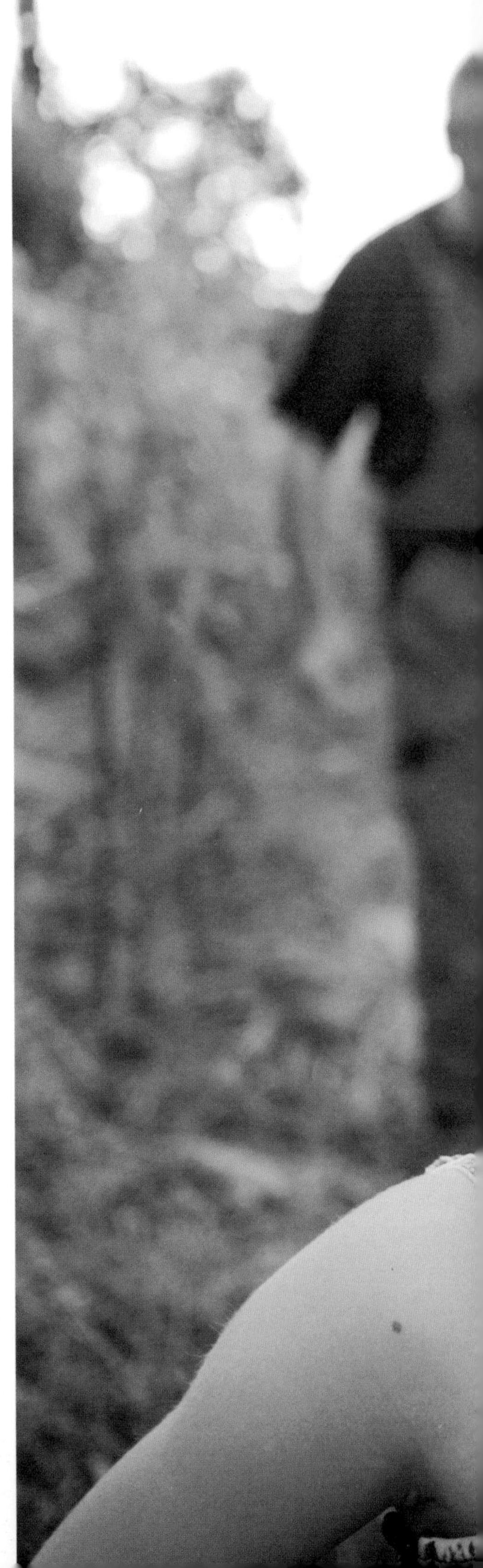

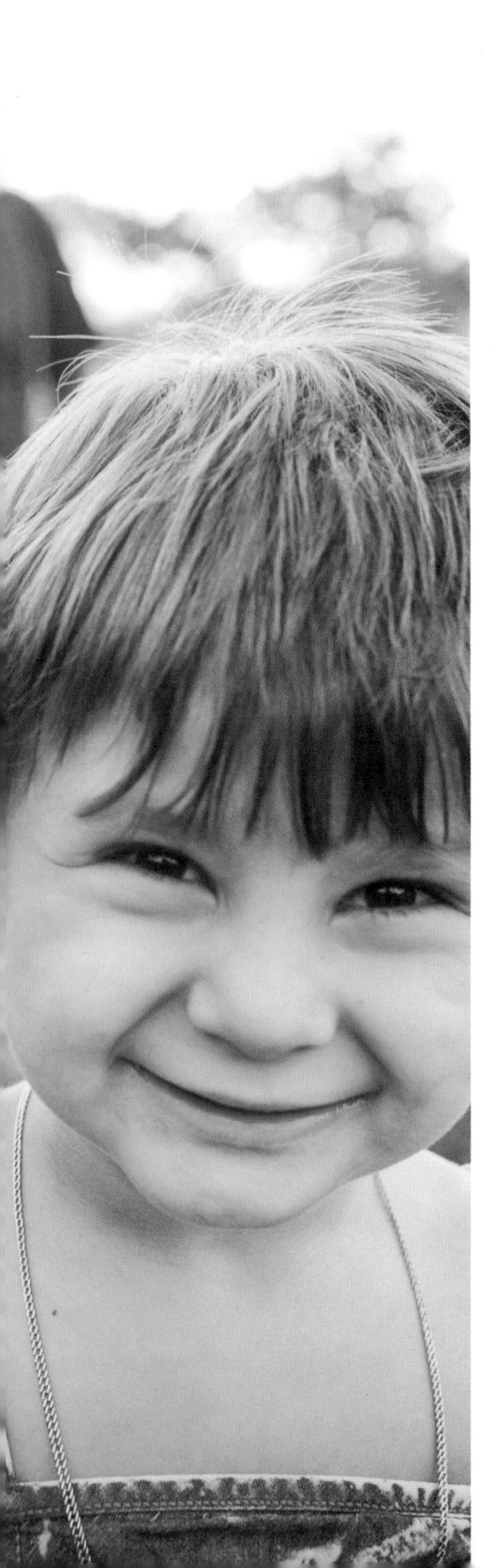

bestseller *The Omnivore's Dilemma* that if CAFOs all had glass walls, they wouldn't exist. He's probably right.

The sheer scale of industrial systems, both farming and processing, often moves far beyond the carrying capacity of the community. Prior to cheap fuel and transportation, no business could amass this amount of plants or animals in a single place because oxen or horses could only move small amounts not very far in a day. But cheap fuel and mechanization changed that, creating for the first time in human history an option no longer bounded by ecological, social, or economic carrying capacity in a community. Instead, these systems could exceed community resources.

Along with the scale came secrecy, from perimeter fencing to patents to special concessions and subsidies from government agencies and politicians. The result is a structure that is fundamentally segregated rather than integrated. Gone is the cobbler who lives over his shop. Instead, he must live in the residential zone and travel to his shop each day in the commercial district. The backyard chicken flock can't eat home-generated kitchen scraps. The scraps go to the landfill and the eggs come from a CAFO 1,000 miles away. The CAFO stinks up its neighborhood and the landfill creates problems in its neighborhood. Integration solves both problems and lets each community function better.

No discussion of community would be complete without appreciating common resources. Community accountability means that we respect shared resources like air, soil, and water. If my food production depletes water resources, or erodes soil, or fills the air with noxious fumes and particles, I'm degenerating my community's wealth over the long term.

The history of civilization too often is the history of ecological pillage and rape. But it doesn't have to be. Although humans are endowed with the very gifts that make us the most efficacious destroyers on the planet, these gifts also make us the most efficient at remediation. The problem is not humans; the problem is our mentality. Are we conquistadors or caretakers? Are we exploiters or nurturers? Community builders or community destroyers?

These are not academic distinctions. We live on a planet created to give abundantly, to heal after abuse. This is not a place of scarcity. It is a place of plenty. We can live responsibly in community in a way that honors the greater world. By focusing on our neighbors, we create a framework for how we'll treat those far away.

SEVA = SELFLESS SERVICE

I am of the opinion that my life belongs to the community, and as long as I live, it is my privilege to do for it whatever I can. I want to be thoroughly used up when I die, for the harder I work, the more I live. Life is no "brief candle" to me. It is a sort of splendid torch which I have got hold of for a moment, and I want to make it burn as brightly as possible before handing it on to the future generations.

—George Bernard Shaw

Seva is the concept of selfless service. In practicing seva, we give for the sake of giving. The action is one of an open palm, an extended arm, a helping heart. In practicing seva, you are devoting yourself to others, to helping the community. If you are not sure where to start, look around and see where the needs are but also look within to see what life experience and gifts you can bring to the table. You may even find your wounds and challenges to be of assistance here, for where we have been hurt we are also understanding and open. Use your life's energy to make the path easier for others.

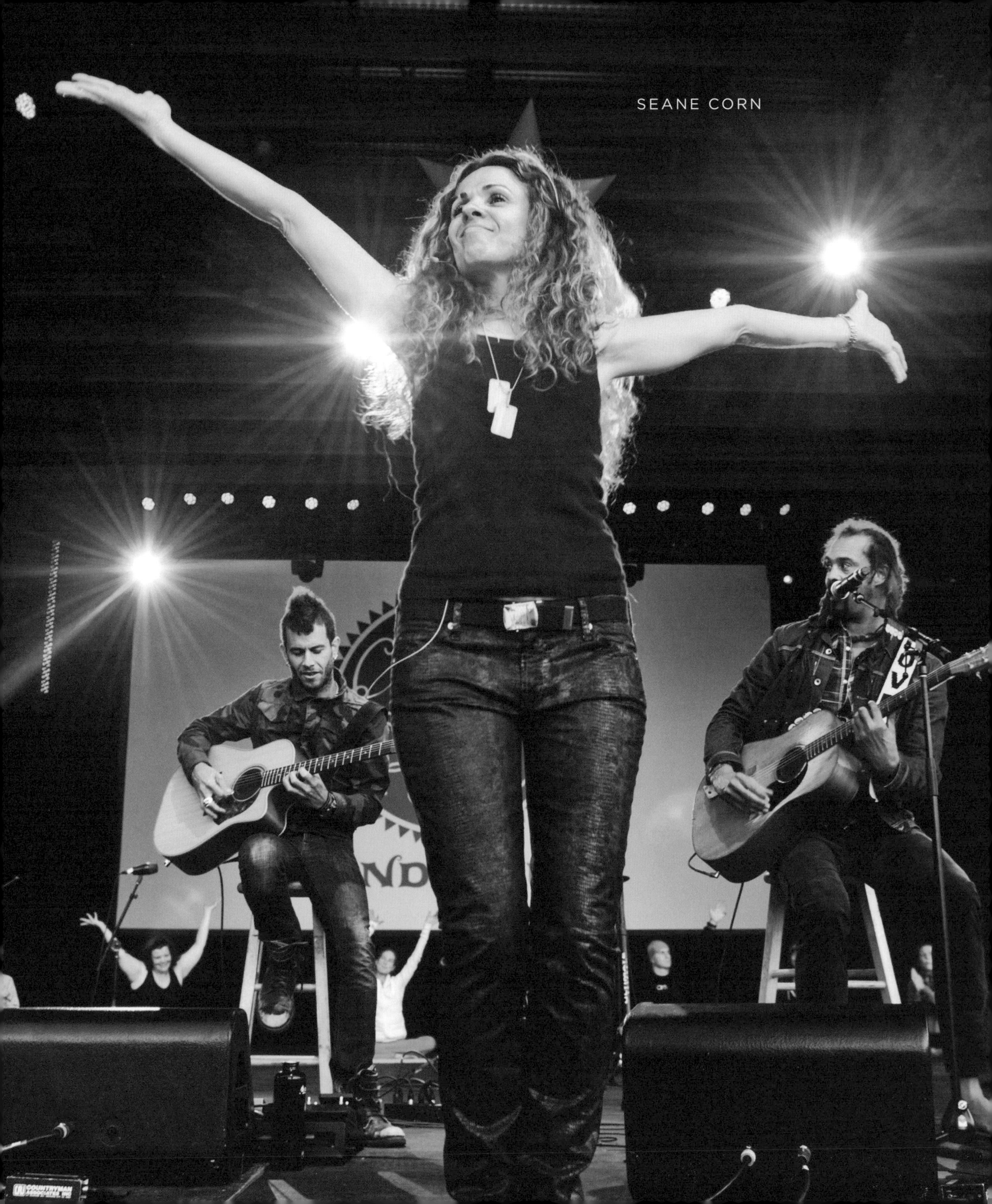

SEANE CORN

Serving Instructions

To be of service—to devote your time, energy, and actions to the health, happiness, and well-being of another person, crisis, or circumstance—is an act that allows us to be engaged and connected and to participate in creating emotional and practical change for the benefit, empowerment, and even survival of others. Sometimes this change occurs in someone else, but almost more often in you.

SERVE BECAUSE:

1. You want to experience and understand the world beyond the bubble of your own culture, privilege, and belief systems.

2. You recognize that everything in the universe is interdependent and ultimately interacts. As human beings, it is our inherit nature to do the same, but we often resist this natural impulse because of fear, ignorance, apathy, or entitlement. Service creates the opportunity to be in relationship with an "other" and deepens our capacity for connection with each other, the planet, and Spirit.

3. At this time in your life you have the time, space, money, or opportunity.

4. At this time in your life you have NO time, space, money, or opportunity.

5. It is an extension of your love. Serve because of your own life experience. Serve because someone once served you. Serve because you want to create balance in your life. Serve because it shifts consciousness. Serve because it is important to understand life outside your comfort zone. Serve because you are grateful. Serve because you can witness someone else's experience with empathy based on a shared understanding or experience, even if your gender, ethnicity, sexuality, economic circumstance, or political affiliation is different. Serve because it is a significant way change can truly occur both inside and out. Serve because you must. Serve because you can.

Although there are many ways we can get involved with service and help, there are also many ways that—even with good intentions—we can hurt or create more harm. Never get involved in service with the intention to "fix" something or somebody. We must focus on our own unhealed places and make certain that the decision to help or serve another is not a way of denying or avoiding our own disowned self. So if you want to serve:

1. Make certain that you are committed to your own inner work. Make this a priority. Also, be open to learning about important issues like racism, ablism, systemic oppression, power and privilege, sexism, gender differences, cultural sensitivity, etc. There are many ways to be of service. Know yourself and choose to participate in a way that is safe for you and helpful to others, especially if the environment you are serving is a "trigger" for you and your own unhealed trauma.

2. Reach out to programs in your local community and ask if they need help. Already know your skills and interests, so that you are not creating more work for them by asking them to figure out what you can do to participate.

3. Know where you are at in your own life and what is truly sustainable. It is easy to overcommit and burn out as a result. Commitment and consistency are critical to many organizations, especially those working with children. Know your capacity and don't make promises you can't follow through on.

4. Visit your city's website. There may be a list of volunteer opportunities in your area. Contact your library, religious or spiritual institutions, yoga studios, community colleges, or local hospitals to learn about different ways to get involved that may interest you.

5. Go online. There are countless organizations worldwide that serve our planet in a variety of ways. Consider what is important to you at this time. It might be animal rights, social justice, domestic violence, HIV/AIDS, environmental sustainability, gay rights, etc. Take a moment to consider what calls to you. Do the research and think about the ways in which you can be involved. Reach out to these organizations and see what local affiliates they may have and take initiative by being proactive, getting informed, and assessing your availability and skills. Also, recognize that service can look different at different times. It doesn't necessarily make sense to run off to a third-world nation to help the children there and neglect the children you have in your own home! Perhaps conscious parenting is the best use of your service right now.

Regardless of what you do, the most important contribution we can make in our service to others is to show up from a place of compassion and love. If we can succeed in this, then peace, happiness, and goodwill for all isn't just possible . . . it's inevitable.

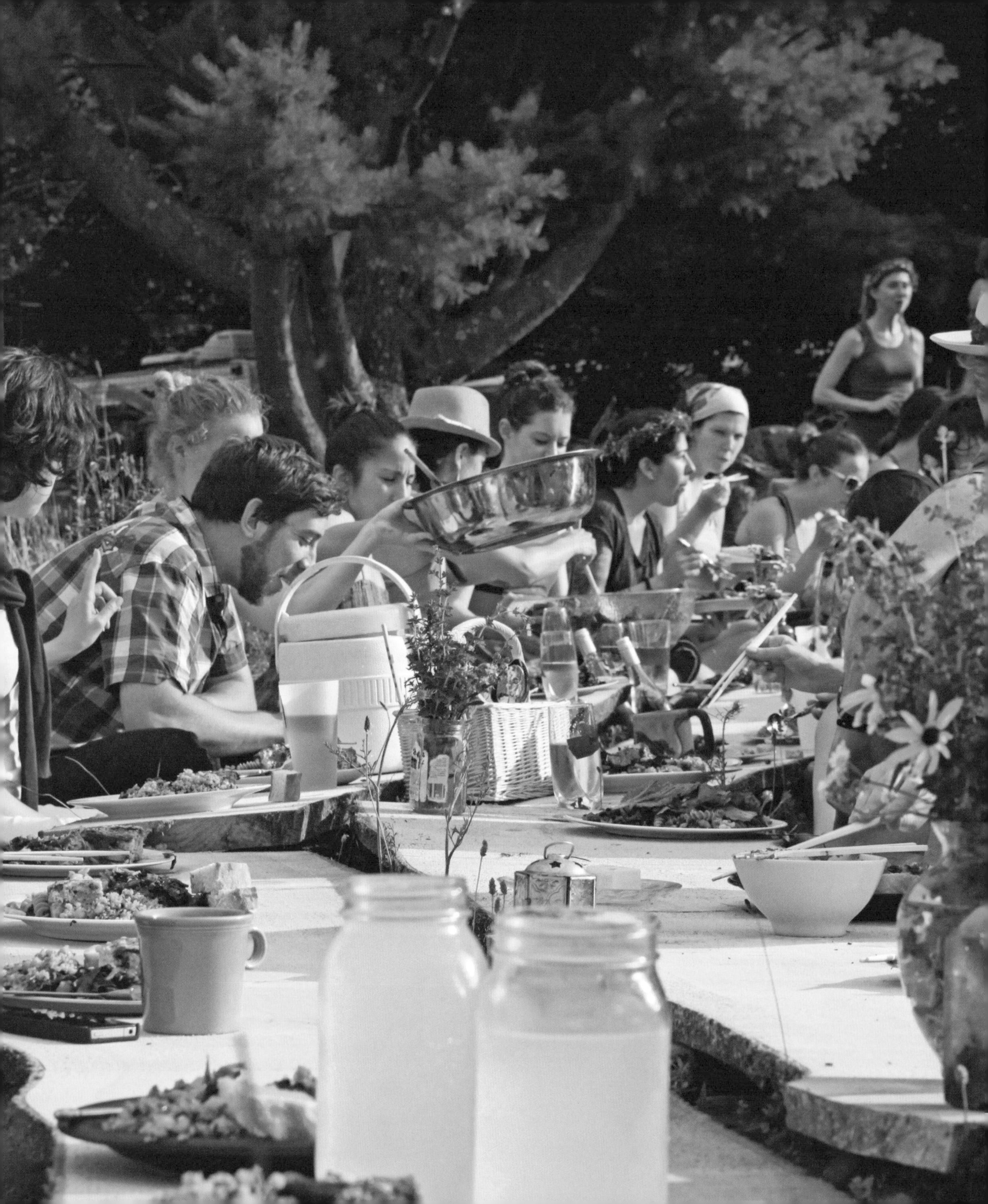

MOVEABLE FEAST: FARM TO YOGA

ABBY PALOMA

Shortly after I began living at Growing Heart Farm, I remembered Thich Nhat Hahn's story of interdependence.

When a student asked a wise woman what she saw in a piece of paper, the woman replied, "I see the clouds."

The student asked, "How do you see the clouds in this piece of paper?"

She answered, "I remember the person who made this paper and his family. I remember the tree from where the paper was harvested; I see the sun that fed the leaves with sunlight and the rich soil that nourished the roots. I see the water that rained down from the clouds to grow this tree. This is how I see the clouds in this piece of paper."

The earth is an extension of our bodies. The health of our soils is the health of our blood. The well-being of our air is the well-being of our breath. The vibrancy of the individual is the vibrancy of the collective.

The current food system is suffering. An increasingly large amount of food is being sourced from faraway lands. American farmers are being paid less and less for their crops. Our water, soil, and entire ecosystem are threatened by chemical fertilizers and pesticides. But solutions are in our hands. Today, the most radical things you can do are to grow your own food, know the person who grew it, and share "happy" food with your community.

I gave one of my first farm tours to a group of visiting friends and yogis. There was fascination and laughter as I told stories of these edible plants. I remember the moment when I pulled a carrot from the ground. There was silence, then cheering. Just as the wise woman saw the clouds in the paper, I saw a wave of realization cross my friends' faces. It was that thing they always knew, but might not have remembered: "Food comes from the ground!" This reminded us all that *we,* as people, as friends and neighbors, could grow food. Whether on a windowsill, in a backyard, or on a farm, the power of growing food is in our hands.

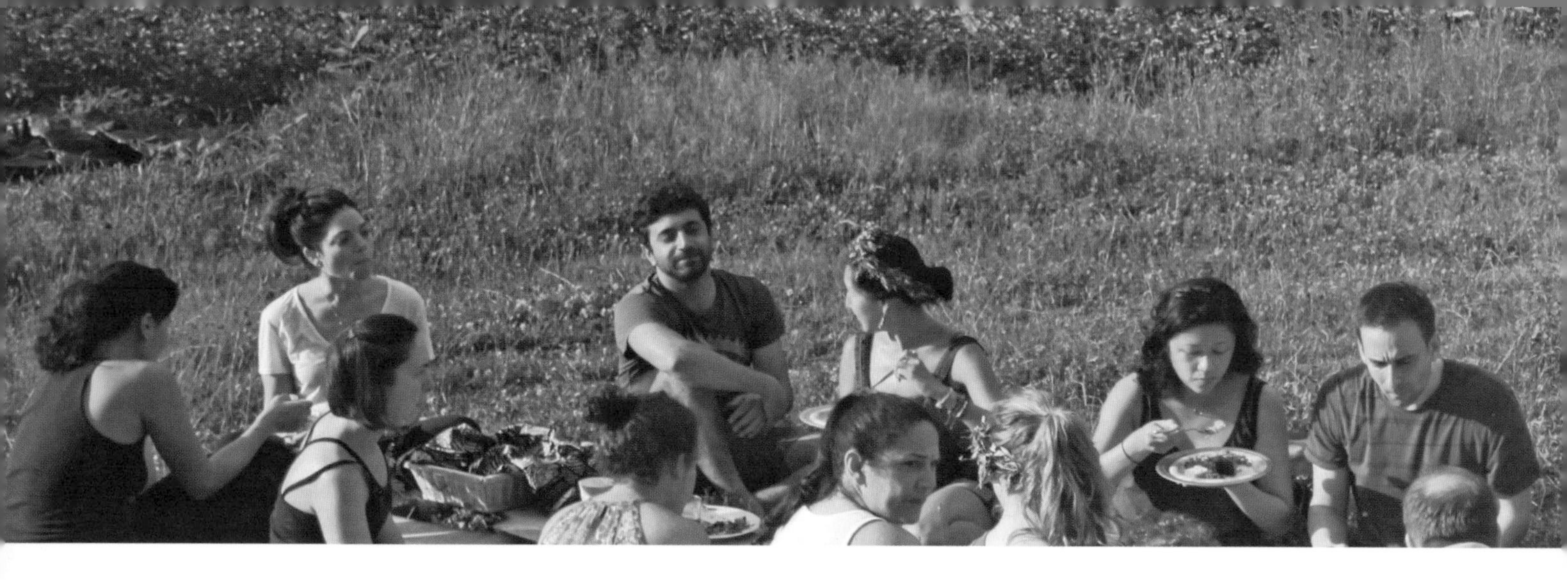

COMMUNITY-SUPPORTED AGRICULTURE

There is an ongoing migration of a younger generation heading back to the land to grow food the way their grandparents did. Many of these farmers grow food in a Community-Supported Agriculture (CSA) model. CSAs give communities the opportunity to support farmers at the source. Members help cover farmers' overhead costs and provide financial security for the season. This shared-risk model accounts for the will of Mother Nature, sometimes generous and sometimes devastating.

Once the season begins, members pick up weekly CSA "shares," a box of seasonal vegetables. There's little time between when the veggies leave the ground and when they arrive in a member's kitchen. Many CSAs include a volunteer program where members can volunteer on the farm and truly support their farmers while connecting to the earth.

The CSA model provides stability for farmers while providing members the highest quality food, in the closest reach to where they live. Any business venture that will succeed in the current times must maintain the mantra "win-win-win," acting with a triple-bottom-line mindset. A win for the business is a win for the customer and a win for the larger community. We see the clouds in our paper, the welfare of our farmers and the health of ecosystems on our plates. These models oppose cutting corners, oppose taking more than what is offered, and oppose capitalizing on the loss of others. In a CSA, every aspect of the seed-to-plate journey is handled with respect for the land and the people on the land!

So where do the yogis come in? As a strong community, we know how to congregate. We practice together at studios. We have tools to organize: structure, infrastructure, and flexibility. We are like a CSA in a box, all ready to go, minus the veggies. Hence, we are perfectly matched to support our farmers. Win-win-win opportunities are endless. Yoga studios can double as CSA pickup locations.

Growing Heart Farm's CSA members include my yoga students and fellow yoga teachers. People constantly recipe-swap and share excitement about the bounty of their CSA boxes. Sharing the same food, from the same soil, connects people at a cellular level. Communities literally begin to move together.

Our CSA members are all running on the same fuel, the same kale and tomatoes: local, not chemically overloaded grocery store food.

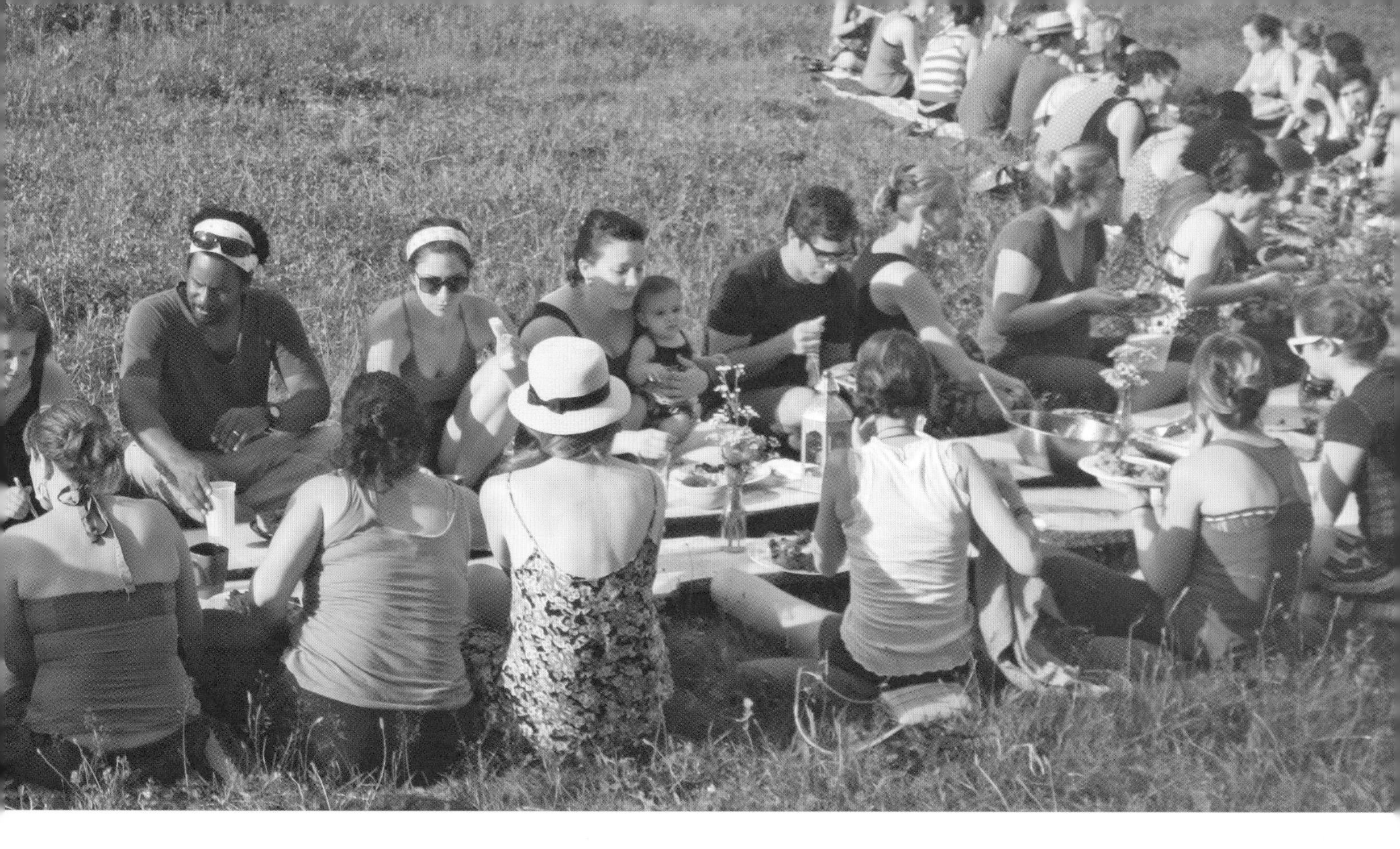

FARM TO YOGA

Collaboration with farmers does not end at the yoga studio. My yoga community now joins me on the farm. Farm to Yoga is a model I developed with friends at Growing Heart Farm over the past five years. Throughout the growing season, we host Farm to Yoga dinners where dozens of yogis congregate at the farm for a glorious gathering. The day before the gathering, our chef and I tour the farm to design the menu based on produce so ripe it cannot even wait for the farmers' market or CSA box. The day of the gathering begins with another farm tour; yogis experience the field by seeing, touching, smelling, and tasting the vegetables straight from the source. The walk through the fields is always a way to come back down to earth and reexperience the profound and simple truth: Food comes from the ground!

This opening sets the stage for a deep yoga practice, literally grounding. We gather in our outdoor yoga classroom among the grass, trees, and big sky. After yoga, we return to the field, where our dinner table is set, overlooking the rows of squash, heirloom tomatoes, and basil. While experiencing the delicious and mindful creation of our chef and farmers, the overwhelming feeling is one of interconnectedness. At this point, everyone has touched the plants that are nourishing them and shaken hands with (or hugged) the farmer who tended those plants, while surrounded by their kula, their community who treks the humble human path, seeking balance together. Here, we remember who we are at our essence.

SEED TO SEED

How can our actions lead to better choices for our selves and our planet? I dream about win-win-win ways of being and knowing. As yogis, we have the tools to organize and already value the importance of being in community. Local farmers need our support. The new food system we consciously create needs our action.

I am here to invite us to take our practice a bit deeper . . . to practice mindfulness bite by bite. We choose every day—multiple times a day—what we put inside our bodies. How can we see the clouds on our plates? How can we see our farmers with the seeds for our future? How can we see the communities that are thriving because of our actions?

Imagine when we as a community are running on the same fuel, operating at the same vibration, because the food we eat is grown with love, close to home, by people we trust. The good news is this is already happening; we are already what we want to become.

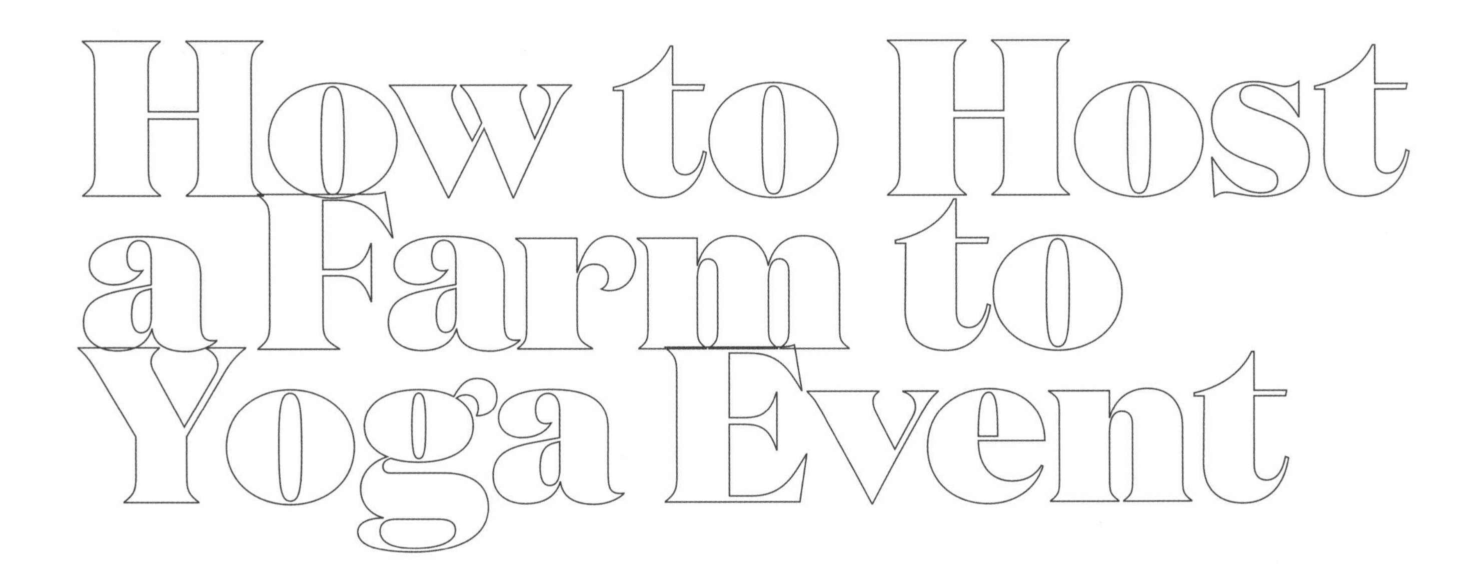

How to Host a Farm to Yoga Event

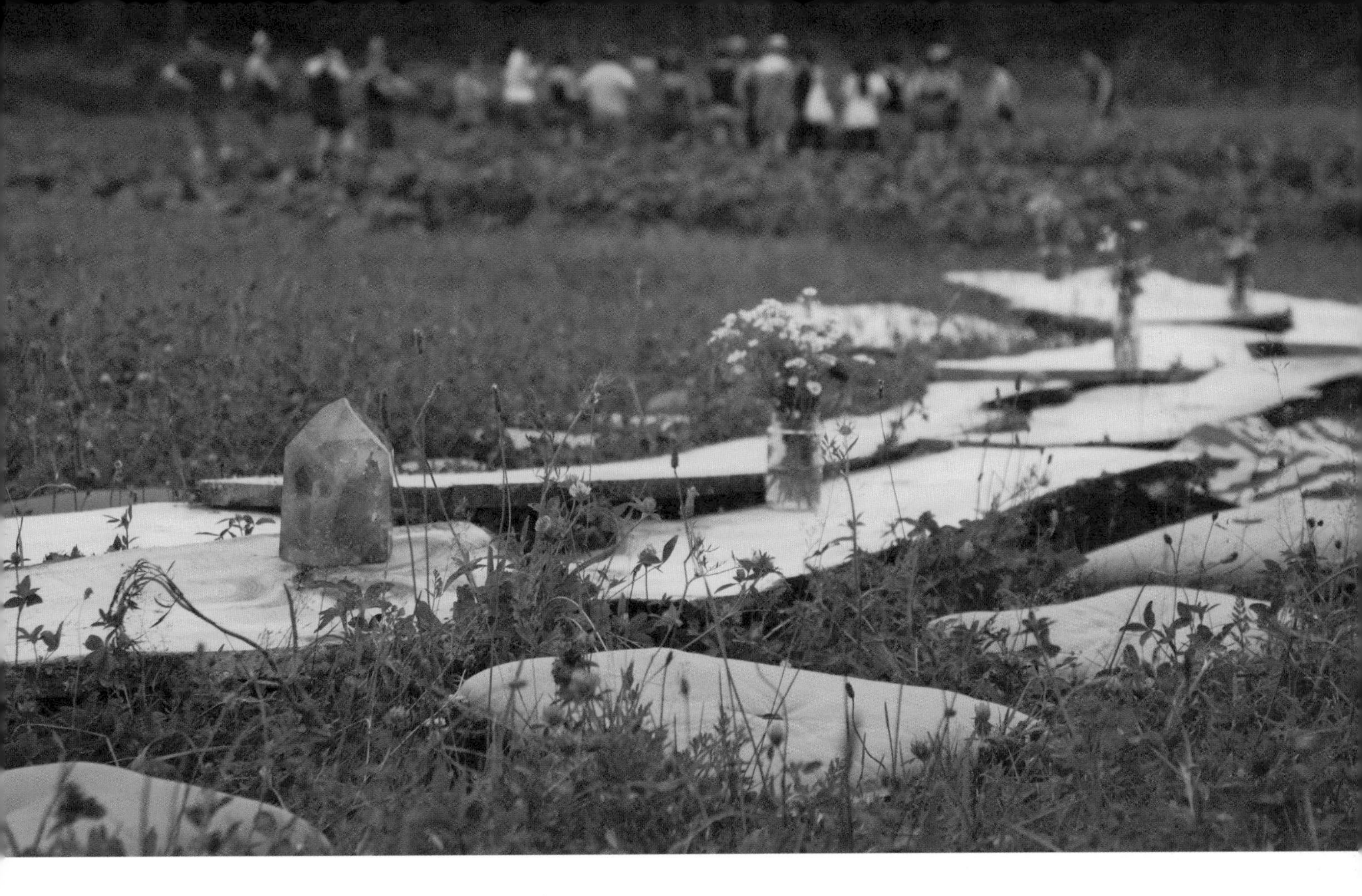

Special ingredients:

Find local farm or venue with space for yoga and dining.

Invite an inspired yoga teacher.

Invite a holistic/locavore chef.

Promote through your local yoga and food community.

Too Daunting to Host a Farm to Yoga Dinner But Still Want to Get Your Hands Dirty?

Join your local CSA.

Volunteer at your local farm.

Visit a local farm with friends and attend farm events.

Start a window or backyard garden.

Join a community garden.

Shop at the farmers' market.

Save your seeds/support seed libraries.

Every breath we take is an exchange between what is inside us and what is outside. Our carbon dioxide is exhaled into the vastness of this world, and we inhale the oxygen that our ecosystem so generously provides. And the process continues. Our atmosphere may consist of oxygen and carbon dioxide, but it also includes the flow of our own thoughts, attitudes, and feelings. What we send out interacts with the world and is sent back. If what we send out is kind and tender, we usually get that back. We reap what we sow. Some call it karma.

Thomas Merton, the famous Trappist monk, said, "A man who is not at peace with himself necessarily projects his internal fighting into the society of those he lives with. And spreads a contagion of conflict all around him." This captures the idea that who we are, what we are, and what we do ripples out into the world. Just like our breath.

Knowing and understanding this ripple effect idea makes it important for us to develop the skills and capacities that can allow us, from moment to moment, to make the best possible decisions. We must train our minds to see clearly and our bodies to be grounded and relaxed in the present moment. This centering is fundamental to achieving the objective of bringing more peace and justice to our world. Our state of mind, our anxiety levels, our fearful or loving thoughts and actions all register in the greater collective of our nation. If we slow down, breathe, and relax, we will raise our level of awareness and begin to see our internal thoughts. We will see the space we have between our thoughts and thus we can see the possible actions available based on those thoughts. We will begin to see that we have the ability to make choices, and not merely reactions.

When faced with obstacles, we may see that we become frozen, overwhelmed with fear, and we make no choice at all. Only when we can see this reality can we possibly muster the courage to overcome it. We can develop the skill to allow ourselves to reclaim power over negative thinking and fearful thoughts, which make us apathetic, strap us in chains, or fill us full of excuses. By slowing down and raising our consciousness, we can become fearless and see that we call the shots, not our fear.

In yoga, we learn that we can cultivate the ability to slowly stretch our bodies; we can also cultivate the ability to stretch our world. We overcome fear on the yoga mat by nudging ourselves past where we were the day before. We look fear in the eyes and conquer it. But as we learn this through practice with our bodies, we can also apply this same process with the body politic. Just like with the body, it takes slow, gentle, yet courageous movements. Breath by breath, inch by inch, day by day, we can end up in a place we never believed we could end up. In yoga, we don't get there through sudden jerks in new directions. There's an intention, then some positioning, then a breath and we let go to allow all of the previous actions do the work. Eventually it becomes a movement.

If enough of our citizens can take this approach, we all, both yogis and nonyogis alike, can set a new intention for the body politic and begin to reposition society. We can then breathe new life into our nation and slowly create a movement that will transform America into a nation of openness, creativity, and love instead of a nation of the stiff, fearful, paralyzing polarization that we see today. Like a new yoga pose, this begins with a touch of courage. This is not a pipe dream, although there will always be people of differing political persuasions that refuse to stretch or open themselves to the possibilities that come with transcending a current position. That probably won't change. They have every right to be that way, and we should not judge.

But I believe a majority of us are longing to stretch ourselves physically, emotionally, socially, and spiritually. We can transcend the fears that tell us not to move into a new asana or to get off the meditation cushion when an uncomfortable series of thoughts arises or to not participate in the political process because we feel our vote doesn't matter and our voice is a lone one. We have overcome fear, anger, and apathy before; we can do it again.

If you believe that you are in a constant state of interaction with the world around you, then you should have ample motivation to put out into the world exactly what the world needs. As you open your heart, the national heart will open just a little bit more. As you open your mind, the nation's mind will open just a little bit more. As you become more tolerant of others, especially those you disagree with, so our nation and world will become a little less judgmental. There's a well-known expression, "Be the change you wish to see in the world." And if we embody the love, compassion, resilience, and creativity that lie within us, then our education, healthcare, and economic systems will embody those characteristics as well. If we come from the deepest part of who we are, the part that connects us to all that resides outside our skin, then we will change the poisonous discourse in our country. We will listen. We will empathize. We won't judge. In short, we will elevate our country and world to the next level that is our destiny. We can do this together, one amazing human being at a time. It all starts from the inside. Our inside . . . not somebody else's. Be the change!

Most mornings I start my day with breathing exercises to calm and balance my nervous system. Then I spend anywhere from twenty to forty minutes in complete silence. My intention is to keep my attention gently focused on my breath, which trains my mind to be in the present moment. Aware of the breath coming in, aware of the breath going out. Inevitably, my mind will wander to the past and future. Once I become aware of this, I gently return my focus to my breath. And as crazy and chaotic things happen throughout the day, I take moments periodically to quietly recenter myself back to the present moment.

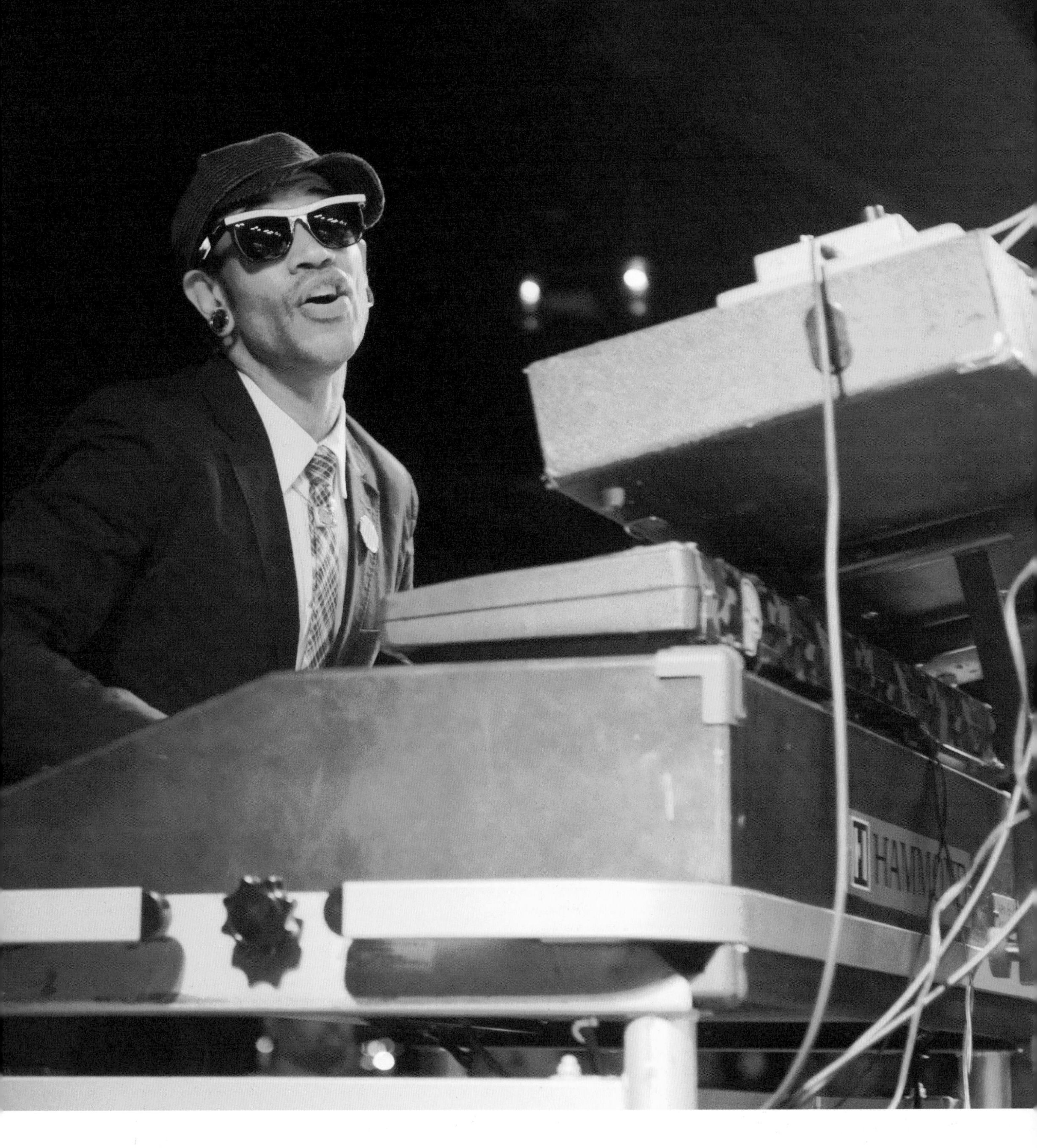

The floor of the club undulated with the synchronous movements of the crowd. Fifteen hundred pairs of feet landing and elevating in perfect union. Hands in the air, swaying, like a choreographed exercise class. Neal was feeling it.

Neal Evans is the best Hammond B-3 organ player in the world. If you think I don't know what I am talking about, then you've never heard Neal. This night, he was in complete control. Neal plays all the bass lines with his left hand and has rigged his organ to produce subsonic frequencies. He was toying with the crowd now, dropping the bass out and holding a cluster of ever-ascending high notes. This is how he builds the tension.

In the best music, something changes while something stays the same. The beat grooved on, the guitar chanked rhymthically. Up and up Neal went, adding higher extensions to the chord. But with no bottom, you're on a roller coaster. You're climbing the ascent. Instinctually, you know what's next, but when is it going to happen?

I've always thought there were two kinds of musicians: the creator and the conduit. The creator generates all the music from inside his body. You see the emotion in the contortions of his face as he summons the notes. The conduit is empty, open to God's grace to pass right through him, onto his instrument, and into people's hearts.

Neal is a conduit, his face placid. He moves on his instrument like an athlete. No one can take their eyes off him. To watch effortless mastery is truly divine.

He takes it to the high C on the organ and just holds it, the beat relentless beneath him. He raises his left hand, like an emperor greeting his subjects. Hold on! You know it's coming. You're at the apex.

Holy fucking shit! He plays the lowest subsonic bass note you have ever heard. The pint glasses are shaking off the tables. And everyone, EVERYONE, loses their mind. I know people think the floorboards are going to buckle as the crowd jumps up and down in perfect harmony and joy.

Adam Deitch, the drummer, tugs my sleeve. We're standing on the side of the stage. He leans into my ear, "That dude makes everyone feel the same."

This is the reason why people come to a concert, for this transcendental shared moment. A moment when nothing matters except what is happening right there and then. Briefly, you access the inaccessible.

Nothing compares to the primal power of music to bring people together and collectively share emotion. And the greatest musicians know this.

Music expresses that which cannot be put into words and that which cannot remain silent.

—Victor Hugo

DJ DREZ

Everyone responds to music. There is something about the vibrations of sound that helps us remember our truths. Yoga is about that same practice of constant connection to truth. Because yoga asana can really impact how energy flows through our bodies, I feel that careful consideration must be taken when creating a playlist for the practice.

People have commented on how much they enjoy the instrumentals I play during a class. Although the individual track may be a very special creation, it has more to do with the emotional connection to the actual melodic tones and bass as well as the drums. That's why lyrics are tricky. They can trigger memories that can reflect any emotion and throw someone outside themselves. When that happens, we can even forget we are on our mats in practice. That is not really the yoga practice, to be living in a memory outside the body all while struggling to breathe and balance with the body. With fewer words or no lyrics, it is easier to create a space for a person to experience that moment of being with self. This is why it is very rare to hear me play straight up hip-hop, rock, or pop in a classroom.

Most of the students and teachers I play for are entering the yoga studio from city life. Having to then sit in a quiet room and be quiet can be maddening. When I fill the room with music, even with a simple drone, it allows them to hug in the prana so that they can begin to feel themselves and remember they are not all of those outside things. It's as if the music vibrations calm the mind and this allows the body to soften and follow. Please don't hold me responsible for what takes place when that happens. I have seen people jump for joy, laugh, get angry, and uncontrollably sob all during the same song. That's the beauty.

If we take a closer look at my "For What It's Worth" remix on *Jahta Beat*, it is a perfect example of giving a little bit of the familiar, but combining it with Indian instrumentation and mantra to give this song a new power. The old gives birth to the new and the new is built upon the old. These cycles reflect the cycles of life, and I offer this whole experience and spirit through the roots music and traditional sounds of roots people from all over the world.

Do you remember the first time you asked yourself, "Who am I and why am I here?" This question is the seed of change. The ancient yoga texts and enlightened teachers for millennia have said this inquiry is one of the first steps in discovering our dharma, or our duty or purpose in life. This question can help us apply our knowledge, understanding, and gifts to serve something greater than ourselves.

For me, growing up around an entrepreneurial engineer father working in the emerging field of renewable energy created a sense of excitement (and often fear) about what could happen next. He inspired me, but it took a while to find my path. I studied his businesses in college and, a few years later, begged to join him on an innovative project in northern Italy. Young, naïve, and ready to change the world, I thought everyone would be as passionate as I was about turning the world's waste into usable energy. But neither the technology nor most people were ready for this yet. Looking back, I see that these were some of the toughest years of my life, but they were also the beginning of the journey into a deeper understanding of my dharma, working at the intersection of sustainability, finance, and philanthropy. I then went on to build and contribute to companies that advance clean technology, renewable energy, and social enterprise.

In the path of discovering one's dharma, life's events unfold in often mysterious and yet synchronistic ways. In 2011, I teamed up with a young entrepreneur named Kimbal Musk to take our shared knowledge to launch the Kitchen Community, a philanthropic arm of the Kitchen family of restaurants. From there we created the nonprofit organization the Learning Garden as a way to create community through food across America.

Learning Gardens connect kids to real food in low-income schools and communities across the country. In a Learning Garden, kids get to plant and grow, experiencing where food comes from firsthand. We are literally planting seeds of community. The gardens are hands-on learning environments and experiential play spaces. Instead of going into urban schools and tearing up concrete and sidewalk, we use modular plastic containers that snap together to create outdoor gardens. In this way, we don't wait for perfect conditions to grow, we work with the environment as it is. Learning Gardens foster childhood nutrition, socialization, community, and student achievement in underserved neighborhoods across the country. They are designed to be places in which kids want to learn and teachers want to teach, thereby creating a long-term, positive investment for the school and the community.

The very first Learning Garden was planted in 2011 at Schmitt Elementary in Denver. By 2014, the Kitchen Community had created 167 Learning Gardens impacting nearly 100,000 children in schools across the country on a daily basis—in Chicago, Colorado, and Los Angeles, as well as other cities and towns.

My dharma started as a seed of intention and intuition, and grew. Likewise, the Learning Garden began as a seed and blossomed. It only takes a seed.

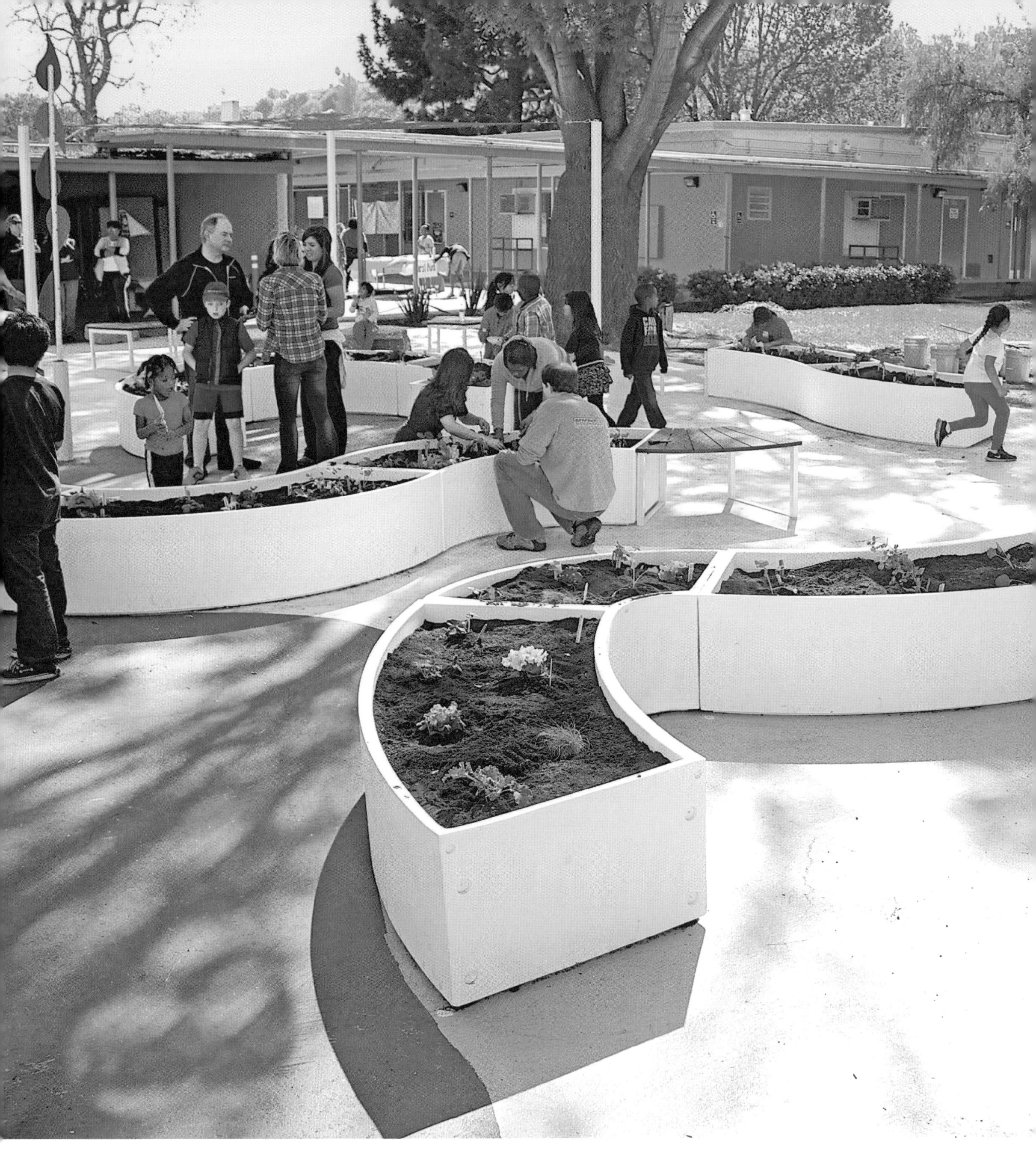

find your community

CHELSEY KORUS AND MATT GIORDANO

Direction Playlist

compiled by Kelly Casey

- **Holograms**—*M83*
- **Intro**—*The xx*
- **Space Walk**—*Lemon Jelly*
- **Halcyon Days**—*Mokhov*
- **Corvette Cassette**—*Slow Magic*
- **Alice**—*Pogo*
- **Always This Late**—*Odesza*
- **Woods and Gives Away (Instrumental)**—*Helios*

wave one *warm up*

Position your yoga Mat's facing each other approximately 2 feet apart.

Taking your time, getting past insecurities into a place of connection.

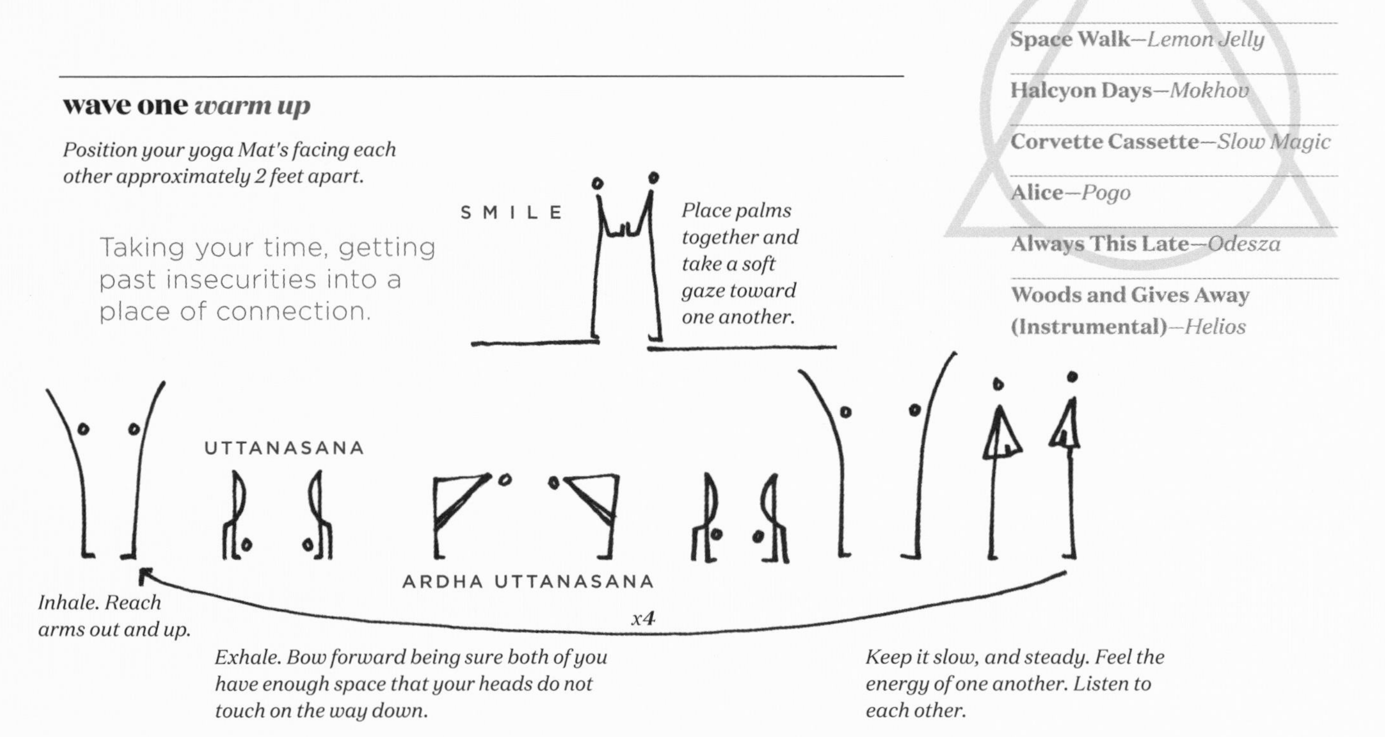

Place palms together and take a soft gaze toward one another.

Inhale. Reach arms out and up.

Exhale. Bow forward being sure both of you have enough space that your heads do not touch on the way down.

Keep it slow, and steady. Feel the energy of one another. Listen to each other.

wave two *trust and lean back*

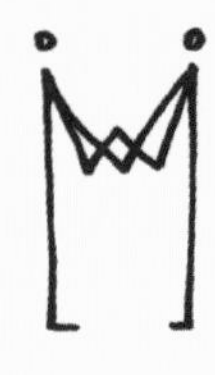

Step a little closer toward each other. Grab hold of each other's forearms by crossing your own forearms on top of each other.

Support and be support.

No folding at the hips.

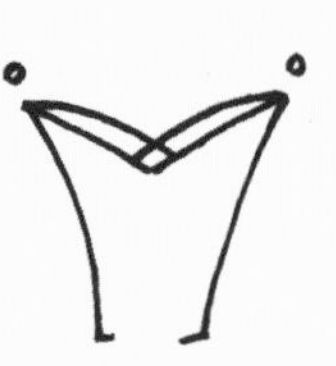

Lean away from each other until your arms are fully straight. The tendency will be to bend the arms to hold yourself upright. Slowly lean back and allow yourself to be supported by each other. Lift the chest up, draw the shoulders slightly up and then back, and take 3 BREATHS.

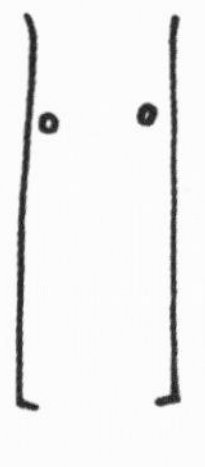

URDVA HASTASANA

wave three *london bridge*

Connect with a softness of palms that welcomes the connection of your partner.

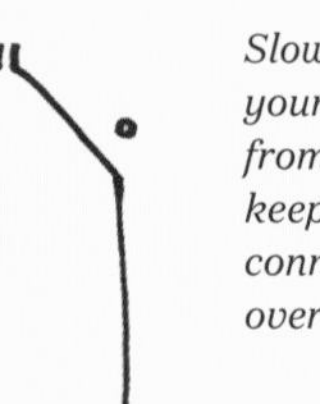

Slowly walk your feet away from each other, keeping palms connected and over head.

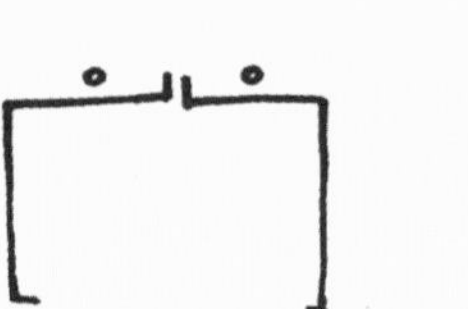

If you are the more flexible of the two, support your friend with your breath and help her feel supported by you.

Turn head and torso to look underneath the top arm. 3-5 BREATHS

Come back up and switch sides.

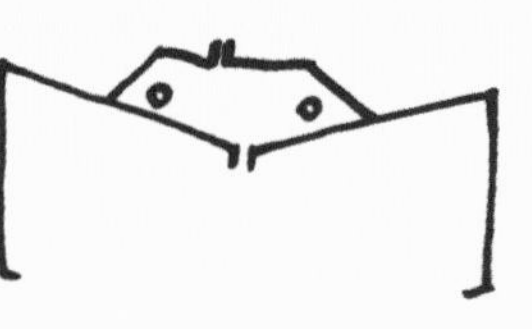

wave four *soaring warrior*

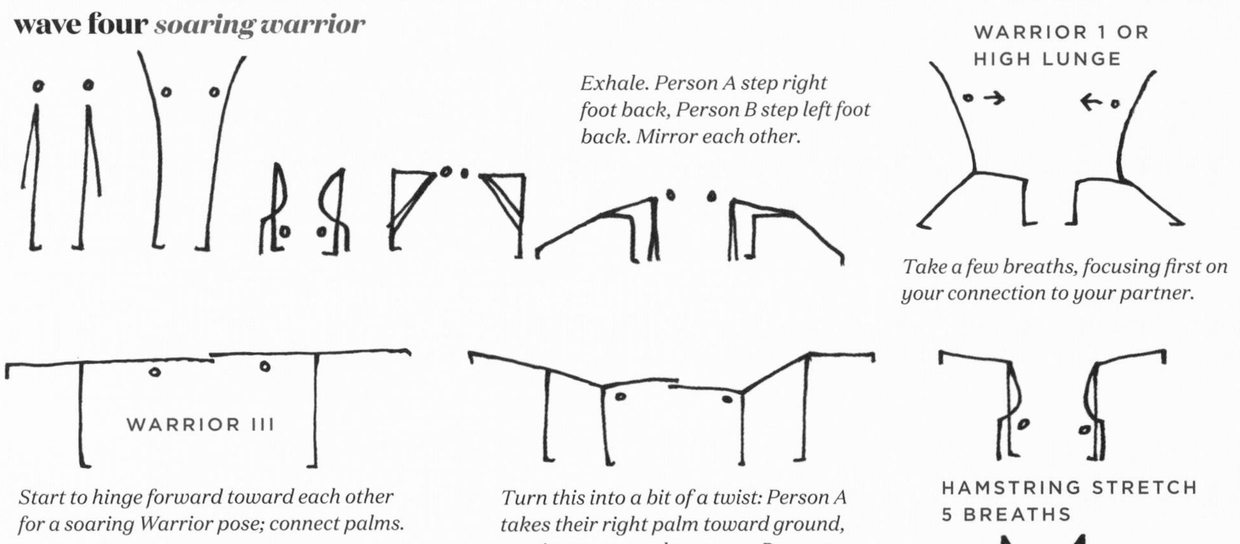

Exhale. Person A step right foot back, Person B step left foot back. Mirror each other.

WARRIOR 1 OR HIGH LUNGE

Take a few breaths, focusing first on your connection to your partner.

WARRIOR III

Start to hinge forward toward each other for a soaring Warrior pose; connect palms.

You can readjust your distance from each other; torso on an upward angle of 45 degrees is recommended.

Turn this into a bit of a twist: Person A takes their right palm toward ground, staying connected to person B as you did in LONDON BRIDGES; *both look under the raised arm.*

HAMSTRING STRETCH 5 BREATHS

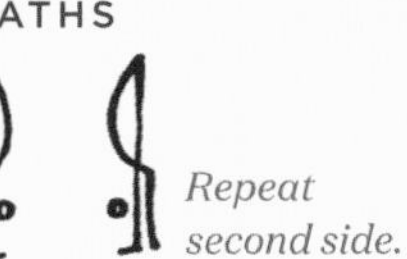

Repeat second side.

wave five *chair counterbalance and twist*

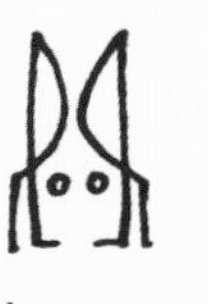

Find an energetic connection to the back of each other's heart.

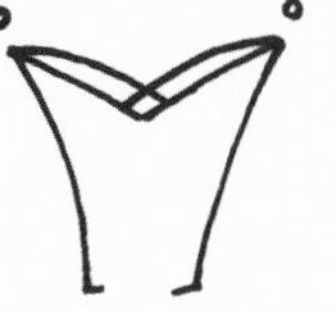

TRUST LEAN-BACK POSE

Keep leaning back, and slowly bend your knees. PARTNER CHAIR POSE

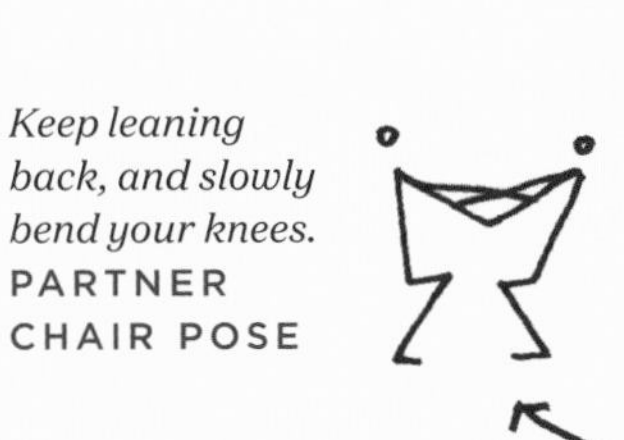

NOTE: *if you have to bow forward, first sit up tall and draw shoulders back; then if you are still bowing forward, walk closer to each other.*

For the twists, you will both be squeezing each other's right arm as a way of silently communicating what comes next.

Once you have checked in with the squeeze, release your right hand and reach behind you for the twist.

wave six *plank high fives*

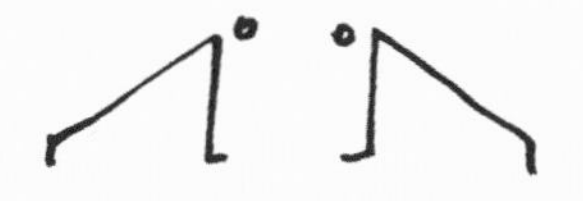

Take feet fairly wide for more stability, keep the hips high and the upper back full (rounded and letting back rib cage expand and contract with breath).

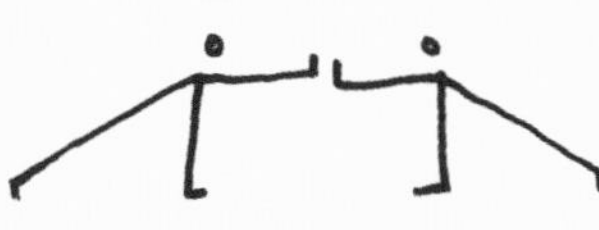

Lean into your right hand, grip fingertips into the ground to strengthen the muscles that keep the hand safe, and see if you can high five with the left hand.

Switch sides, lean to left hand, and high five with right.

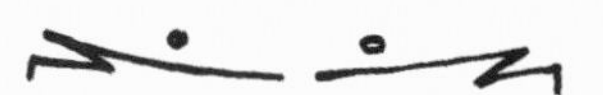

CHILD'S POSE *together*

Resync your breathing

and then come to

DOWNWARD DOG

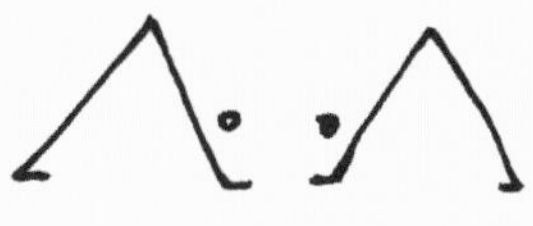

wave seven *standing open hips*

Inhale. Person A takes the right leg up and back. Person B takes the left.

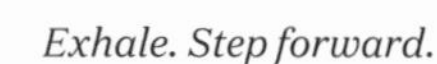

Exhale. Step forward.

Inhale. Come to WARRIOR II.

Take in the beauty of your partner's energy.

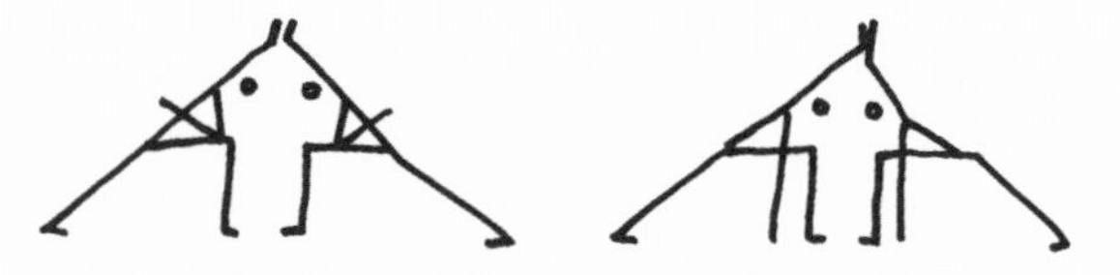

Exhale. PARSVOKONASANA. *Take the front forearm on thigh or outer edge of your front foot. Stretch top arm over head and try to connect to each other. Interlace hands if possible. It is always okay to readjust distance.*

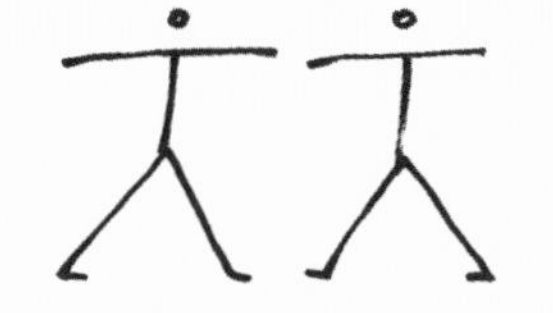

Straighten front leg. Pivot front foot in, till it is parallel to the front of the mat, turn the back foot out so you are prepared to do WARRIOR II *facing the back of your mat.*

Outer edge of you back foot is connected to your partner's outer edge. Hold hands with the hand that is closest to each other, take a breath in. Exhale, bend the knee that is facing the back of the mat.

Work as a team.

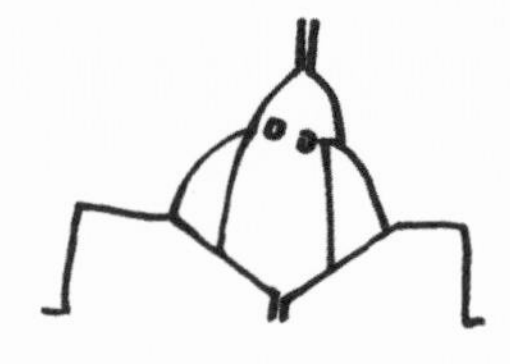

Inhale. Reach your free hand up and over into reverse warrior. Some partnerships might be able to touch top hands, but this requires certain height proportions and quite a bit of flexibility, so simply reach toward each other.
5 BREATHS

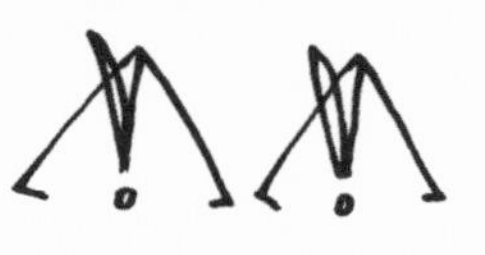

PRASARITA PODOTONASANA

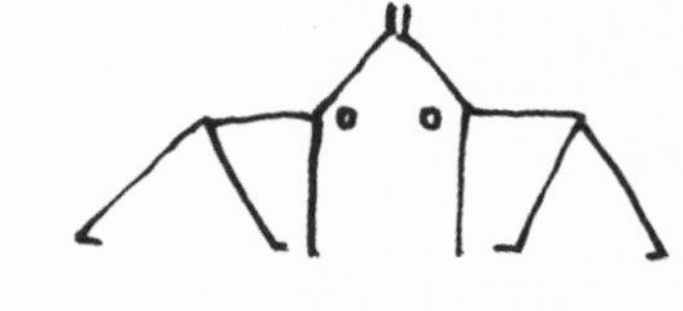

UTTITA TRIKONASANA. *Triangle pose (you may take top arm over your ear and connect to your partner either forearm, interlaced hands, or high five style.*
5 BREATHS

CHATURANGA DONDASANA

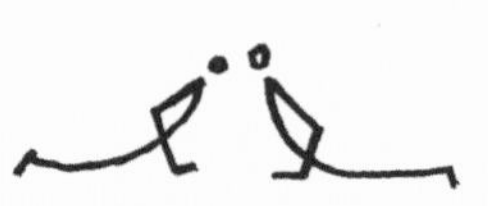

Inhale UPWARD DOG *or* COBRA

Exhale DOWN DOG

Repeat the sequence on Person A's left leg, and Person B's right.

wave eight *cool down*

Person A does pigeon with right leg forward, and Person B with left.

The heart is the energy center that holds our connection to each other.

Once happily situated in pigeon, Person B will give Person A slow squeezes to their forearms, sending healing and loving energy through the hands. After 10 BREATHS *(or more), switch.*

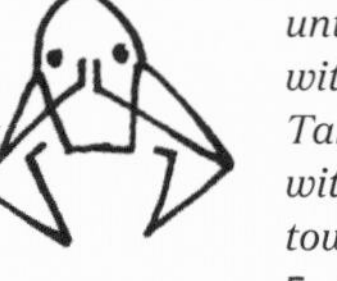

JANUSIRSASANA. *"Scooch" closer together until your foot is connected with your partner's foot. Take the forearm grip with your hands, and bend toward your straight leg.* 5-7 BREATHS. *Come up and switch legs and repeat side bend on the other side.*

PRANAYAMA/ MEDITATION: *Connect backs and allow your bodies to breath together.*

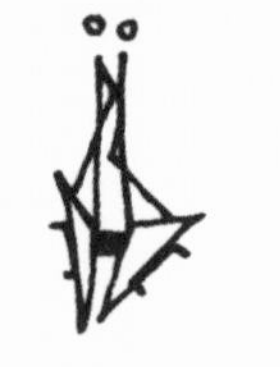

SUKHASANA

SAVASANA

Facing each other, share silence for at least 5 easy breaths. End with a heart to heart hug and a "NAMASTE."

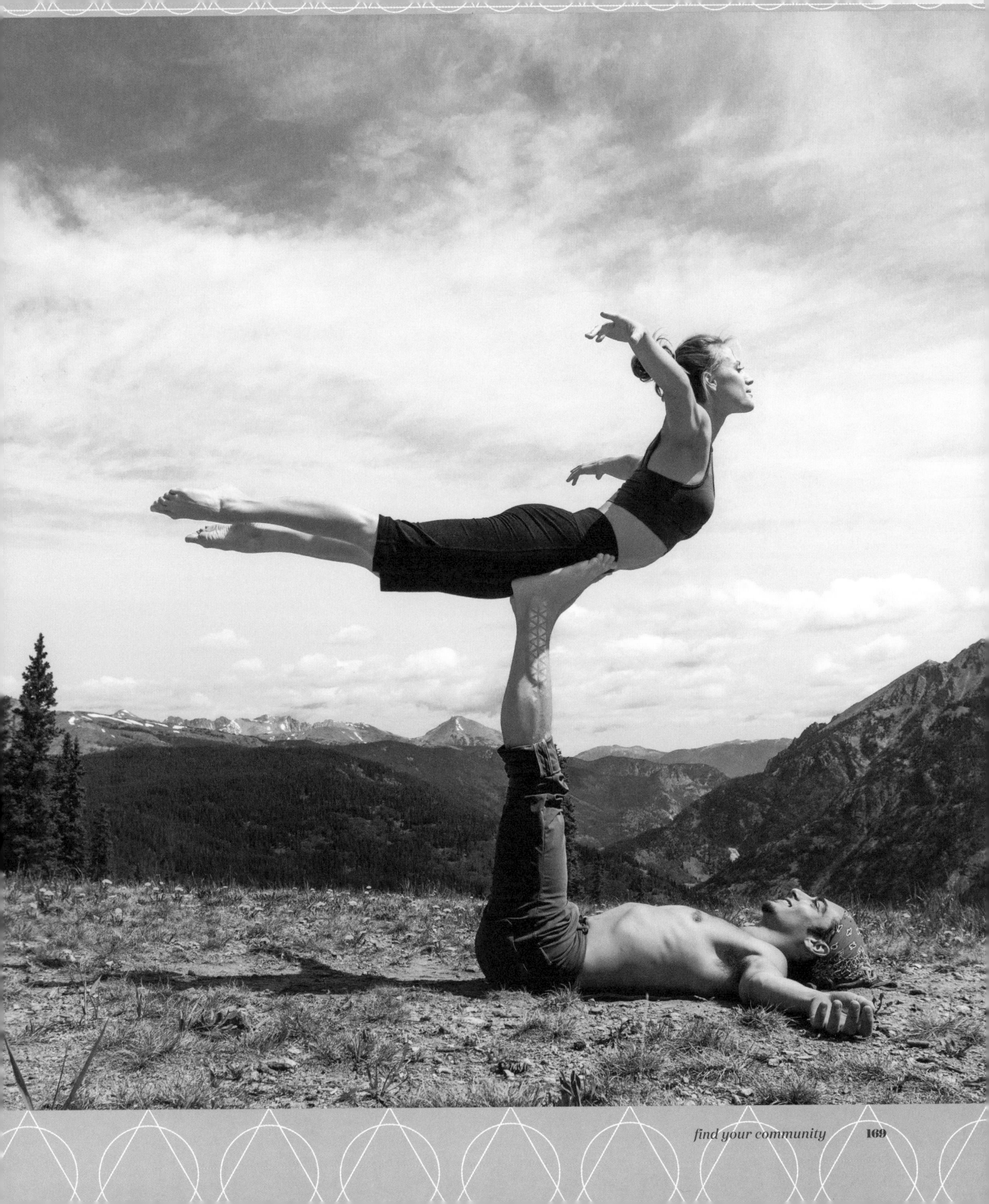

YOUR COMMUNITY: DINNER IS SERVED!

MARA MUNRO

In the Buddhist tradition, your community is called *sangha*. There is no greater place to cherish sangha than over a meal. Start with a moment of gratitude and bring a new level of intention to your sangha. Take this time to honor the life of the plants and animals that have been given and appreciate your loved ones.

"May we receive this meal with gratitude for the Earth and sacrifices that were made to feed us. May we be open to the hearts and needs of this community and all beings. May all beings have food, shelter, love, and community."

Meal Prayer

DURATION:
Five minutes

LOCATION:
Kitchen

MINDSET:
Appreciative

TOOL:
Pen

1. Make a list of what you value most about the food you are about to eat and the people you are about to share your meal with.

2. Record the feelings you experience when you eat with people you love.

3. Craft a prayer that unites the food with the people and your feelings.

4. Before your meal, share your prayer with the table.

Food unites us, enlivens us, nourishes body, soul, and community. As our society slowly remembers our connection to the Earth and what it yields, food, from garden to table, once again becomes a hub for our communities.

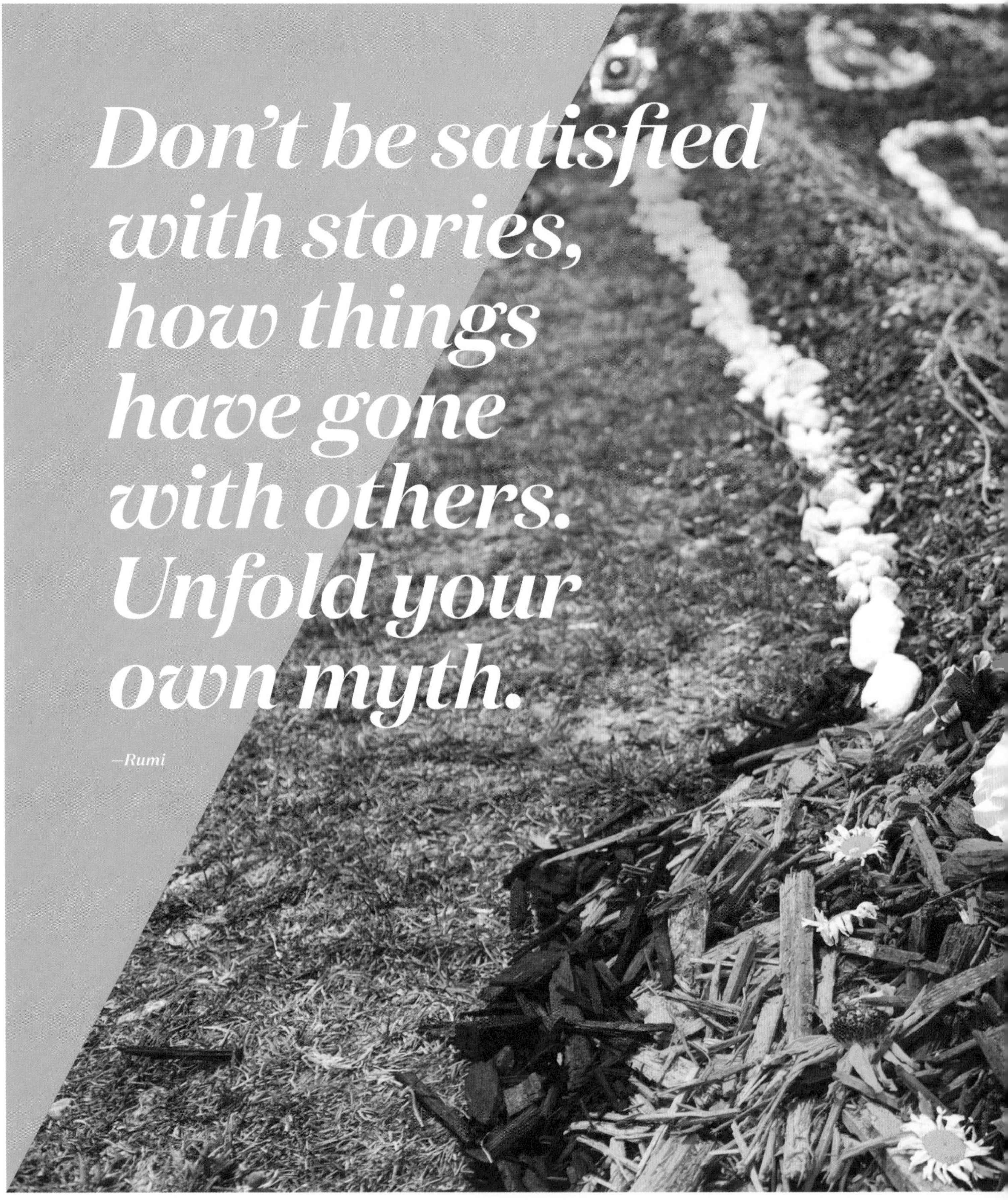

Don't be satisfied with stories, how things have gone with others. Unfold your own myth.

—Rumi

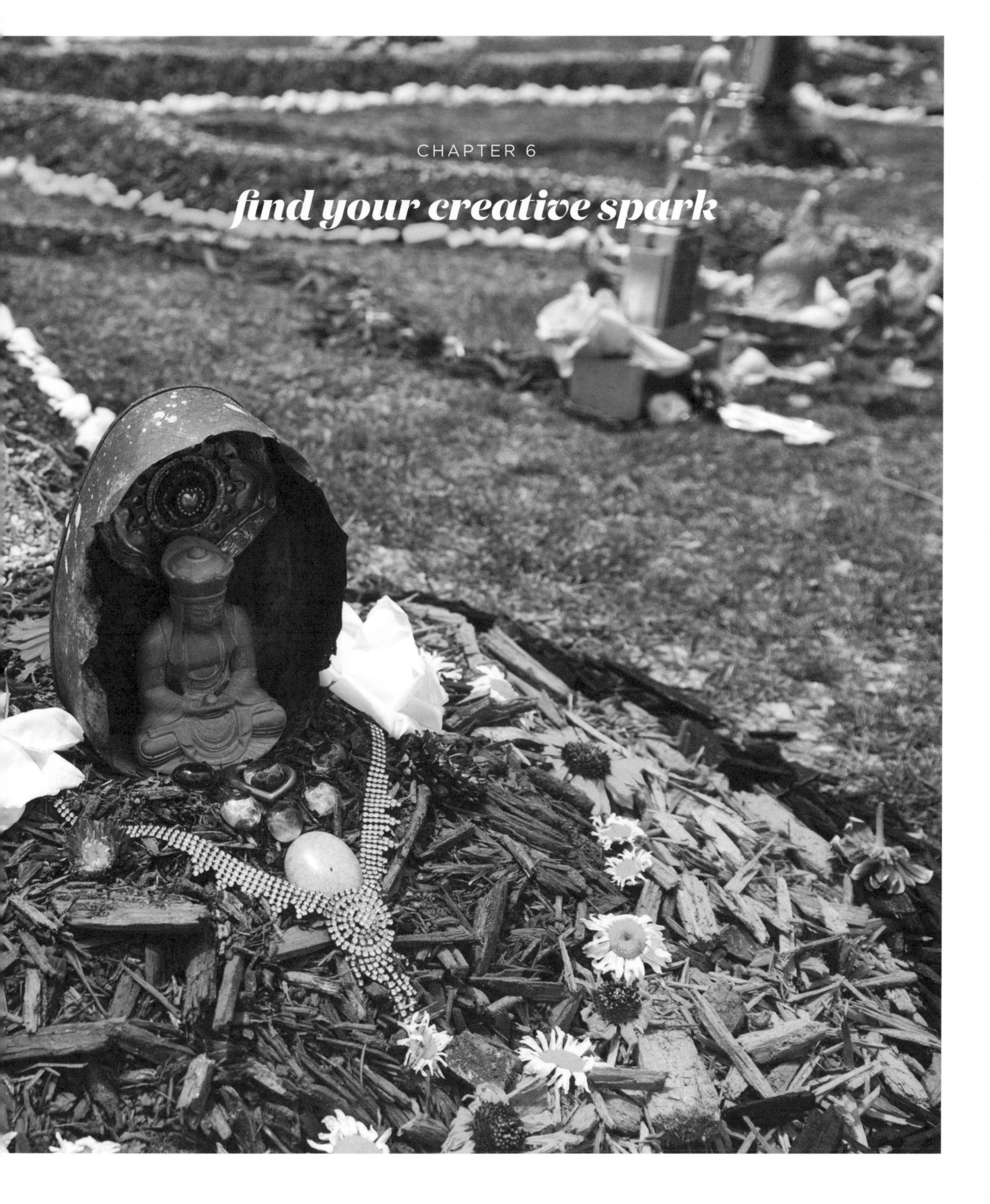

CHAPTER 6

find your creative spark

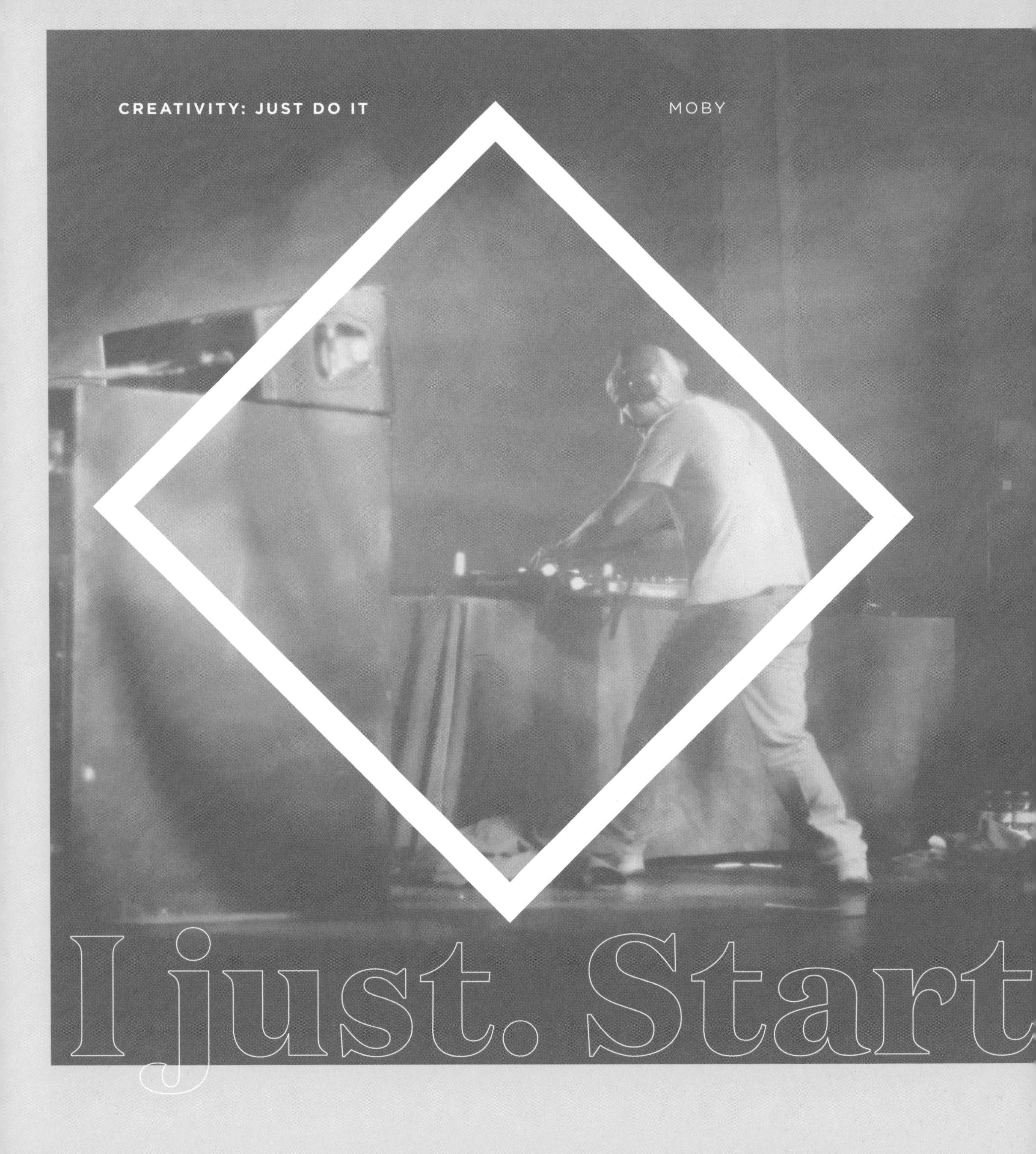
I just. Start

I just. Start. Doing it.

I was brought up by artists. My mom was a painter and pianist. My uncle, a photographer. Two of my aunts are writers; my grandmother was a watercolor painter. Everyone in my family had some weird creative outlet. There was never a stigma around creativity and there was no pressure. From an early age, my family just sort of asked me, *"What do you want to do? Here's a piano, do you want to learn piano? Here's a guitar, here's a typewriter, here's paint. Go do whatever you want to do."* No one ever said: *"Is it good? Is it bad? Should you be doing this?"* This really prepped me for a lifetime of art. It's just what I do. It's freedom. I don't really prepare myself. Now, I go into the studio, turn on my equipment, and start playing around.

I think this can be really similar to yoga. I do yoga five times a week by myself, and I have for years. When I tell friends of mine about this they ask, *"How do you find the discipline?"* I always think, *"You just do it."* For the first six months, it took discipline for me. But I find the more you do something, the easier it becomes to do.

For me, it's the same with art, the same with everything. There's a lot of magic in just beginning.

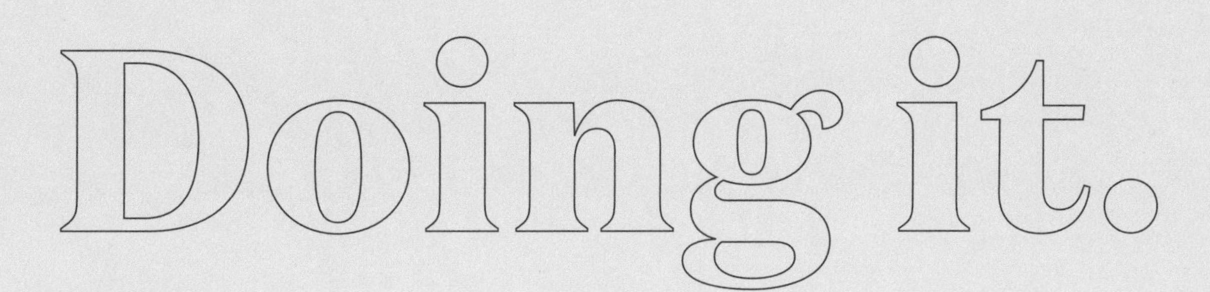

You can't use up creativity. The more you use, the more you have.

—Maya Angelou

Most of us were taught that creativity comes from the thoughts and emotions of the mind. The greatest singers, dancers, painters, writers, and filmmakers recognize that the most original, and even transformative, ideas actually come from the core of our being, which is accessed through an "open-mind consciousness."

In ancient traditions, open-mind consciousness was considered to be a spiritual awakening, the great enlightenment that dissolves the darkness of confusion and fear and ushers in peace, happiness, clarity, and contentment. Today, the notion that there's one formulaic way to achieve this spiritual awakening and creative vibrancy has been blown apart. You don't have to run off to a monastery or practice meditation for thirty years before attaining a breakthrough.

"Open-mind awareness" is also known in the West as a "peak experience," "being in the flow," or "being in the zone." I call it accessing your core creativity, because I believe that deep inside every person lies this potential for connecting to a universal flow of knowledge and creativity that's boundless and expansive. Our individual thoughts and memories are a part of this greater, larger resource.

And it's about practice.

Just as an athlete who's in condition has the muscle tone to be able to spring into action instantly, someone who regularly accesses this core creativity becomes creatively toned. For this person, the faucet to this remarkable flow of inspiration opens up easily, naturally, and often, allowing spontaneous and dramatic breakthroughs. When you're creatively toned, instead of merely dipping your toe in the water and playing it safe, you're willing to be utterly daring. Knowing this, you can navigate through a sea of self-limiting thoughts and transform such unwholesome beliefs as "I had my chance and blew it," "It's too late; my time is over," "I'll never be happy again," and "I can't."

In Buddhism, there are three states of consciousness, defined as wise mind, big mind, and open mind. They serve as metaphors for the stages we go through in the process of tapping into our core creativity, or what's called "open mind." In this receptive state, you feel a sense of spaciousness, timelessness, and willingness to entertain new possibilities. You're curious, nonreactive, compassionate, and accepting of the present experience, whether it's positive, negative, or neutral. Creative flow occurs here in the main part of the house of self.

Train and Tap In

These states of consciousness mirror the three steps in the art of creative transformation:

1. **LET GO INTO WISE MIND**. By paying attention to your mind flow, you see all the thoughts and feelings that might distract you, but you're wise enough to simply let them go. Opening up, you become ready to tune in.

2. **TUNE IN TO BIG MIND.** As you tune in, you cease focusing on your breathing or your sorting process. All becomes quiet and serene as you melt into bliss, the waters of your consciousness undisturbed by feelings, thoughts, or sensations. In big mind, there's no individual "I" present. There's a vast, spacious, eternal, and pervading sense of pure, pristine awareness that allows you to move forward.

3. **MOVE FORWARD INTO OPEN MIND.** You allow the creativity from your core to flow into you, sweeping you up and sending you in the direction of the unknown. Once you've experienced the mystical and transformative power of your core creativity, you can trust in its currents and let it send you downstream; though surrendering to it at first, you then gently steer it as you begin to recognize which way you'd like to go and remember that you have the power to direct your course.

BEYOND JUST THINKING: HAIKU POWER

ERICK SZENTMIKLOSY
AND DANIEL ZALTSMAN

sensei always said
nothing like haiku to make
a good party great

—Lisa Markuson

Writing poetry is a way to meditate on something deeply. You've got to look close, contemplate, and feel the spirit of something (beyond just thinking about it) to write a poem.

Haiku are bite-size poems from the Japanese tradition, three lines often embodying the idea of juxtaposition. Traditionally, the syllable count is **five in the first line, seven in the second, and five the third.**

We help people write the haiku they already have inside them. We ask people what inspires them and let their thoughts flow through us, transforming into words on paper. The secret is, what we deliver to the readers is very much their own. We see the look of conviction in their eyes and use that energy as fuel for the fire that burns a haiku into our mind. It falls out through our fingers through the soft punch of keys on a typewriter.

You can write your own haiku to drop inside yourself and see what's there. Or you can use it to look closely at the word around you. Writing a haiku catches what is floating in your mind and spirit, placing it on a page as a mindful metaphor.

HOW TO HAIKU

STEP 1: *Sit and give yourself some space to dream and think. Look inside. Look outside. What's inspiring you? What's troubling you? The first thing that comes to mind is a great start.*

STEP 2: *Extrapolate a little bit. If "love" is the first thing that comes to mind, ask yourself, why? Did you just recently fall in love? Did you just witness a couple staring into each other's eyes with a burning passion hotter than the sun? If so, maybe your topic isn't really "love," maybe it's "falling in love," or a couple staring into each other's eyes. Refine the thought; write about that instead.*

STEP 3: *Play with putting your thought into seventeen syllables.*

For example:

Maybe your topic is a couple staring into each other's eyes with a burning passion hotter than the sun. Play with the five-seven-five format:

EYES DO THE TALKING

Five syllables! You have your first line!

You have your first line, but it doesn't really deal with two people. Let's get to that in the second line. We might imagine this couple was sitting quite close to one another, so:

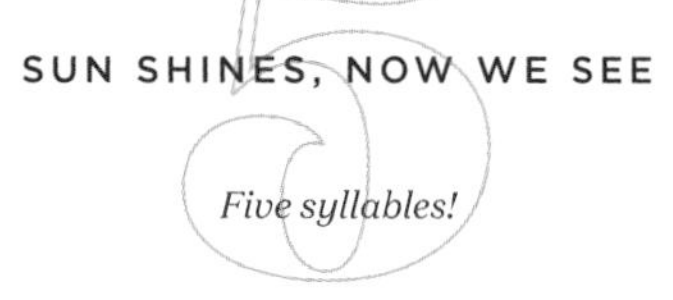

THE BREATH OF ANOTHER NEAR

Seven syllables! Now you have your second line.

There was some mention of burning passion hotter than the sun. Let's close it off with that:

SUN SHINES, NOW WE SEE

Five syllables!

Haiku:

EYES DO THE TALKING

THE BREATH OF ANOTHER NEAR

SUN SHINES, NOW WE SEE

Read it over a few times and make sure you love it. Let it sink in. You might want to switch the first and third lines because you might feel a more thoughtful delivery that way. You might think it's too literal, and want to replace one or two lines with a different metaphor. There are a million things you might think about it. Either way, if you made it this far, you're on your way.

FUTURE HAIKU PRACTICE

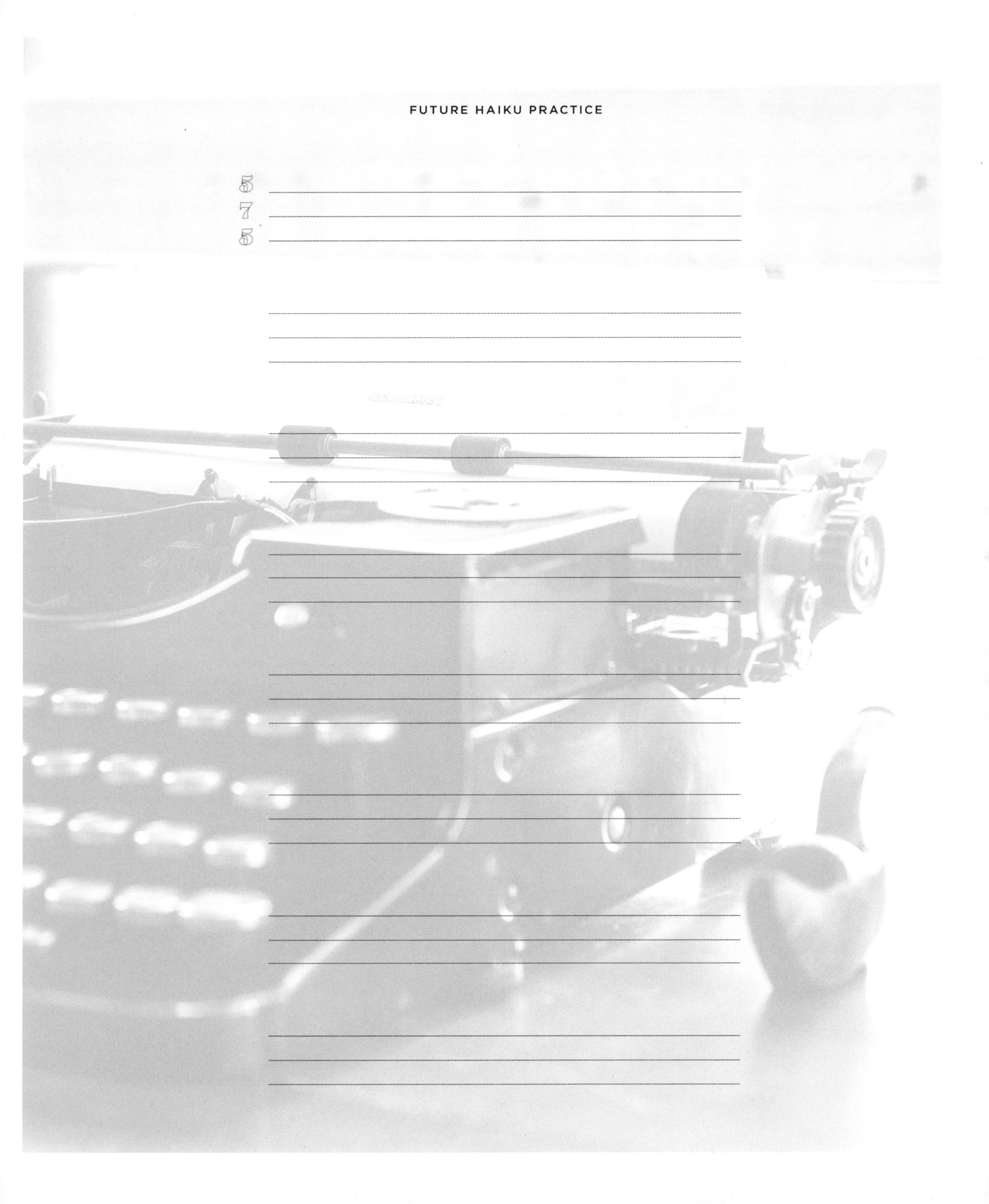

5
7
5

And those who were seen dancing were thought to be insane by those who could not hear the music.

—*Friedrich Nietzsche*

Jumping from boulder to boulder and never falling, with a heavy pack, is easier than it sounds; you just can't fall when you get into the rhythm of the dance.

—*Jack Kerouac,*
The Dharma Bums

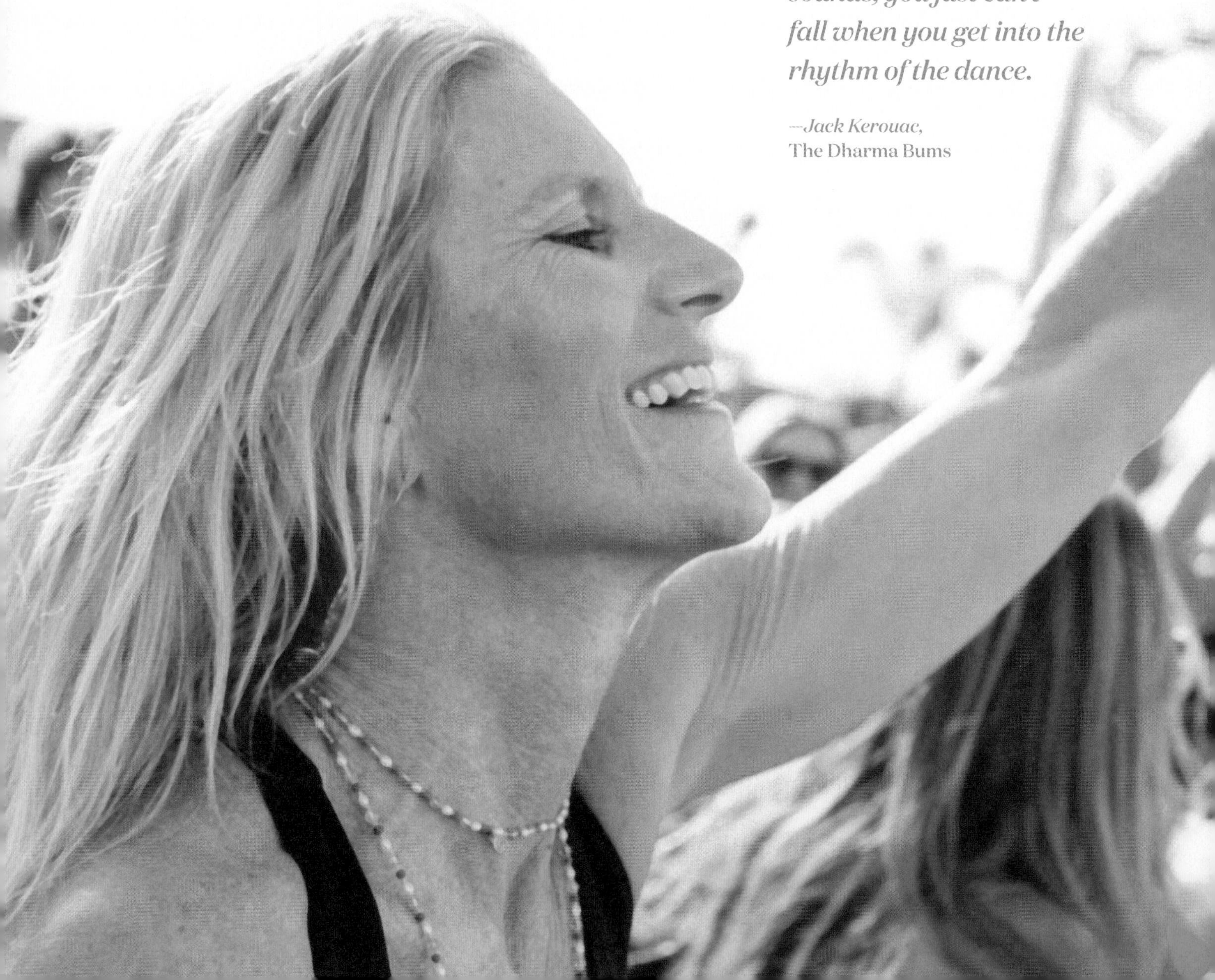

We were born into a world of rhythm. It began in the womb as our whole being developed around the "dum dum" of our mother's heartbeat. Our body is a rhythmic symphony and our heartbeat is the great conductor. Each of the oscillations that we experience from our thought waves to our emotions, stress, and states of flow can all be mapped by their rhythmic signatures.

From shamanic cultures that have worked with the healing power of rhythm to the music therapy in ancient Greece to the classical Indian system of raga and rasa, rhythm and music have been understood and utilized for thousands of years for healing.

We have been gathering around music, breath, movement, and the power of celebratory play under the open sky for a long time.

My theory is that the music-movement complex connects us to our intrinsic source of creative power—the energy that generates ideas, new neural pathways, our greatest joy, and high states of energetic coherence—all for free! Music is medicine. It can be a way to release. It can offer mystic states of communion that are peak experiences of life.

This innate power as movers and shakers, however, has also been systematically repressed for over two thousand years in the little-known global history of dance. Thousands of people have died for dancing, and artistic traditions have been abolished, as in the end of the thousands-of-years-old temple dancing tradition in India during colonial rule. All over the world, drumming and dance have been illegal in the past century, suppressed or controlled to subdue this innate personal power.

Whatever the barrier to our innate flow is—cultural, past conditioning, self-consciousness, awkwardness, lost connection to inner spontaneity—when it dissolves, we see its power—the geyser of nature moving through us.

EVERYONE TO THE DANCE FLOOR

When we dance, and I mean REALLY dance—sweaty, messy, uninhibited, and tranced out—we cannot stay stuck. We can't hold on. Whatever's inside us HAS to move. Through dance, we clear and connect. Dance is one of the most potent healers we know!

1. **Find the beat.**

   Music is crucial. Like a boat carrying you out to sea, a good beat has the capacity to lift you out of your habitual self-concept and usher you into uncharted territory. It gives your limbs something to ride and your mind something to rest in.

2. **Move the feet.**

   Think of it as a traveling tadasana/mountain pose: Your soles meet the earth like a dance partner, and from that connection you become aware of the rest of your body. From the ground up. You might get a little antsy to go faster and do something more fancy and complicated right away. Meet the beat. Feel. Explore. Play.

3. **Shake it out.**

   Wiggle your shoulders, knees, neck, hips, spine, thighs. Notice which places are easy to move and feel, and which ones aren't. Be with the music. Don't force anything. As the music picks up, let yourself drop deeper into feeling. When thoughts come up, say hello and return to sensation. It's just you and the music.

4. **Play with your edge and breathe.**

   Movement is a healer. Moving shakes things up! Notice if you ever feel unsafe. Trauma is stored in the body and moving can stir things up. If this happens, consider a movement therapist or coach to guide you; see it as a gift to wholeness. If you feel safe and good, stay with it.

   Just like your asana practice, it's not a true practice unless you're BREATHING. Your breath connects your mind with your body, and facilitates both the loosening of stuck energy and its removal. Let your dance be a breath, too. Really move.

5. **Make some noise.**

   Like breath on steroids, a holler, groan, or shriek can do a lot to release whatever you've been holding on to. Feel into those places that need to let go, and give them a voice. If you're in a club or other public dance situation, a big WOO-HOO! can often do the trick. And really? Whether we're talking noises or dance moves here, the weirder the better.

6. **Stay open.**

   When we give ourselves permission to break it down and shake it out, we give what we've been holding back to its natural state of movement. And if you keep moving, whatever's happening inside you will fall back into the natural rhythm of healing you were born with, and have no choice but to transform.

7. **Allow, allow, allow.**

   Give it time. Let it happen. Don't interrupt yourself or rush the process. Trust the intelligence dancing within you. It is smarter than you know, and it contains every seed necessary for the full healing and blossoming of the greatest version of you.

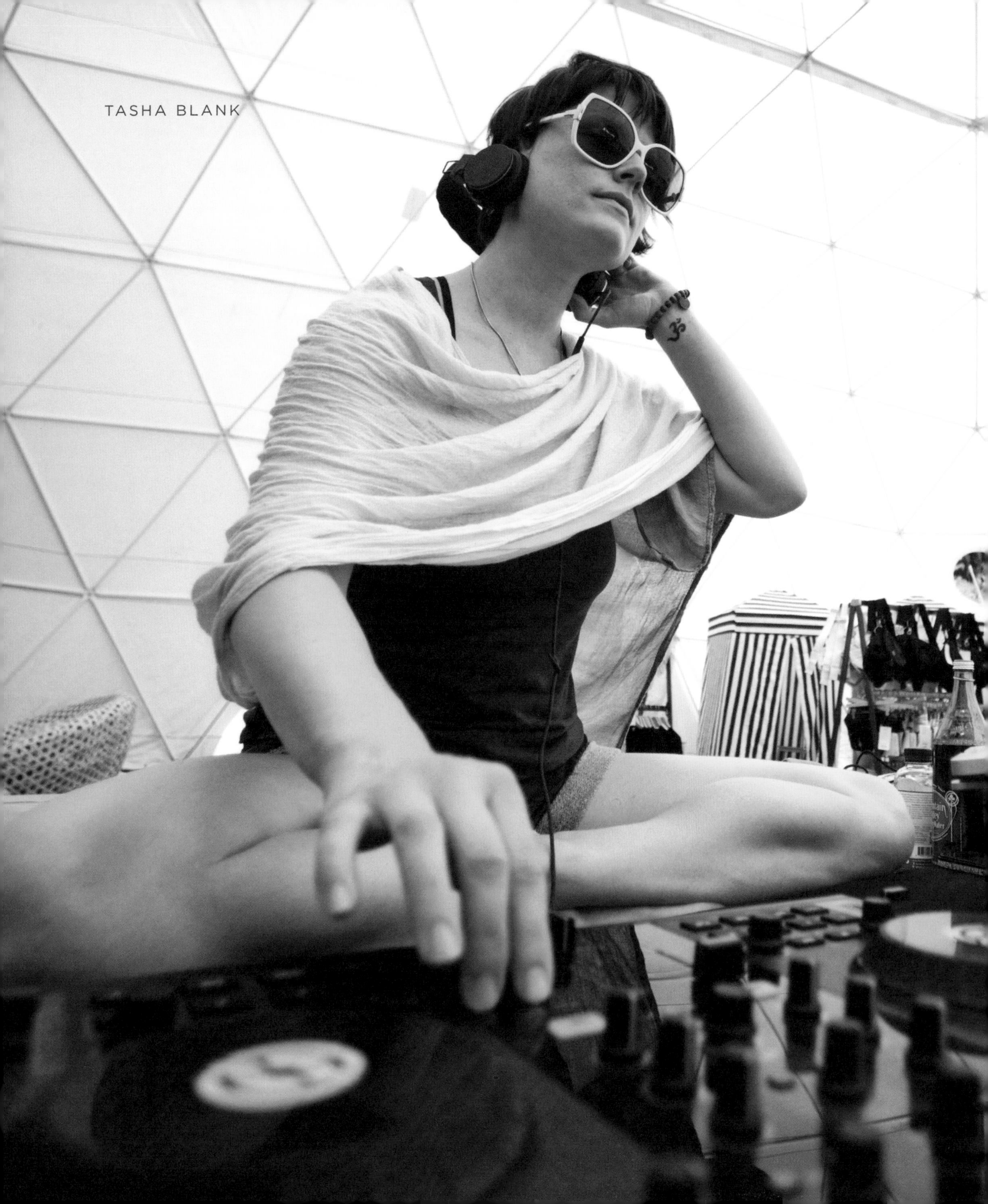

TASHA BLANK

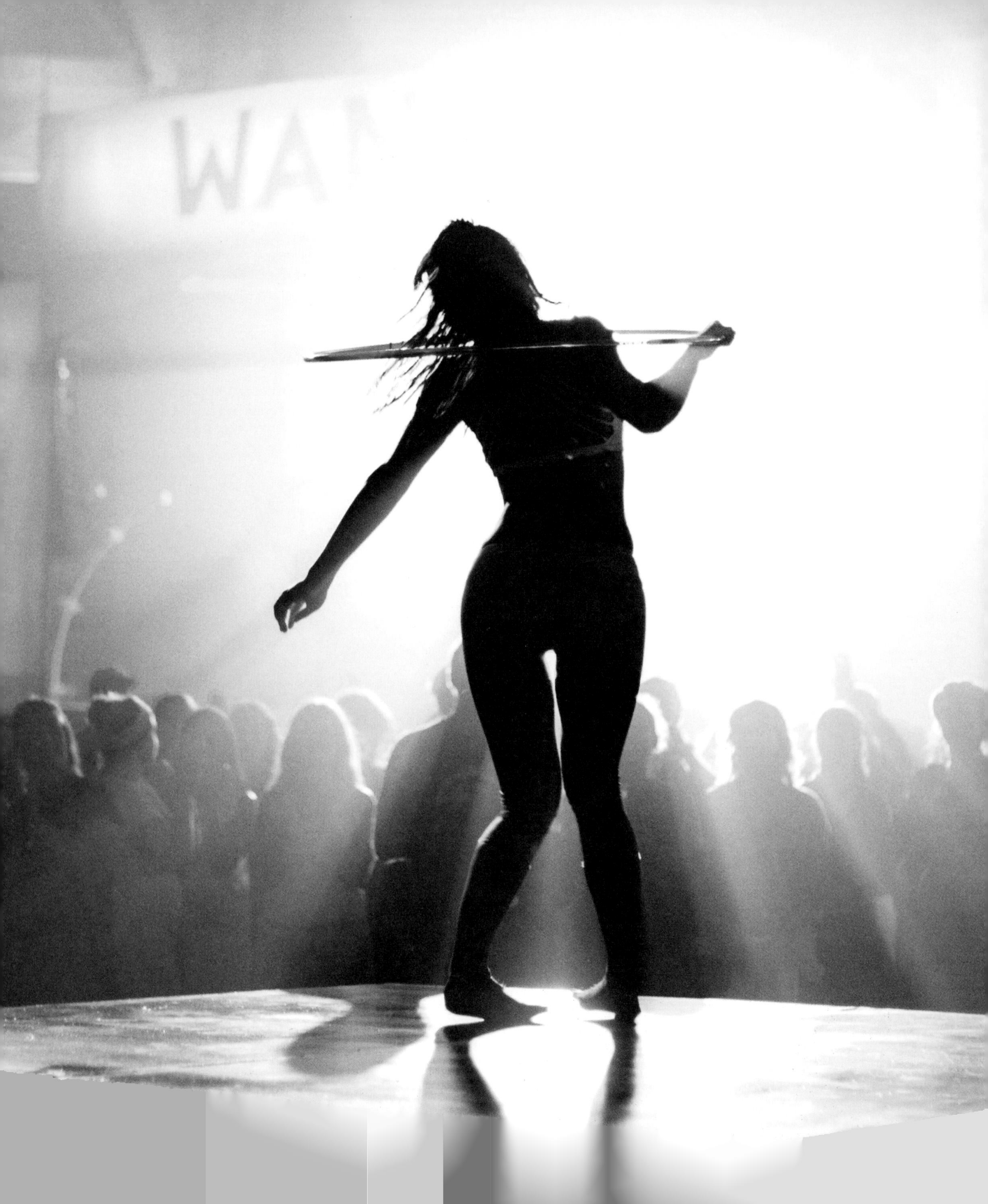

The creative impulse in all of us sometimes needs to be coaxed out. The question is not how do we become creative, but how do we allow our latent creativity to flow again, unburdened, alive?

The answer is not an earth-shattering, revolutionary idea that will take years of practice to master. The answer is something we have carried with us all along.

Play

As children we learned about our vast, new, magical world through uninhibited play. Play is not dependent on success, measurable results, neat choreography, or careful steps. It is complete within itself, begs us to get messy, to be loud and large, to fail and to be okay with it. If we can connect to play, we give our overworked, overwhelmed, self-censoring minds deep rest. This makes play especially important in our adult lives.

Right now where you are, allow yourself to remember the last time you played. Feel in your body the sensations: the free movement, the heightened awareness, the beat of your heart—maybe you can feel even the light behind your eyes.

If you can feel into that place, you may somatically remember that play first and foremost calls us into presence and offers us an in-the-moment and unapologetic version of ourselves, free of all the weighty expectations we carry around—both imagined and very real. Without the extra baggage, we tap into a very sacred space where we lose our sense of small self, and—if even for one moment—gain the world.

So I offer you a radical thought. That when you open wide the doors to even the most simple act of play, like walking in nature, singing a song, laughing with a friend, or swirling under the sun with a hula hoop, listen deeply first, then say YES to what arises. Your doing so will be another step toward designing ourselves and our culture whole, sustainable, viable and in alignment with the greater good. It's as simple as giving ourselves permission to simmer in what so many of us seek, but regularly disqualify ourselves for—joy for the sake of joy.

Every child is an artist. The problem is how to remain an artist once we grow up.

—Pablo Picasso

DESIGN YOUR DAY

As adults in the world, we have many responsibilities, and tend to schedule work as the priority. But what if you took out your calendar, right now, and made PLAY a priority?

SCHEDULE IT IN: Fifteen minutes in the morning for stream-of-consciousness writing or perhaps a haiku or two. In the afternoon, schedule in half an hour of "free" time to go for a walk, or dance it out to your favorite song. It may feel "frivolous" at first, but know that play is essential for health and can keep us vibrant in our lives. Keep to your play schedule for a week, then extend it. Play may be a muscle you need to rebuild!

MORNING PLAY:

7:00

8:00

9:00

10:00

11:00

12:00

FREE TIME:

1:00

2:00

3:00

4:00

5:00

6:00

7:00

BRAINSTORM IT OUT

If you're rusty, you may not be sure what to do in your playtime at first. Take some time to brainstorm a list of activities, your very own "Play Idea Bank." Then use the list in the future. Think of some joyful things you can have in your back pocket that are free, accessible, and fun. Of course, in the moment, you may spontaneously think and feel even more ideas as the spirit strikes you, but you'll have a play savings account to fall back on.

Saraswati is the goddess of the arts. She floats on water, reminding us that creativity needs to move, like a river, to be healthy. Her white swan symbolizes her purity and also the ability of the arts to purify the mind and help us rise above mundane ways of seeing the world and ourselves.

I have been painting and making art for as far back as I can remember. By my late teens, I was studying art seriously in school and interning at a posh San Francisco gallery. Then a health crisis in my sophomore year of college led me to my first yoga class. Yoga quickly became my lifeline, and the only place where I felt healthy and at peace. I started to look at the art world as narcissistic and competitive. I began to devote myself to yoga and turned my back on my ambitions as an artist.

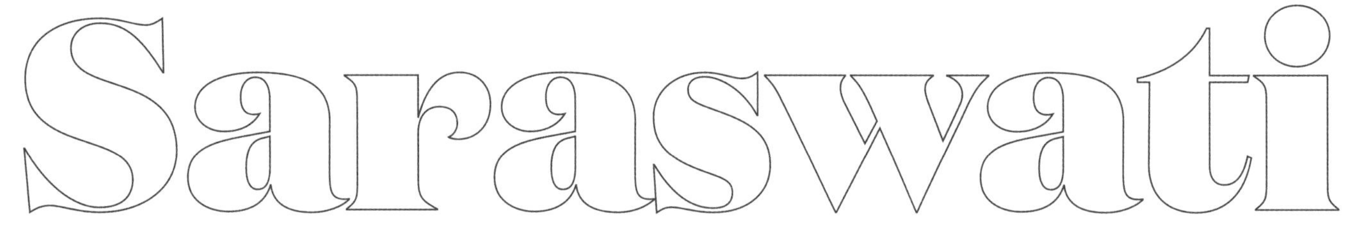

I met my husband, MC Yogi, in my yoga teacher training, and he is one of the most creative beings I have ever met. At the time, I was renting a tiny studio in a basement where we would paint together, even going back and forth on the same canvases. A year later, we traveled to India. India broke me wide open. The colors, the smells, the energy, and everywhere I looked—in rickshaws, sari shops, temples, restaurants, train stations—there was magical, mystical art. Gods, goddesses, saints, sages, and holy animals—I never imagined that art could be so integrated with spirituality, and so integral to daily living.

Upon our return to California, we opened our own yoga studio. And while most of my time was spent teaching, practicing, and running the studio, slowly but surely, the desire to make art crept back in. I became fascinated with the ancient Buddhist paintings in the caves of Ajanta and with the calendar art of the Hindu gods and goddesses and wanted to make my own versions of them. I learned that in India, there were yogis who created art with the same intention they brought to other yogic practices: to transcend suffering. These yogis made art to uplift the viewer and to give others the experience of enlightenment. This gave me infinite hope, to think that my art and my yoga could be combined in this way. I remember suddenly feeling that these two sides of myself that had long been in conflict had now found a place of deep union within me.

Over the years, however, my inspiration came in fits and starts. I wouldn't paint for months, and then paint like a madwoman getting ready for exhibition. When I was engaged creatively, I would be filled with vitality, inspiration, and energy. Then there were times when the creative stream would seem to run completely dry. I would start to lose my confidence, and an insidious self-doubt would start to take root.

"Do I have anything of value to offer the world, anyway?"

I would wonder.

I started to recognize a correlation between my happiness and if I was making art or not. But how could I get reinspired once the inertia of a creative slump had set in? I decided to turn to yoga for answers.

The yoga tradition is amazing. It gives us Saraswati, and we can contemplate her, and chant her name, and maybe all our latent inspiration will come rushing back to us. But if this doesn't do the trick, we can go a step deeper. For the ancient yogic texts also describe a trifecta of goddesses, or shaktis, who represent the different aspects of our creative nature.

JNANA SHAKTI is the goddess of the intellect. Good art has intelligence, and creativity is the root of all intelligence. Coming up with good ideas, discernment, and problem solving are all part of the artistic process, and if we leave the intellect out of the picture, we can be sure our expressions will lack the clarity to be really powerful or meaningful.

Journaling and reading sacred texts would be some ways to enliven the mind and spark the light of intelligence. On the flip side, too much mindless TV, video games, trashy magazines, or gossiping would diminish our Jnana Shakti.

KRIYA SHAKTI is the goddess who governs our senses. She reminds us that great art requires refinement of the senses. Making art requires a more sensitive way of seeing and hearing, and yogic control over our movements in order to express ourselves with accuracy.

We want to nourish our senses with good food, loving touch, amazing art and music. We want to get our energy flowing with yoga, dance, singing, and chanting. But if we overindulge the senses, then the whole thing backfires. Because sleeping too much, too much sex, too much drug use and alcohol will numb our senses and will ultimately create an energetic dead end for our creative inspiration.

ICCA SHAKTI is the goddess of our will. She gives us the power to take action, and to turn our dreams in reality. Without her, we are just living in an opium-like haze of creative fantasy. Engage in sangha, or sacred community. There is nothing that fires up my own will like being around other powerful creative manifesters. Just being in their presence, or even reading about their triumphant acts, sparks the desire to create within my own being.

Abhyasa, a Sanskrit term for steady and consistent practice, is also helpful. It is one thing to have the burst of creative energy at the beginning of a project, but the will to see it through takes abhyasa.

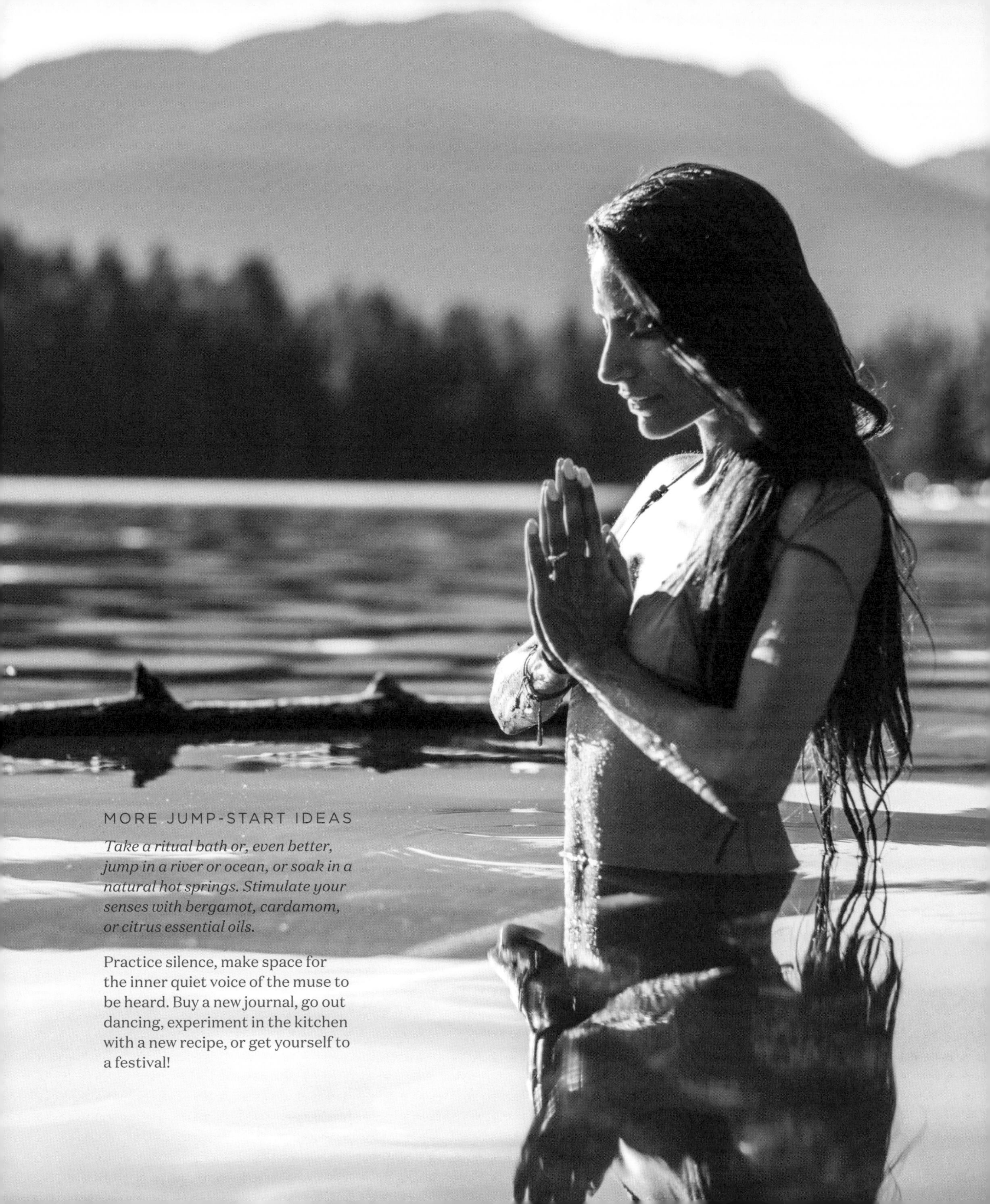

MORE JUMP-START IDEAS

Take a ritual bath or, even better, jump in a river or ocean, or soak in a natural hot springs. Stimulate your senses with bergamot, cardamom, or citrus essential oils.

Practice silence, make space for the inner quiet voice of the muse to be heard. Buy a new journal, go out dancing, experiment in the kitchen with a new recipe, or get yourself to a festival!

YOGA + CHOCOLATE

DAVE ROMANELLI

I have dedicated my life to infusing the ancient practice of yoga with modern passions like exotic chocolate and fine wine. Some of the purists have grumbled, "That's not yoga!" to which I respond, "The more people doing yoga, the better the world is." And when there's chocolate and wine, you better believe there are more people doing yoga.

It all started with a Yoga + Chocolate retreat I led with Katrina Markoff, the founder and visionary behind Vosges Haut-Chocolat. We went to Oaxaca, Mexico, during the Day of the Dead ceremonies. Oaxaca is the birthplace of chocolate, where it is consumed not just as a dessert but as an offering to the gods. On this retreat, I led people through flowing yoga classes in mystical courtyards, after which Katrina guided them through tastings of her Vosges chocolate creations. It was a hit, and for the past ten years, I have shared the Yoga + Chocolate experience all over the world.

Without a doubt, people's favorite is the Barcelona Bar, a milk chocolate infusion with hickory-smoked almonds and fleur de sel sea salt. In a postyoga heightened state, one's experiences amplify flavors as the salt accentuates the chocolate's sweetness. The message behind Yoga + Chocolate becomes clear ... everything is richer, sweeter, and better when experienced in the moment!

In today's world, presence is a precious resource. Too many days go by without a single memory. And it's only getting worse. Do you remember what you did a week ago Wednesday or two weeks ago Saturday? Life has become a big blur, and it is imperative to our peace of mind that we take time each day to slow down and be present. No one will do this for you. You have to take a stand and live in the moment!

My mantra: A beautiful, funny, and delicious moment each day keeps the stress away. Whether it's a street musician you encounter on your way to work, or a beautiful full moon in the night sky, or a favorite meal you always eat too fast ... at least once each day, will you stop and savor life? And here's the catch, will you do it without technology?

Our greatest moments and most powerful memories are recorded via sensory perception. The smell of pine trees can transport you through time and space and right back to the yard you played in as a kid; the taste of homemade pomodoro sauce can trigger memories of childhood dinners with your grandparents; and how can you ever forget the touch of your very first and very favorite yoga teacher's hands giving you the perfect adjustment?

Those are the things we remember best. There is no app on your phone to replicate sensory experiences and the way they touch your soul.

Next time something important happens, before you take out your phone to post it on social media, get down on your knees and smell it, touch it, taste it!

That's the idea behind Yoga + Chocolate: to remind us of our capacity to experience life as a feeling, a sound, a sight ... and not just a bunch of words and images.

Oscar Wilde said, "Nothing can cure the soul but the senses, just as nothing can cure the senses but the soul."

When we really need to show up fully for our partner, kids, and co-workers, we need to be our most vibrant, empowered, SOULFUL selves. We need qualities of spirit like intuition, compassion, and courage to find our way through life, to navigate the dark days, and celebrate the bright ones. While yoga ignites the spirit, it's not always possible to roll out the mat when we need a lift. In those scenarios when a physical yoga practice is not realistic, I ask you: Is there any feeling you can experience on the yoga mat that cannot also be experienced in one deep, rich, slow, delicious bite of exotic chocolate?

That is why I believe so strongly in integrating everyday passions with yoga. Chocolate, wine, and music are a bridge between the ancient practice and the modern world.

Try it. After your next practice at home or at your studio, indulge in your favorite piece of chocolate. But do it mindfully. Break the chocolate into two pieces. Listen to the soft break. Place a piece on your tongue. Feel the symphony of flavors on your palate. Engage your senses completely, while keeping in mind the three guiding principles behind the Yoga + Chocolate experience:

CELEBRATE LIFE NOW

We are always waiting for something to happen to give us permission to be happy. Waiting to get a promotion, waiting to lose weight, waiting to fall in love. If you are waiting now, you'll be waiting ten years from now. Enough with the waiting. Unleash your love and passion in this very moment! If not now, then when?

CHOCOLATE IS RICH IN FLAVONOIDS

When you look at the lives of supercentenarians (people who live to be 110 or older), they generally are not vegans or yogis or health freaks. They share qualities like a great sense of humor, resilience to life's challenges, and joie de vivre. The oldest woman in the history of the world, Jeanne Calment, lived to be 122. She ate two pounds of chocolate per week. If you ever wondered about the true meaning of joie de vivre, there it is!

HAPPY IS THE NEW HEALTHY

I often ask people the question, "Are you enjoying your life?" It's such a simple question, but usually people have to think. The answers range from "Hmmm, not so much" to "Not as much as I'd like" to "Sometimes." If the answer is anything less than a resounding "YES!" then we have to come to life differently.

My friend's sex education advice to her kids is: "If it doesn't feel good, you're not doing it right." And so it goes with living. Before you put all this time, energy, and money into getting healthy, losing weight, being better at yoga . . . make sure you are enjoying your life. Take a moment today to feel blessed, to walk in the sun, to crank up the tunes, and for crying out loud, eat a piece of chocolate.

DESIGN YOUR OWN SEQUENCE

ERICA JAGO

This is a practical yet deeply intuitive methodology for designing a sequence that provokes intertwined experiences of our creativity and spirituality. This process will help you develop your voice and be expressive in your instruction as a teacher. Design a group class, or a solo sequence just for you. Check out the example here, then grab your favorite pen and fill in the grid on the following spread. Let's begin.

YOGA BY DESIGN: STEP-BY-STEP

1. ***Sankalpa***—*Begin by writing three to five sentences, in the form of a sankalpa, which can be used at the opening of your sequence to clearly communicate the mood or intention of a particular theme. I find it helpful to think of one word or use a quote or poem to inspire the theme.*

Sankalpa:

Our task today is to cultivate an awareness around the heart that is healing.

The more heart awareness we have, the greater our connection with others, with ourselves, and with the pure feeling of delight.

2. ***Anatomical focus***—*Next, define the anatomical focus in a short bulleted list. This becomes the alignment you will cue in every pose.*

Anatomical focus:

1. Lengthen sides of waist upward
2. Heads of the arm bones, back and down
3. Bring bottom tips of shoulder blades into back of heart
4. Expand collarbones

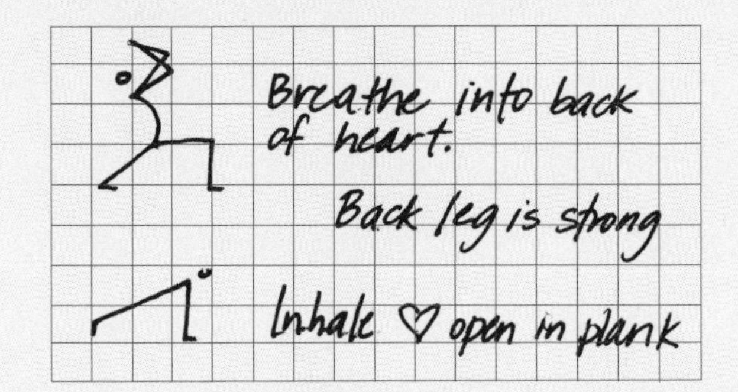

3. ***Sequence***—*Next comes the sequence. By drawing out the sequence using asana glyphs, you can record the progression of poses you want to flow through over the course of the class.*

4. ***Peak pose***—*Consider the highest point of activity.*

5. ***Three-wave grid***—*That progression of poses is mapped out over a three-wave grid that warms you up, takes you to the peak pose, and winds you down for savasana. For a thirty-minute sequence, each wave represents ten minutes; for a sixty-minute sequence, each wave represents twenty minutes; and so forth.*

Peak Pose:

chopasana

Aim: 60min sequence for ♡-opener

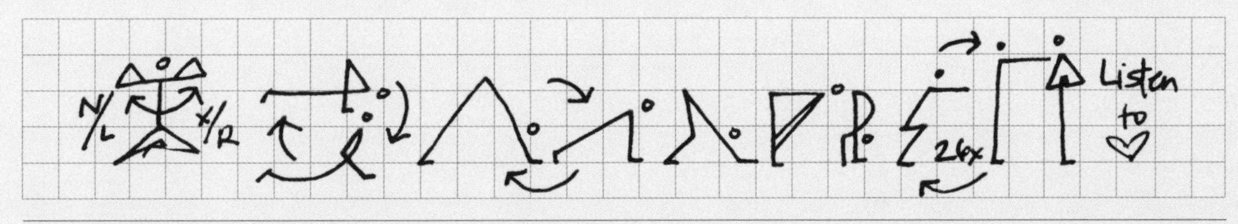

WAVE ONE TIME: 20 MINS

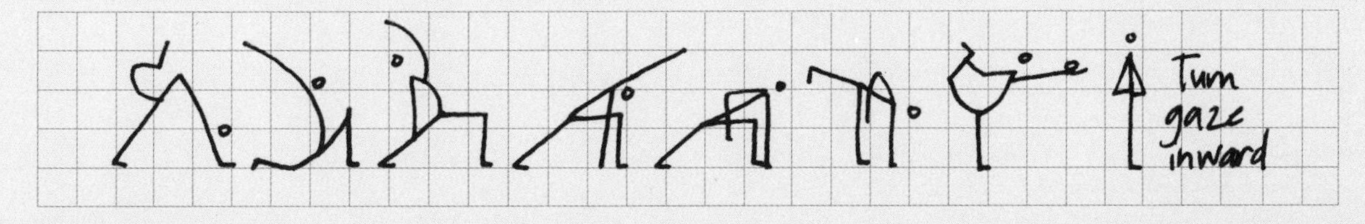

WAVE TWO TIME: 20 MINS

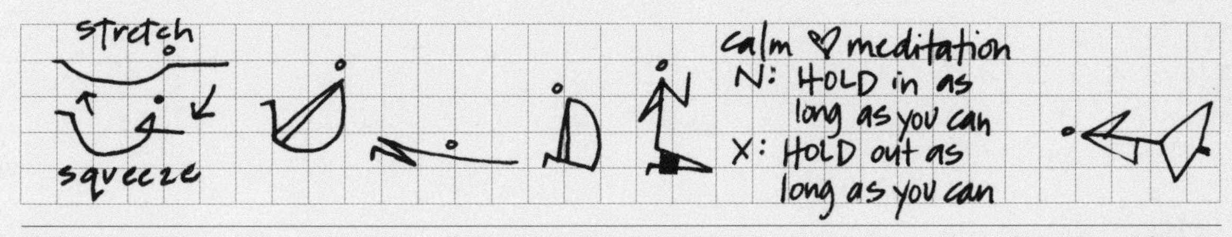

WAVE THREE TIME: 20 MINS

6. ***Talking points***—*Last, further develop the theme by writing down bite-size talking points that can be used sporadically to help deepen the meaning of the poses.*

TALKING POINTS

Every time you breathe, you give the ♡ a voice.

Smile across the chest

Lift your ♡ out of your belly

Be willing to sit in the seat of the ♡ and witness it all

DESIGN YOUR OWN SEQUENCE: YOUR TURN

YOGA BY DESIGN: STEP-BY-STEP

1. ***Sankalpa***—*Begin by writing three to five sentences, in the form of a sankalpa, which can be used at the opening of your sequence to clearly communicate the mood or intention of a particular theme. I find it helpful to think of one word or use a quote or poem to inspire the theme.*

Sankalpa:

2. ***Anatomical focus***—*Next, define the anatomical focus in a short bulleted list. This becomes the alignment you will cue in every pose.*

Anatomical focus:

1.

2.

3.

4.

3. ***Sequence***—*Next comes the sequence. By drawing out the sequence using asana glyphs, you can record the progression of poses you want to flow through over the course of the class.*

4. ***Peak pose***—*Consider the highest point of activity.*

5. ***Three-wave grid***—*That progression of poses is mapped out over a three-wave grid that warms you up, takes you to the peak pose, and winds you down for savasana. For a thirty-minute sequence, each wave represents ten minutes; for a sixty-minute sequence, each wave represents twenty minutes; and so forth.*

Peak Pose:

Aim:

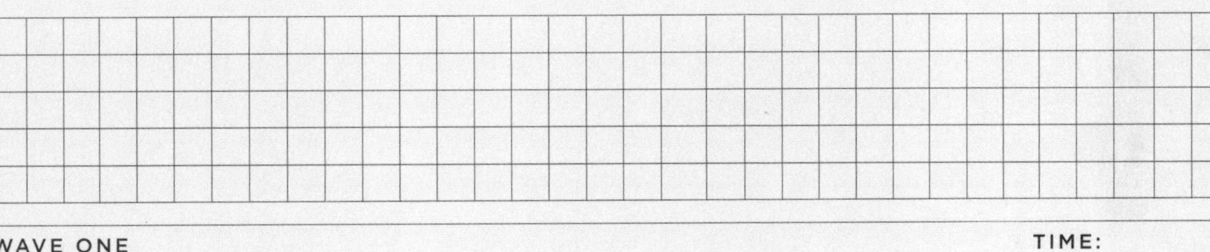

WAVE ONE TIME:

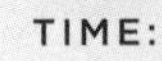

WAVE TWO TIME:

WAVE THREE TIME:

6. ***Talking points***—*Last, further develop the theme by writing down bite-size talking points that can be used sporadically to help deepen the meaning of the poses.*

TALKING POINTS

find your creative spark

IF YOU WANT TO FLY, TAKE YOURSELF LIGHTLY!

GINA CAPUTO

Let's cut loose and embrace our wildness! We'll liberate any stuck boogie by going into fun variations of standard asanas that require you to focus less on precision and more on creative generation of high vibration and laughter!

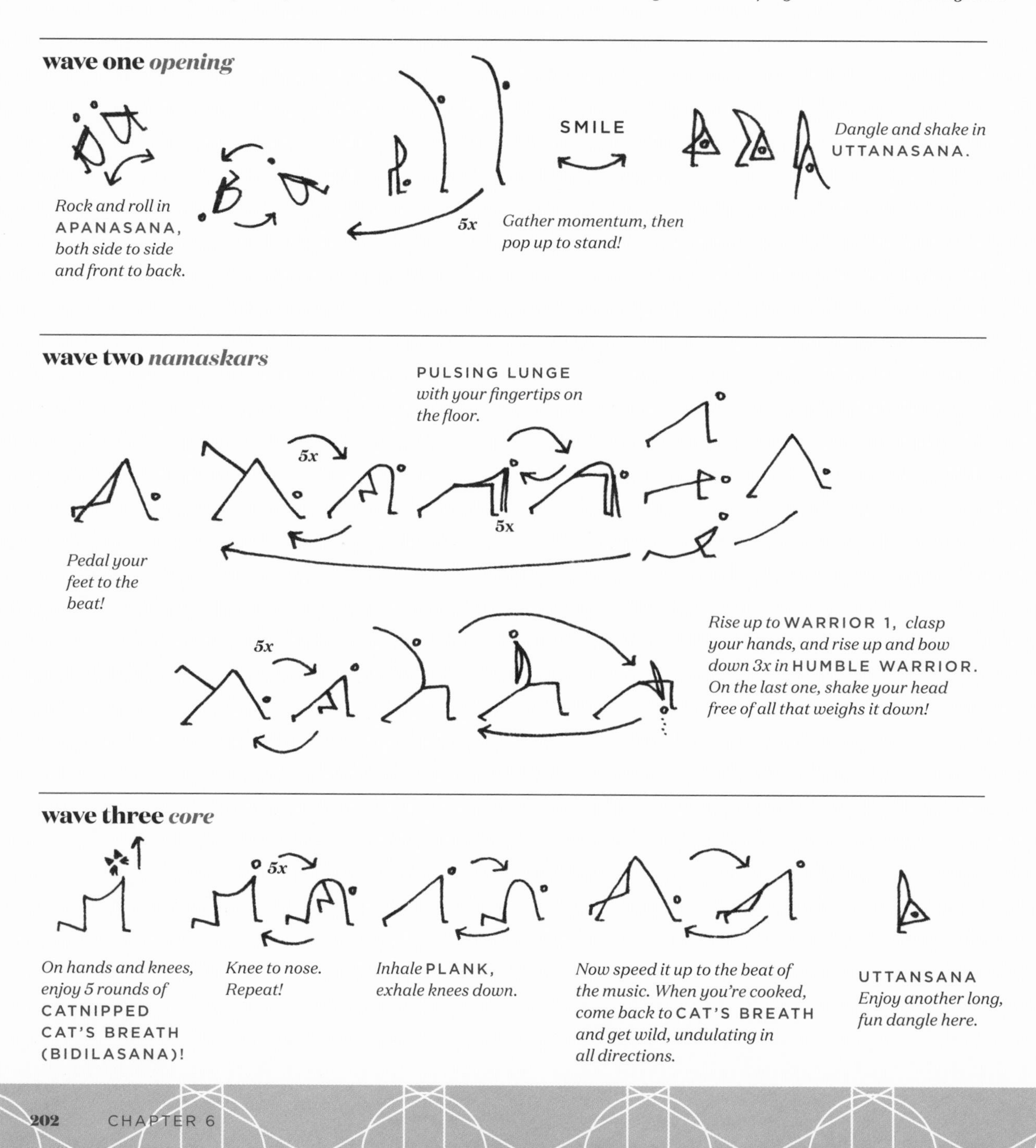

wave one

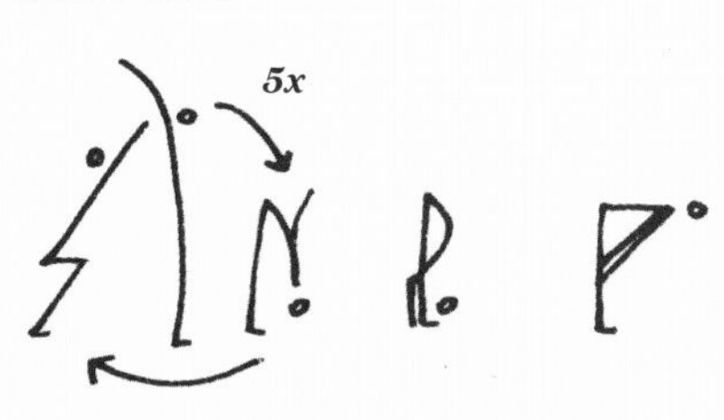

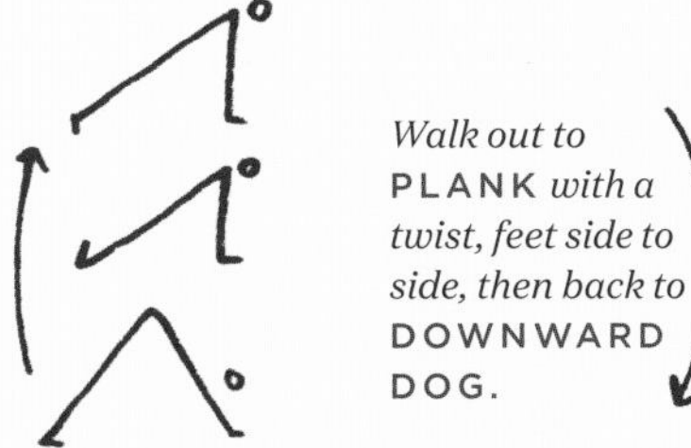

Walk out to PLANK *with a twist, feet side to side, then back to* DOWNWARD DOG.

From the back of your mat, feet together for UTKATASANA. *Sweep your arms up and then down and back* ***5x*** *with the biggest breaths you've ever taken.*

3x

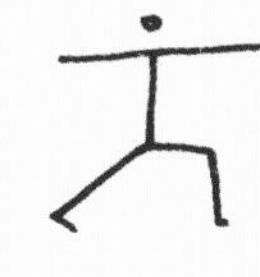

Right leg up and through to a WARRIOR 2 *base. Inhale up to* REVERSE WARRIOR, *exhale out to* HALF TRIANGLE.

TRIANGLE *for* 5 BREATHS

Inhale back up to WARRIOR 2, *and then turn both feet out for* TEMPLE/ GODDESS POSE.

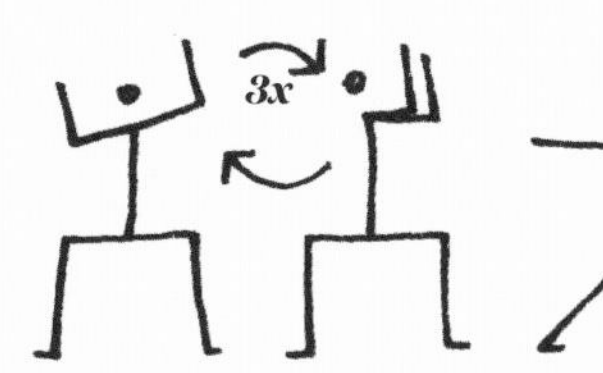

Raise your arms like goal posts—inhale and open them wide, exhale and squeeze them together powerfully.

From there, return to WARRIOR 2. *Release both hands to the floor to* LUNGE, *drop your back knee, and shift back to* HALF SPLITS.

From here, come back forward to lunge and step back to Downward Dog for the second side.

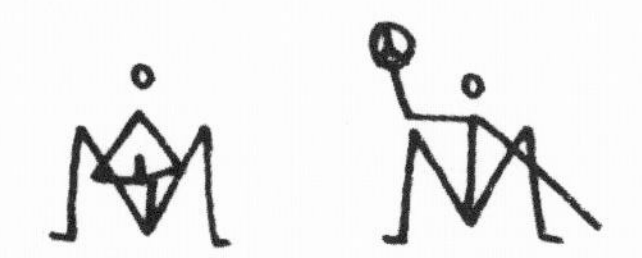

After the second side, jump your feet forward around your hands and drop down into HIPPIE MALASANA*—a deep squat throwing* PEACE SIGNS *on both sides!*

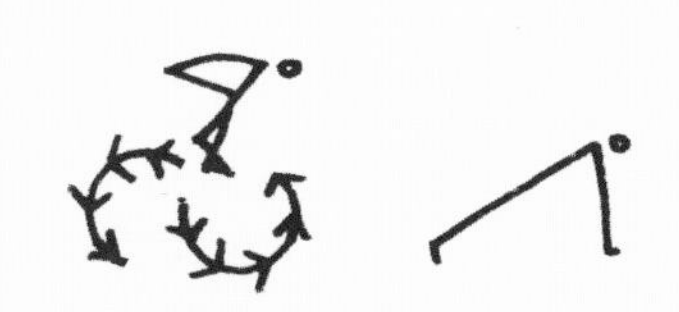

From here, lift your hips and try to tuck your shoulders behind your knees. Hang onto your ankles and try to SUMO WALK *around in a circle—stop to shake your rump!*

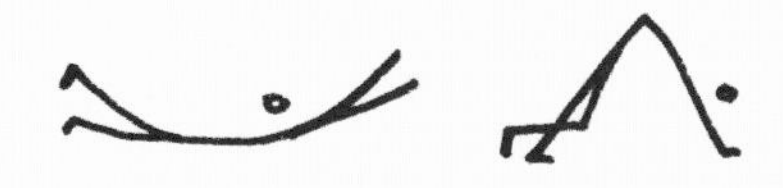

Once you make it back home, enjoy a connecting vinyasa of PLANK *to* CHATTURANGA *to* SWIMMING LOCUST *and end in* DANCING DOWNWARD DOG. *Cut loose!*

wave two

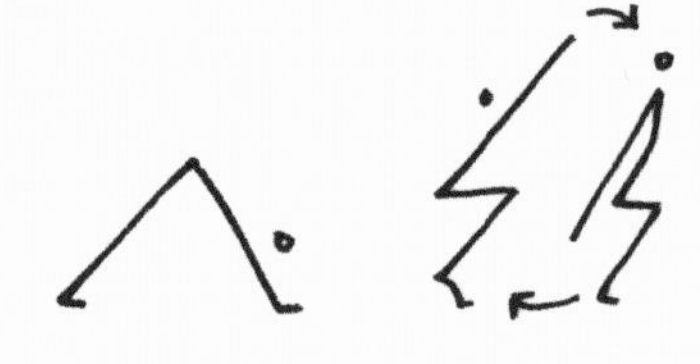

Walk your hands back to your feet and step your feet together again. This **UTKATASANA** *is with sweeping arms but on your tiptoes this time! Whoosh!*

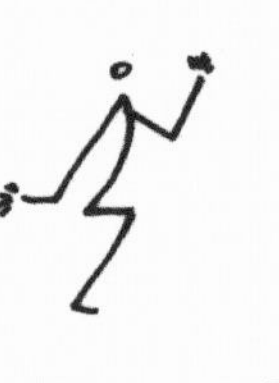

Hold the last one and give it 20 snaps up!

Enjoy a nice long **SASSY UTTANASANA** *with arms clasped overhead, bending your right and left knee to turn your chest to the sky!*

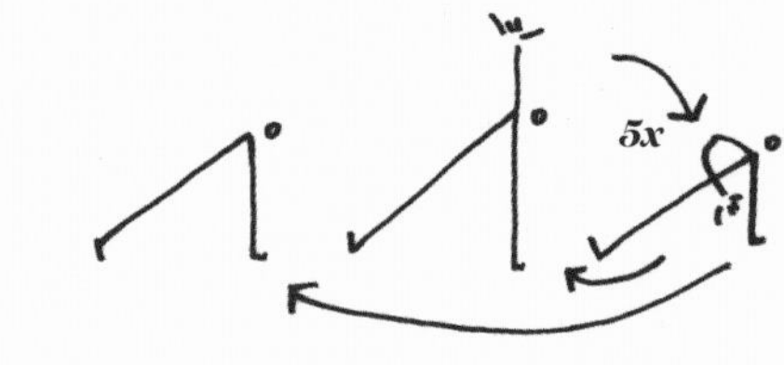

Walk your hands out to **PLANK**—*drop both heels to the right, inhale your left arm up and take* **DISCO MUDRA—STAYIN' ALIVE ARMS** *reach up and down in a diagonal! Switch sides.*

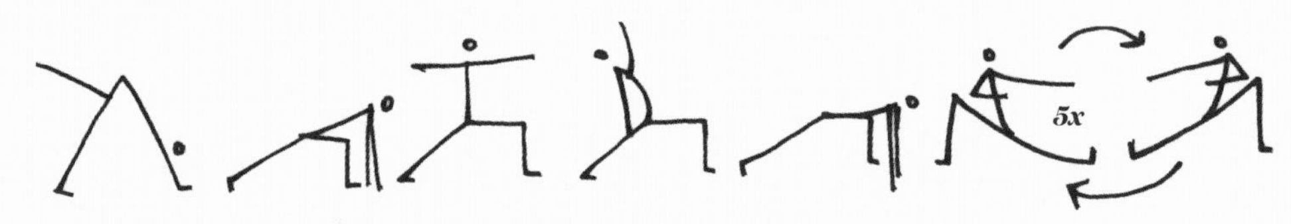

From **DOWNWARD DOG**, *inhale your right leg up, exhale to a* **WARRIOR 2** *base. Inhale up to* **REVERSE WARRIOR** *and then come down and shift over to* **FLOWING NINJA SKANDASANA** *on the left, then to the right.*

Look forward, not down!

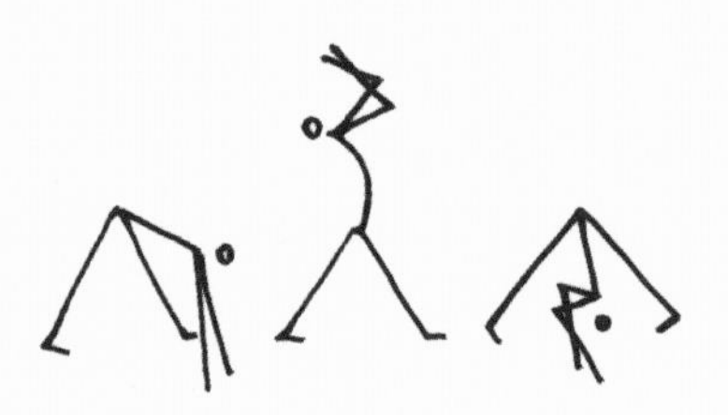

End with both legs straight facing the side for **PRASARITA PADOTTANASANA**. *Inhale your arms out and up overhead, cross them into* **GARUDASANA** *arms, and fold forward again. Repeat 2nd side.*

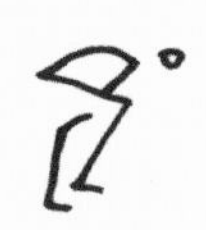

MALASANA
Lift your hips to tuck your shoulders behind your knees like you did for sumo circles. Place your hands behind your heels on the floor or on blocks.

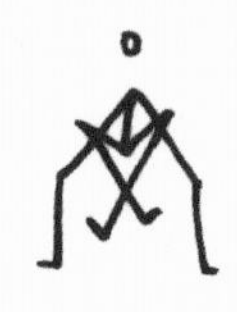

Bend your elbows so you can sit on the backs of your own arms. Squeeeeeeze your legs into your arms and see if you can cross your feet and lift your butt!

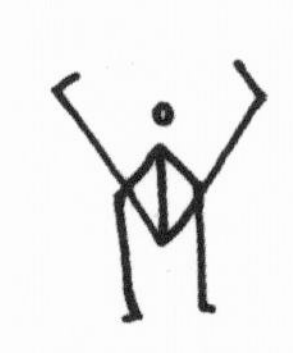

Once you get it, try kicking one leg out at a time, then go for both legs out in **TITTIBHASANA**. *Each time you fall, laugh harder! In the end, we all end on our butts—try to keep your arms behind your knees!*

wave three

Still on your butt, try bringing your heels together. With your arms still wrapped under your legs, grab the arches of your feet like motorcycle handlebars.

VROOM
VROOM

Play with extending your chest out and then bowing forward.

Turn up the corners of your lips.

Try to wriggle your arms and shoulders under your legs more and begin to straighten your legs out, smooshing yourself into SMILING KURMASANA.

Take arms and legs into the air and shake vigorously for UPWARD FACING WET DOG.

finishing

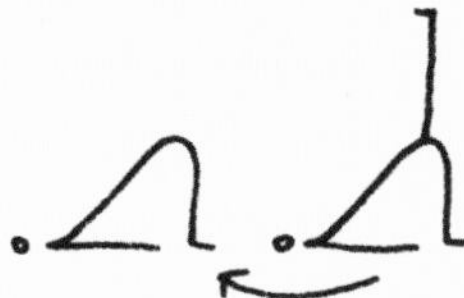

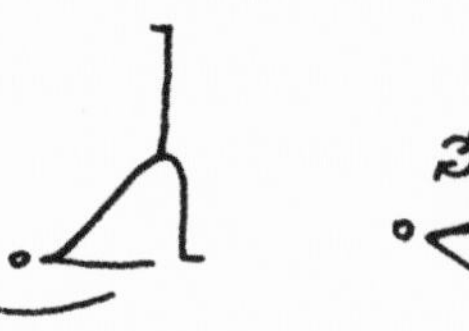

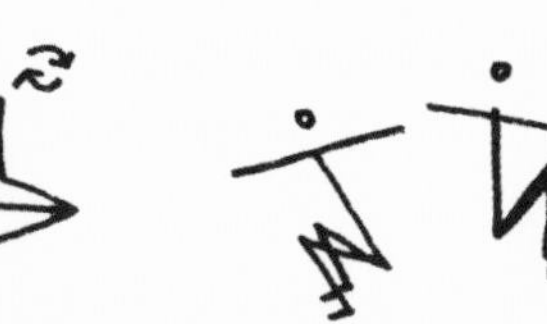

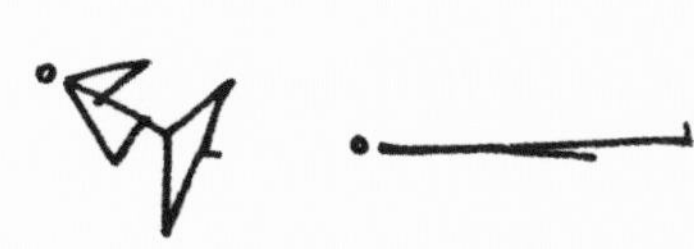

Release feet down for BRIDGE POSE. *Take right leg straight up into the air until you start to quiver. Repeat with left leg. Lower everything down and come into* BICYCLING HAPPY BABY*—hold feet for Happy Baby and then start pedaling your legs to massage your back and to keep the spirit of an actual happy baby alive. Cross thighs for a* SUPINE TWIST *and repeat second side. 5 breaths each side. End with soles of feet together and knees out in* SUPTA BADDHA KONASANA *with left hand on heart and right hand on belly. Dissolve into a blissfully happy* SAVASANA.

Creative Spark Playlist

compiled by Kelly Casey

All songs by Michael Franti & Spearhead

Hello Bonjour —*Yell Fire!*

Say Hey (I Love You)—*All Rebel Rockers*

The Sound of Sunshine—*The Sound of Sunshine*

Hey Now Now—*Yell Fire!*

I'm Alive (Life Sounds Like)—*All People*

What I Got - Look At ALl the Love We Found—*A Tribute to Sublime*

See You In The Light—*Yell Fire!*

Love Is Da Shit—*Home*

Ganja Baby—*Songs From The Front Porch—An Acoustic Collection*

Stay Human (Stereo Steambath Remix)—*Traveler '02*

Life Is Better With You (Acoustic Mix)—*All People*

Have A Little Fatih—*All Rebel Rockers*

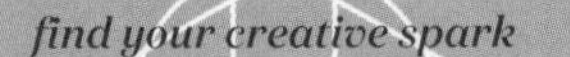

MARA MUNRO

One of your most important tools is the ability to hone, hear, and trust your creative intuition. Your asana practice is the perfect place to sharpen this tool and tap into the innate creativity that lives in your body, not just your mind. Give yourself permission to play, explore, and see the possibilities.

You don't have to be an artist to be creative. Everyone can express themselves with color and form. Think about visual art not as learning how to draw but as unlearning how to not draw.

Color Your Pose

DURATION:
Thirty minutes

LOCATION:
A quiet and open space

MINDSET:
Expansive

TOOLS:
Colored pencils, markers, crayons

1. Get on your mat and drop into one of your favorite poses.

   A. Notice how your body feels in this pose.

   B. Where is there tension?

   C. Where is there ease?

   D. Where does your breath flow?

2. Come out of the pose and choose a couple of colors that you are attracted to.

3. Draw a rough outline of your body, both front and back, and capture what you felt in the pose by using the colors.
   A. Was there a shape or current of energy?
   B. Where did you feel the pose most in your body?
   C. Feel free to write any words, or draw any images, shapes, or textures.
4. Sit back and have a look.
   A. What colors did you choose?
   B. What do these colors mean to you?
   C. Do some research into chakra colors and symbolism.

The most important relationship we will have in our lives is with ourselves. Learning to listen to our bodies, our inner voices, and embrace everything we encounter with compassion is the greatest love affair we can create and nurture in our lives.

SELF-PORTRAIT

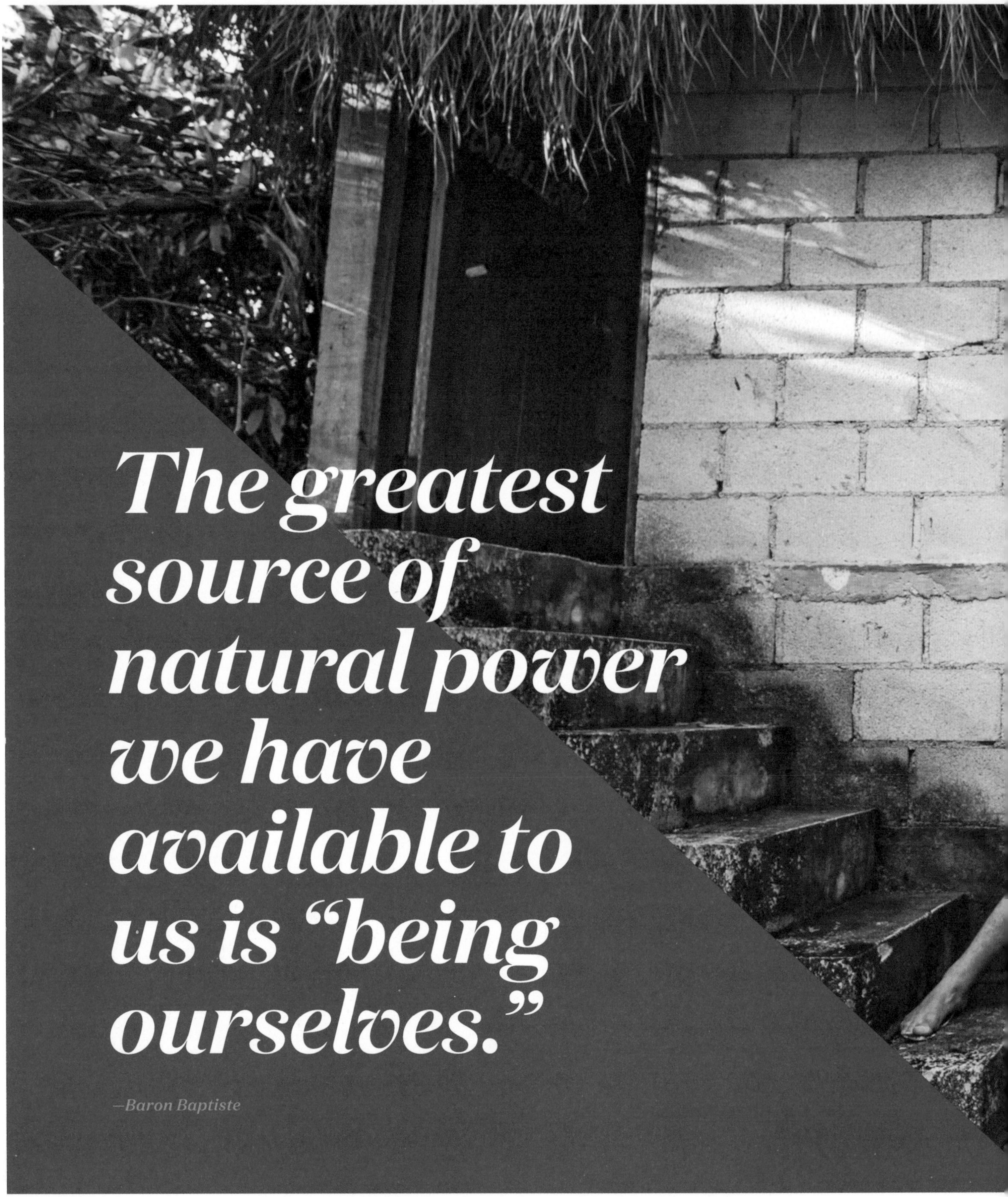

The greatest source of natural power we have available to us is "being ourselves."

—Baron Baptiste

CHAPTER 7

find your center

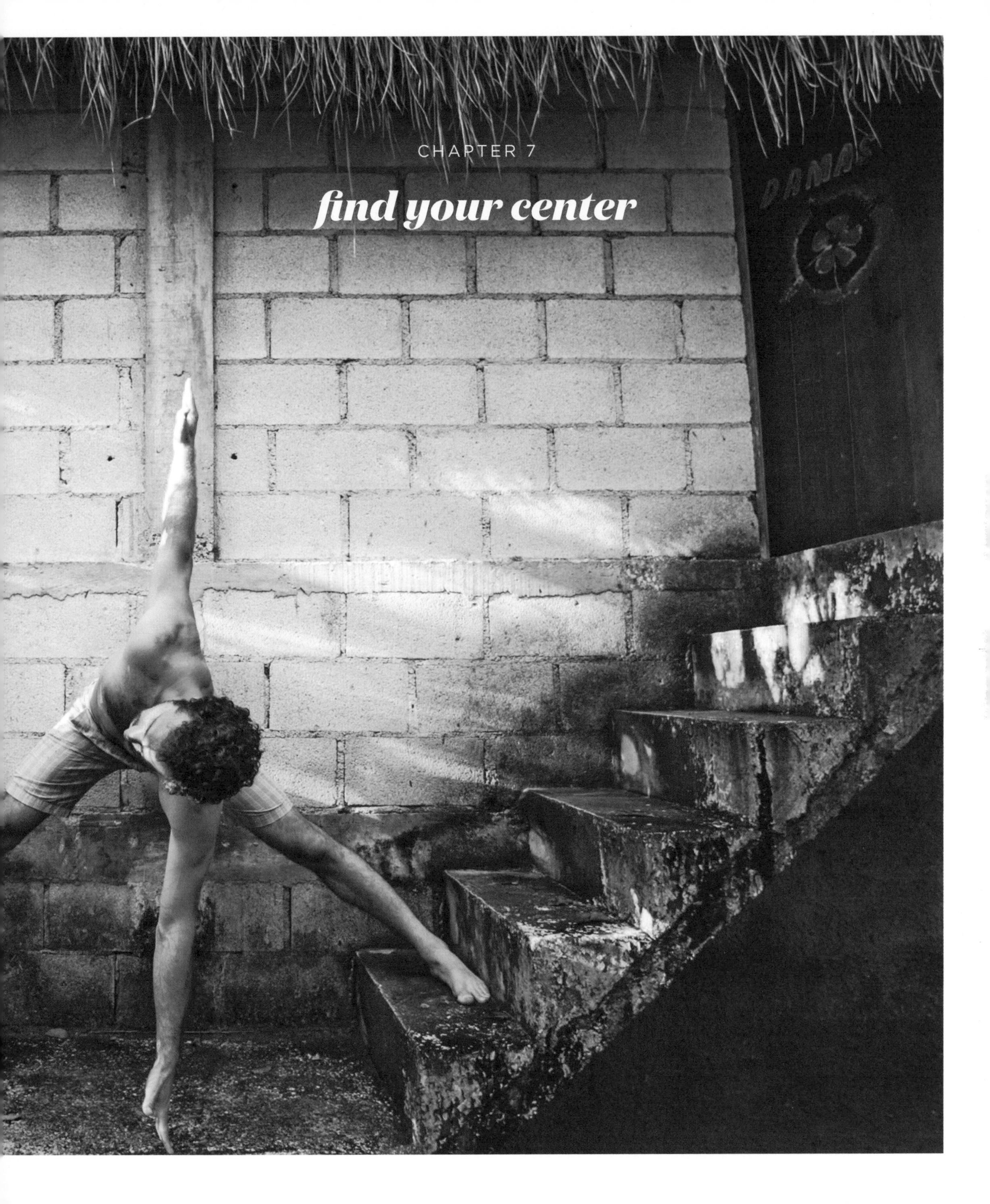

FIND YOUR CENTER AND SEAL IN THE BLESSINGS

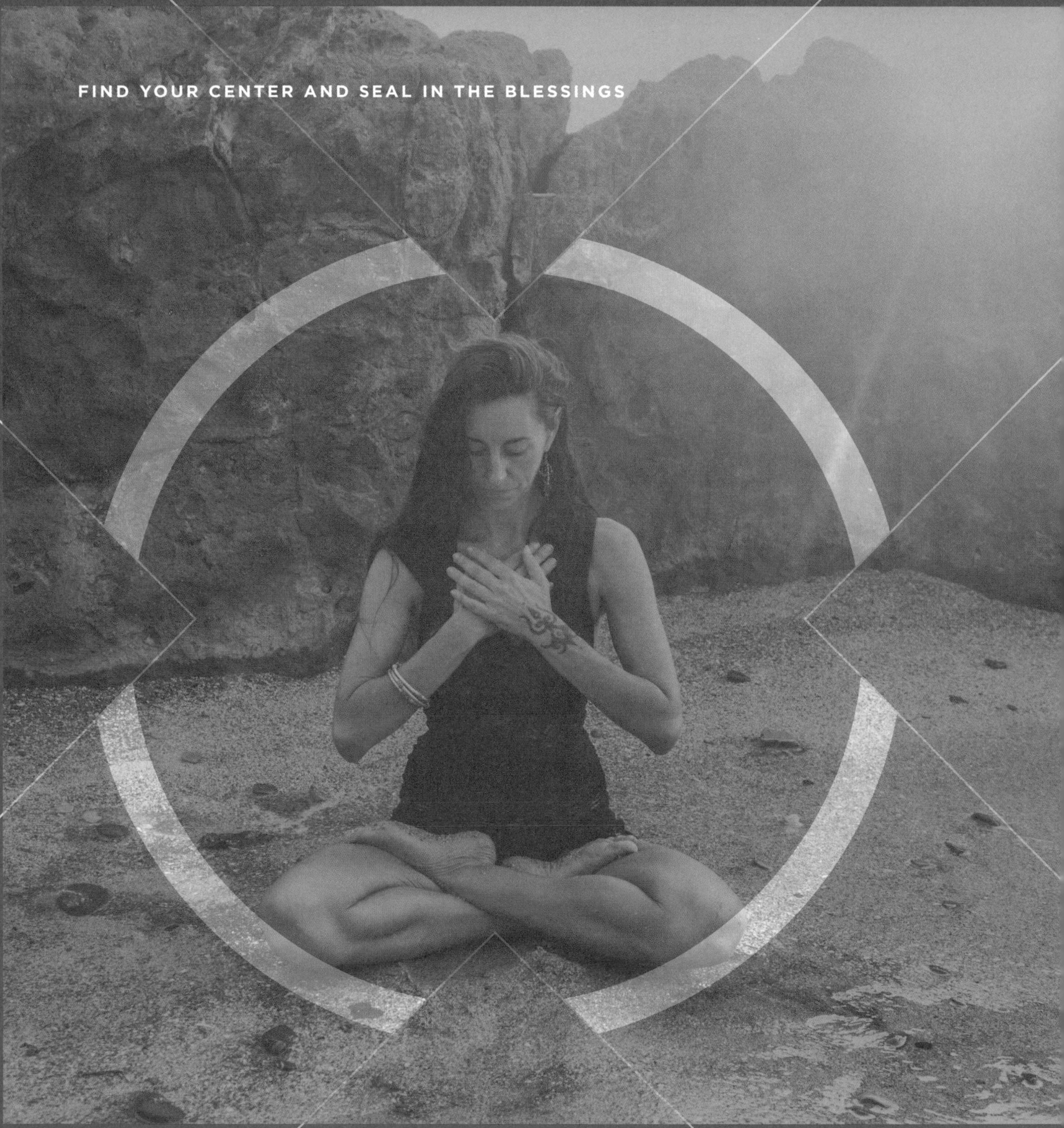

NICOLE LINDSTROM

Along this journey we have the ability to, at any given moment, find our center. The singular point from which everything revolves, from which everything radiates. This nexus of connection to the truest self holds the power to turn dreams into reality and thoughts into life.

Our center is always present amid the chaos, and to find it takes practice. It takes patience, perseverance, gentle listening. It requires being present and letting go.

When we tune out what no longer serves us and tune in, our center is there. It is from this place that we can honor ourselves and the completeness of who we are, maintaining balance and equilibrium. Here, we recognize that our words, thoughts, and actions come from a place of truth.

Take a seat.

Close your eyes.

Find your center.

Seal in the blessings.

Proceed from your center and allow your highest aspirations to take shape and flourish. From the inside out, live with deep compassion, clear consciousness, and genuine intent, honoring the good in yourself and all others.

You've arrived. Welcome.

FIND YOUR CENTER: THE QI GONG PRACTICE OF THE THREE TREASURES

THOMAS DROGE

The Three Treasures in ancient Taoist thought are the heavens (the sun, moon, and stars); the Earth; and human beings, who are at the center. These treasures are repeated over and over: For example, in people, the Three Treasures are the essence (congenital health), the qi/energy or breath, and the spirit/consciousness.

What is unique and amazing about the Taoist viewpoint is that being centered isn't about achieving a static space or some kind of arrival at a singular point; it is, rather, a dynamic consciousness of maintaining the center that aligns us with heaven and Earth.

The First Treasure:

THE HEAVENS

Imagine for a moment the sun, in all its fire and power. The sun's gravity drawing in all around it. The very mission of the sun is to create heat and light; to incinerate and explode—endlessly devouring and expressing life. The sun is using all of its force to draw in the Earth, to literally pull it in and, like Shiva (the god of creation and destruction), transform it into energy.

The Second Treasure:

THE EARTH

Meanwhile, the Earth is rocketing through space at 67,000 miles per hour, determined to continue throughout the universe on its own trajectory. The Earth and sun tell an age-old story of attraction, a balance of forces in harmonious opposition, the sun endlessly trying to draw the Earth into its forge of transformation and the Earth spinning away trying to break out across the cosmos. Yet the very nature of these two, their gravity and velocity, keeps them in a seemingly infinite state of balance.

The Third Treasure:

HUMAN BEINGS (AND LIFE ON EARTH)

Humans can only exist in the potentially explosive yet balanced state of the sun and Earth in orbit. It is here in the dynamism of these two celestial lovers that human life is born and thrives. To find balance is to practice feeling the energy of these two great life forms as the sun and Earth resonate in our own bodies, and then to bring these forces into harmony inside ourselves.

We find our center by discovering the Three Treasures:

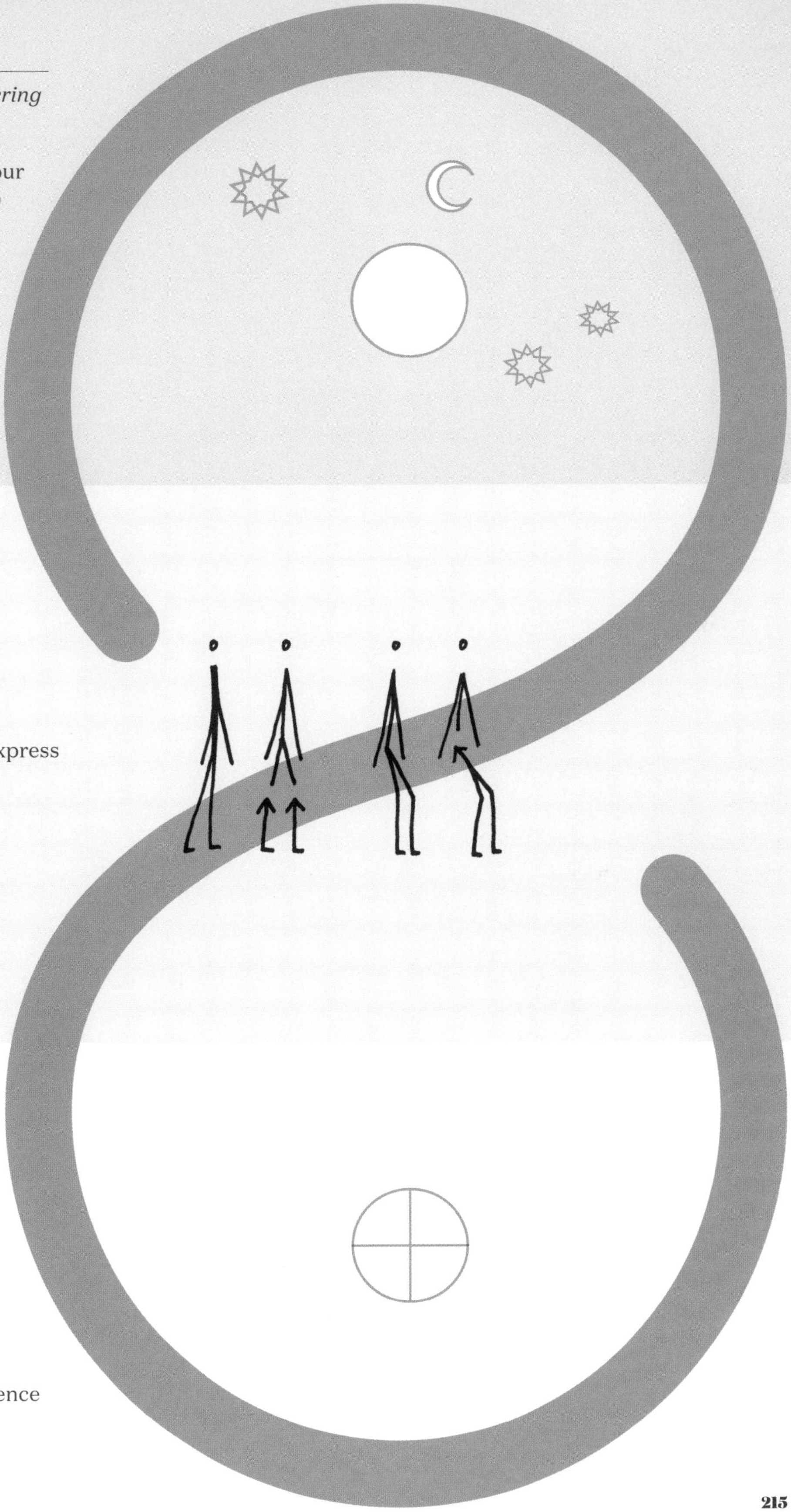

THE HEAVENS, which hold our wisdom and our spirit (shen)

HUMAN BEINGS, who can express creativity and living energy through breath (qi)

EARTH, which holds our essence and physical form (jing)

STANDING POSE:

Stand with your feet about shoulder width apart. Make the outer edges/sides of your feet parallel, soften the ankles, and unlock the knees.

To unlock your knees, straighten them into a full lock by lifting the kneecap and then release until there is just the slightest bend in the knee.

Unlocking the knee in this pose allows the energy to easily rise up from the ground through the legs.

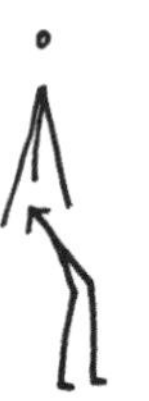

Gently engage the pelvic floor; try to feel the connection between the inner thigh and the pelvic floor reaching up into the hips and lower abdomen.

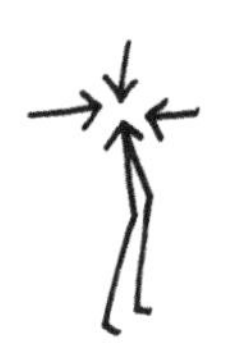

Relax the lower back and contract ever so slightly in the core muscles so that you feel a dynamic tension in the front of the pelvis connecting with the lower back.

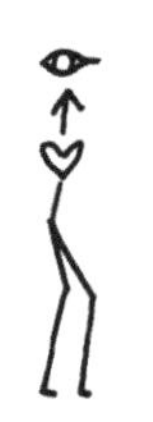

Soften the chest, drop your shoulders, and feel the energy rise up from your heart, opening the throat chakra and allowing your heart spirit to merge with the third eye, what the Taoists call your upper elixir field.

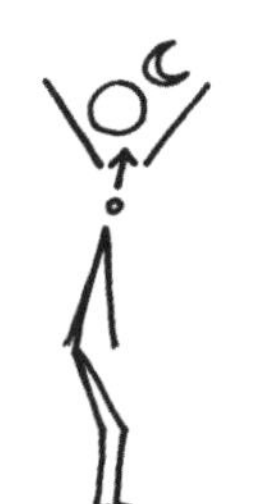

Open your celestial gate or crown chakra (at the center of the top of the head) and connect with the energies of the sun, moon, and stars. Your arms hang loosely by your sides.

Take 3 deep cleansing breaths and let the tension from your body release. Bring your consciousness into the present moment, and inhabit your practice space. Take a moment to turn your focus inward, observe your breath, look within, and listen within.

EARTH POSE:

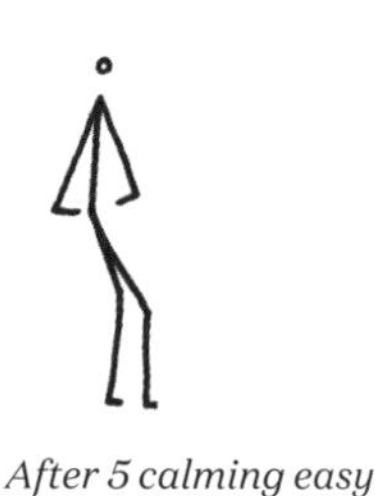

After 5 calming easy breaths, inhale and slowly migrate your hands forward, placing your palms in front of your lower abdomen.

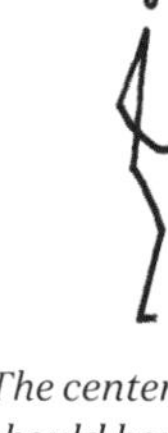

The center of the palm should hover a couple inches in front of the center of the pelvis.

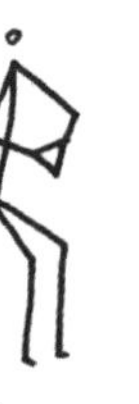

Your fingers are all touching except for the thumb and index fingers; they come together lightly touching at the tips and forming a triangle.

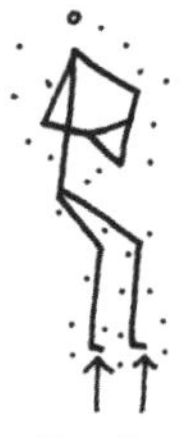

Visualize the nurturing energy of the planet rising up through the center of the arch of your feet. This spot in the center of your foot is called the bubbling well acupuncture point.

Feel throughout your body the deep-rooted stability of the mountains, the flexibility of the forests, and the fluidity of the rivers and oceans. This is the power and calm of the Earth. Take 5–10 easy calming breaths or as much time as you like.

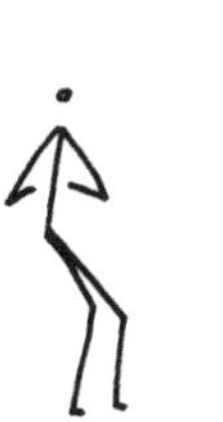

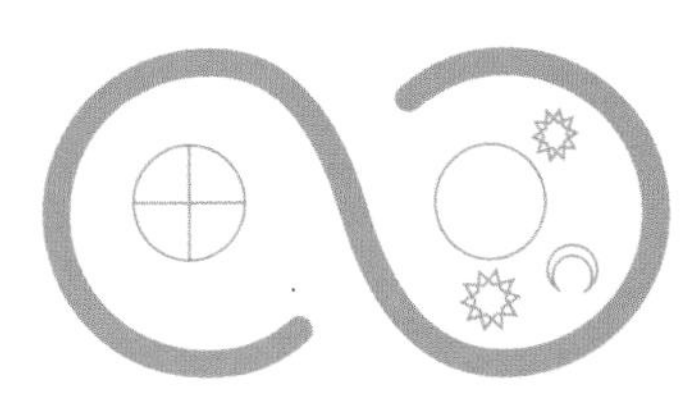

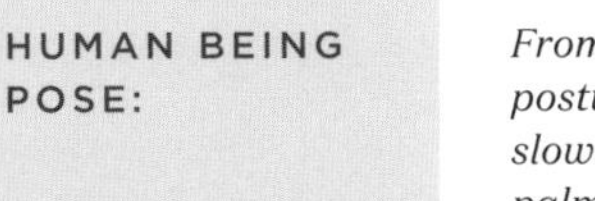

HUMAN BEING POSE:

From the current posture, the hands slowly rise up, the palms face the body and continue to rise until they reach the level of the heart.

The shoulders should be relaxed and down, the elbows slightly lower than the shoulders, the knees remain unlocked or slightly bent, the lower back still tucked, celestial gate still open and connecting with the sun, moon, and stars.

This posture is the Human Being the Prana or Qi (pronounced chee). This is the posture of transformation, the place where we conduct the change between the Earth's nourishing resources and the wisdom of the celestial bodies.

Concentrate your breath wherever you feel any tension and breathe through it, feel the forces above in the stars and sun and below in the Earth fueling the change through your breath.

Feel the center of the Earth connect with the center of your body and the center of the sun. Take 5–10 easy, calming breaths or as much time as you like.

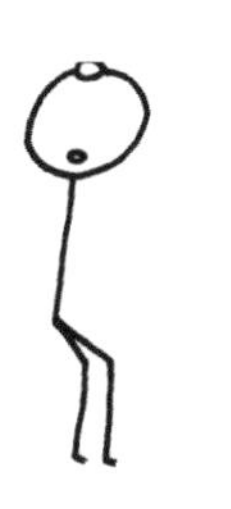

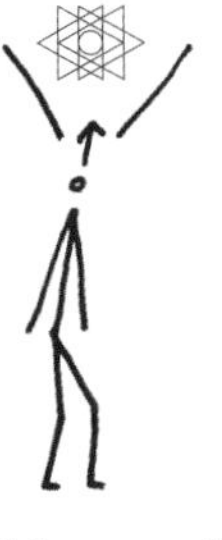

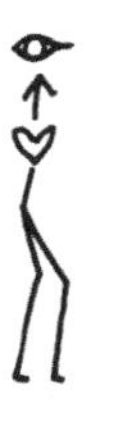

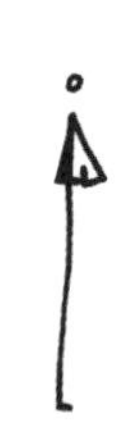

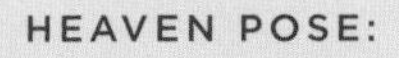

HEAVEN POSE:

Next, raise your hands up toward the sky. Palms turn and face upward; the arms circle up like you are holding a bowl of fruit over your head. The arms are rounded and the shoulders down, pinching the bottom of the shoulder blades together. This is heaven pose, connecting with the energy of the sun.

Feel the warmth of the sun, its activating energy pouring into your hands, warming your body. Open the crown chakra, your celestial gate, and connect with the spirit wisdom of the stars. Focus on your spiritual self, your higher consciousness, your metaconsciousness.

Use your breath to open the third eye and begin to see your inner vision; notice the connection and interdependence of all things and how we are all part of the same universal energy.

Slowly take a deep cleansing inhale and step your feet together with ankles touching. As you exhale, lower your arms down to prayer position at your heart. Take a moment to feel the center of your consciousness and the compassion of caring for each other and our planet. Release the prayer mudra and have a centered day.

Take a moment in this pose, and notice if there are any questions you have been struggling with or decisions you have been having trouble making. Meditate on them for a couple breaths. Allow space for the answer to emerge. Don't worry if it doesn't happen right away, these answers tend to slowly make their way into our consciousness like a flower slowly opening. Take 5–10 easy calming breaths or as much time as you like.

We live in a dualistic culture dominated by conflicts of head and heart, thought and feeling, mind and emotions. This is a culture that knows not that lower and deeper center of awareness—and of will and intent. . . . An ancient Daoist saying tells us: "When you are sick, do not seek a cure. Find your centre and you will be healed." . . . The little "I" reigns in the head alone. The larger "I" is the body as a whole.

—*Peter Wilberg*

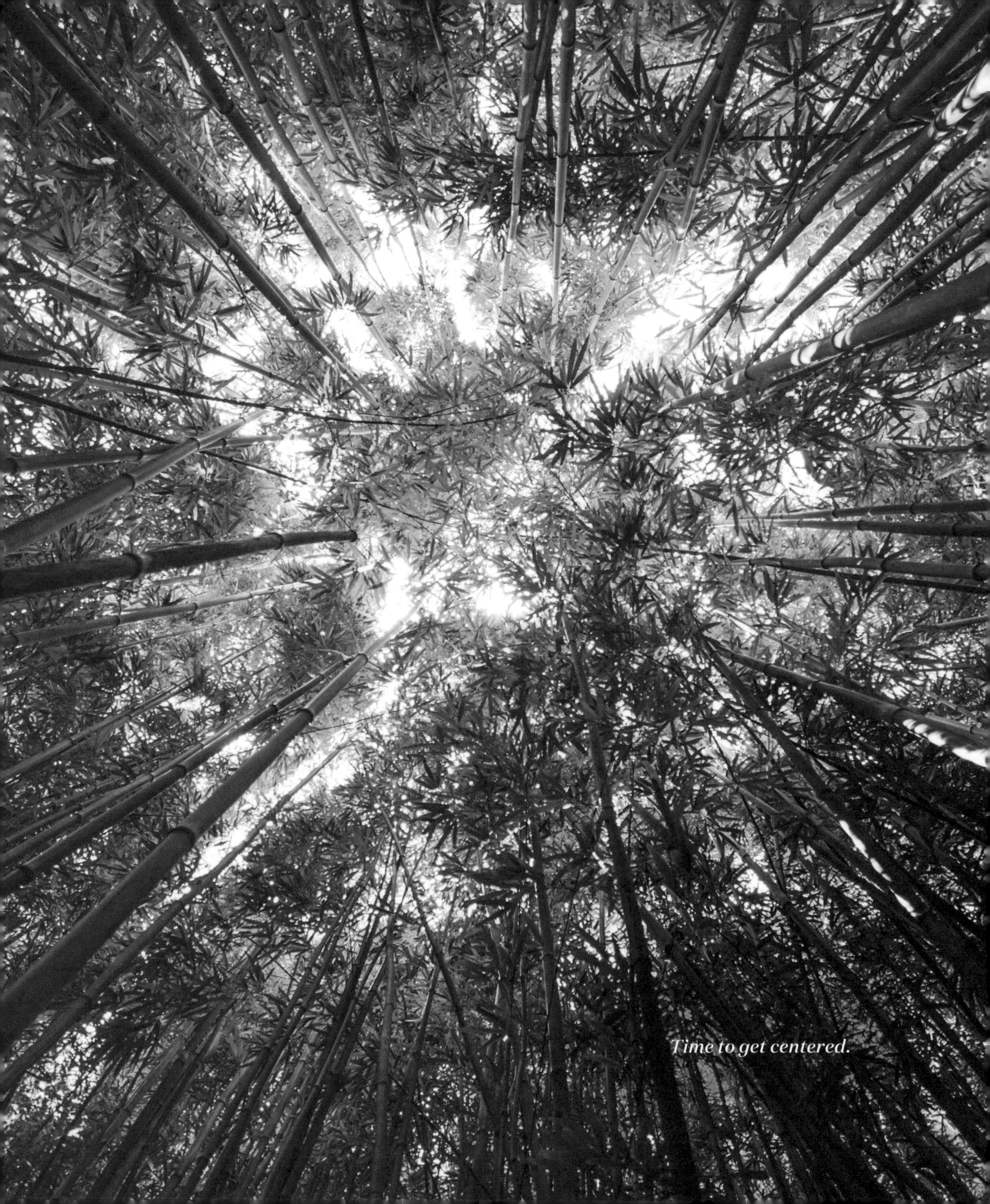

Time to get centered.

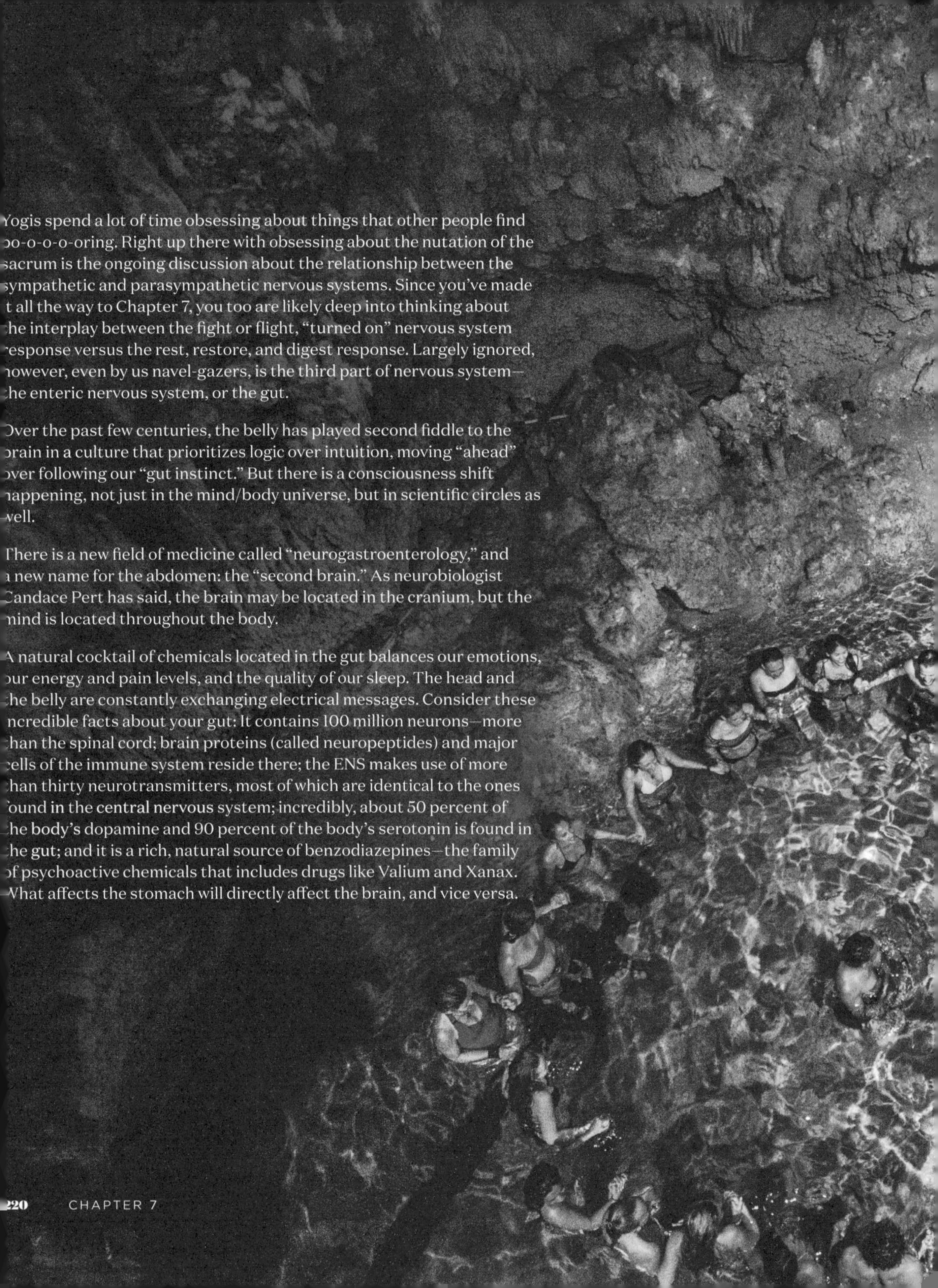

Yogis spend a lot of time obsessing about things that other people find boo-o-o-o-oring. Right up there with obsessing about the nutation of the sacrum is the ongoing discussion about the relationship between the sympathetic and parasympathetic nervous systems. Since you've made it all the way to Chapter 7, you too are likely deep into thinking about the interplay between the fight or flight, "turned on" nervous system response versus the rest, restore, and digest response. Largely ignored, however, even by us navel-gazers, is the third part of nervous system—the enteric nervous system, or the gut.

Over the past few centuries, the belly has played second fiddle to the brain in a culture that prioritizes logic over intuition, moving "ahead" over following our "gut instinct." But there is a consciousness shift happening, not just in the mind/body universe, but in scientific circles as well.

There is a new field of medicine called "neurogastroenterology," and a new name for the abdomen: the "second brain." As neurobiologist Candace Pert has said, the brain may be located in the cranium, but the mind is located throughout the body.

A natural cocktail of chemicals located in the gut balances our emotions, our energy and pain levels, and the quality of our sleep. The head and the belly are constantly exchanging electrical messages. Consider these incredible facts about your gut: It contains 100 million neurons—more than the spinal cord; brain proteins (called neuropeptides) and major cells of the immune system reside there; the ENS makes use of more than thirty neurotransmitters, most of which are identical to the ones found in the central nervous system; incredibly, about 50 percent of the body's dopamine and 90 percent of the body's serotonin is found in the gut; and it is a rich, natural source of benzodiazepines—the family of psychoactive chemicals that includes drugs like Valium and Xanax. What affects the stomach will directly affect the brain, and vice versa.

Of course, Western science is playing catch-up with what Eastern traditions have long understood. All major traditional spiritual practices teach that a solid foundation, located physically in the belly, is necessary in order to progress along a sustainable, healthy path of inquiry. Svadisthana chakra translates as "one's own place or base" in the yogic lineage. The dan tien, or hara, the point below the navel and above the pubis, is considered the undisputed power center of the mind/body in China and Japan. All these traditions stress that you must cultivate strong roots before you can grow toward the heavens.

The West has long had an instinct (a "gut instinct," you could say) about the wisdom of the belly. This is expressed most succinctly in the universally recognized good of being "centered," whether this applies to your personal, work, or spiritual life. Many things feed your second brain—physical and contemplative practices, spending time in nature and with people you love, as well the more literal act of conscious eating. Whereas the brain will often tell you what you *think* you need, if you are able to drop your attention into your gut, you will often *know* what will bring you toward health and contentment.

A daily dose of dedicated navel-gazing is a necessary byway for travelers on the path winding toward true north.

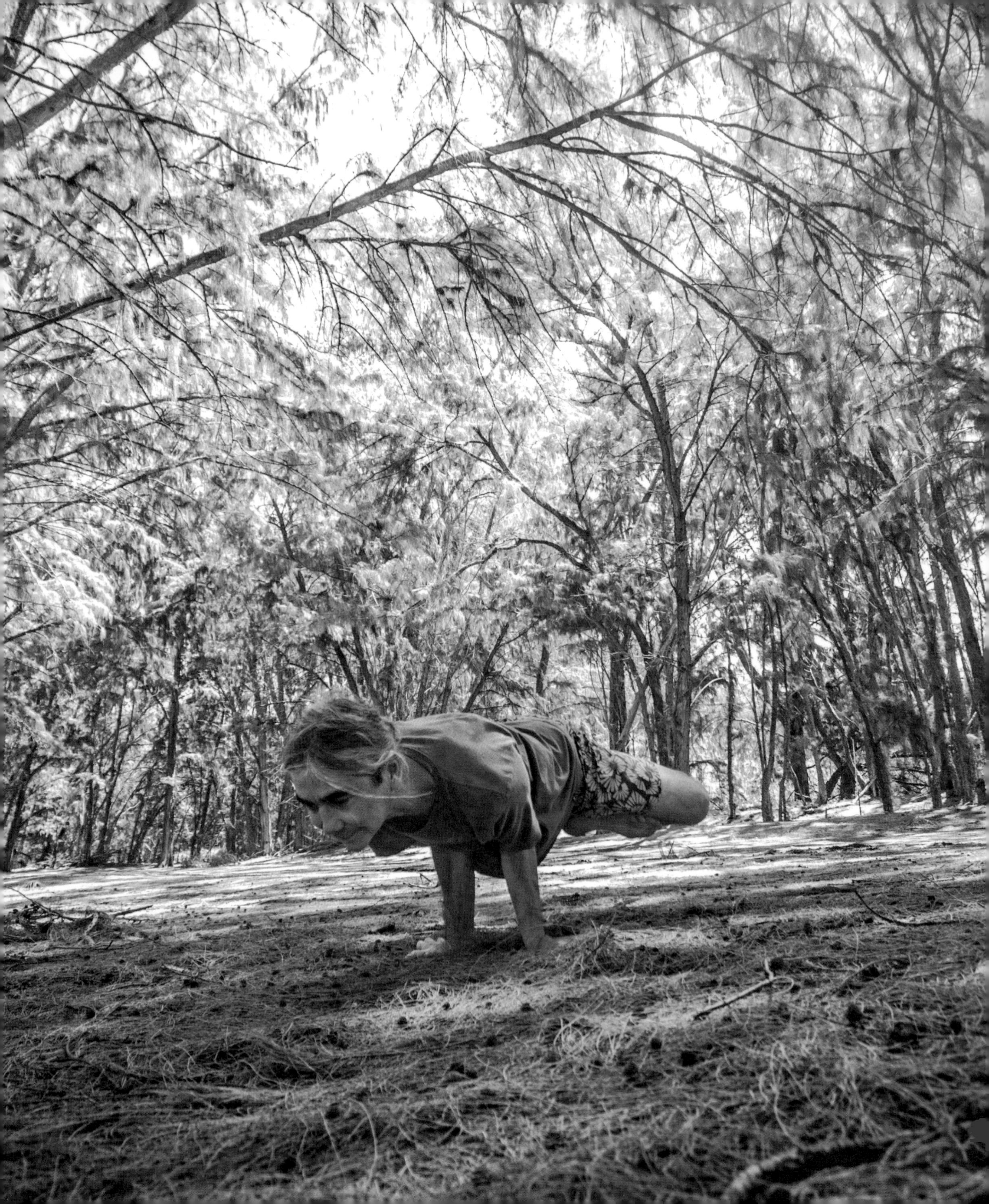

GO WITH THE FLOW

GERRY LOPEZ

The Wave of Life is a long, unpredictable journey. It is one fraught with perils. We encounter jellyfish of doubt, red tides of guilt, and the inevitable rip currents of fear. Sharks, spiny sea urchins, shallow sharp reefs, choppy water, onshore winds, and any number of upsetting factors conspire to cause us to falter or fail. Where do we find the balance to choose the right wave to catch, get to our feet, take the drop, make the turn, and complete the ride?

Yoga teaches us how to live a life in harmony with nature. The most natural thing we do, the simple act of breathing is the foundation of our yoga practice. Whenever we come to our mats, we tune in to the natural flow of the breath, and it is from there that our practice flows. What we learn from our yoga practice we can apply to the rest of life, so that we develop a flow there as well. It's the same when we step out into nature or paddle out into the surf: We tune in to the natural rhythm of the land or the sea to harmonize with these environments. It is only in this manner we can hope to become an integral part of our world as opposed to being apart from it.

Surfing is a very difficult thing to learn to do well because it happens in a world where everything moves and nothing stays still. Success comes when we are able to operate in the present moment and stay focused. A wipeout is the price we pay when we are out of sync with the natural movement of the waves. In small surf, the cost is cheap . . . frustration and some loss of dignity. When the waves are big, not paying attention can be dangerous and painful. The reward of finding one's self in complete harmony with this natural force is a sense of satisfaction and achievement unlike any other.

Surfing and yoga are a beautiful metaphor for life. Life never holds still for us—if we are not able to move with it, life passes us right by. Surfing and yoga teach us how to go with the flow smoothly and to be in the moment spontaneously. Harmony in life comes like waves and yoga sessions, not always perfect but as an ongoing process, moment to moment, following the instructions we set for ourselves and taking what we get.

Creating an altar requires a sacred space, which can be an entire room or simply a small space that is set up with intention. The first step in altar creation is clearing and cleaning. For some, this may be the hardest part of the process. Regardless, it is extremely important to focus your intention for your altar as you choose the sacred space in your home, office, car, or even your garden! Make sure that you thoroughly clear and clean the entire space. Take away anything that is not needed, starting your process with a clean, empty space.

Next, take some time to look inside yourself, seeing what wants to be expressed, honored, or invoked in your life. After you feel that you know, or have an intuition or an idea of your altar, begin the gathering process. I like to think of altars as a three-dimensional expression of a collage, or a manifestation of a dream. You will most likely find that you already have everything you need to create your altar. Choose items that are consistent with what you are intending to invoke in your life. Photographs, crystals, images of deities, fabrics, sacred items, sticks, stones, memorable items, keepsakes, and art are just a few ideas. You really can include just about anything on your altar! I also suggest that you put something on your altar that requires you to tend your altar, or come back to it. This can be a plant, flowers, a candle, or a water fountain. Choose something that represents life to you as you are creating a living altar.

While you are engaged in this process, take time to feel what is happening inside and honor yourself, acknowledging the feelings that are occurring. There is no set timetable for this process, although it is imperative to maintain your intention and focus from start to finish.

Begin by placing your altar table in a central location in the space you have cleared and cleaned. As you are arranging the items that you have gathered and assembled for your altar, don't be afraid to experiment and play with what you are working with!

Look at the nature of the relationships of all that you have gathered to put onto your altar. I have also found that creating different heights on my altar through the use of small fabric-covered boxes, plastic risers, overturned pots, baskets, etc., helps to create dynamic movement in the overall feeling of the altar.

Trust yourself with the choices that you are making, knowing that you will get results consistent with the intention that you have used during the entire altar creation.

Resist the temptation to overthink your process; stay centered in your heart.

When you feel satisfied with your creation, take time to sit, meditate, and be with your altar. Appreciate and acknowledge the beauty within yourself that you have expressed, allowing yourself to receive all of the gifts and abundance that the universe has to offer you in return!

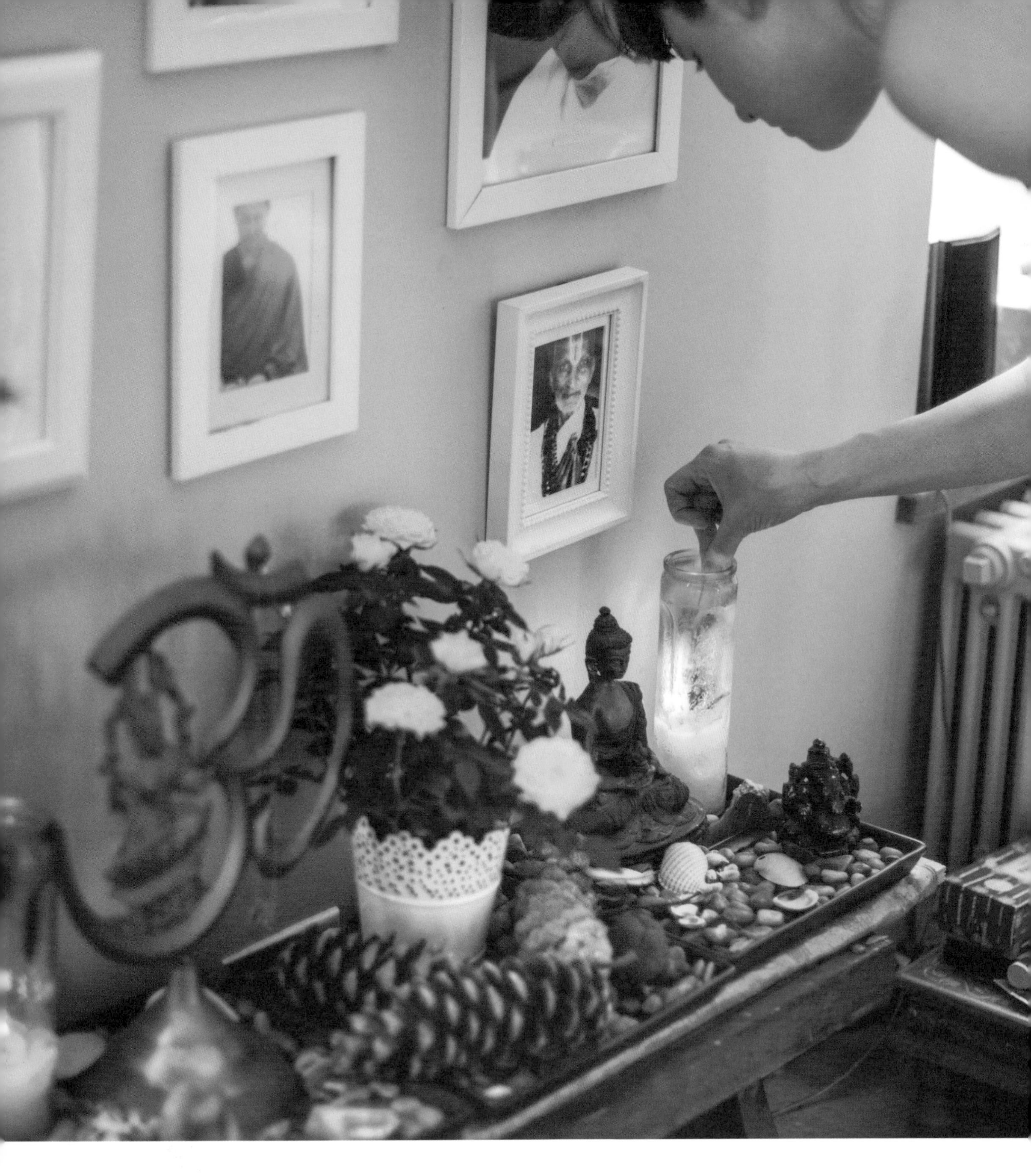

THE UNIVERSAL LANGUAGE

Music is sometimes referred to as a universal language, allowing people from opposite ends of the world to communicate although they have no common verbal language. Some may think this is a result of globalization and technology, with music being accessible internationally through phonographs, cassette tapes, CDs, radio, television, and most of all the Internet, but music has been a universal language for centuries before the first recordings were ever made. How is it that there is a common thread between music from all over the globe, the similarities far outweighing the differences? I believe mankind's oldest influence, nature, and all of its sounds, is the thread.

MUSIC OF NATURE

I grew up in Kelowna, British Columbia, a small town in the Monashee Mountain range between the Rockies and the Pacific. We lived in a rural area bordering a provincial park. As a boy I had no idea all this time in nature would have such a profound impact on my life and music. After high school, I moved to Boston to attend Berklee College of Music. For the first two years, all my time was spent studying jazz and classical music, playing in bands, and practicing my bass hours a day in my apartment or in the rows of practice booths at school. I missed being in nature, so I bought a car and started exploring the wilderness in the Northeast. That summer, I left the booths and took my bass to the woods at Walden Pond every day to practice.

At first I kept up with my regular practice routine of playing scales and classical music and working on being a better jazz bassist, but I soon realized that none of this music seemed to fit with the feeling of being in the woods. It felt like the music was imposed and was not of the environment. I asked myself, "What does the music of nature sound like?" I had no idea, but was keen to explore.

I put the bass down and listened to the sounds of the environment with the same focus and attention I used to study my favorite symphonies or jazz albums. I tried to take in everything I heard: wind, the leaves moving, birds, chipmunks, the creek. Then I closed my eyes and focused on where the different sounds were coming from and from what

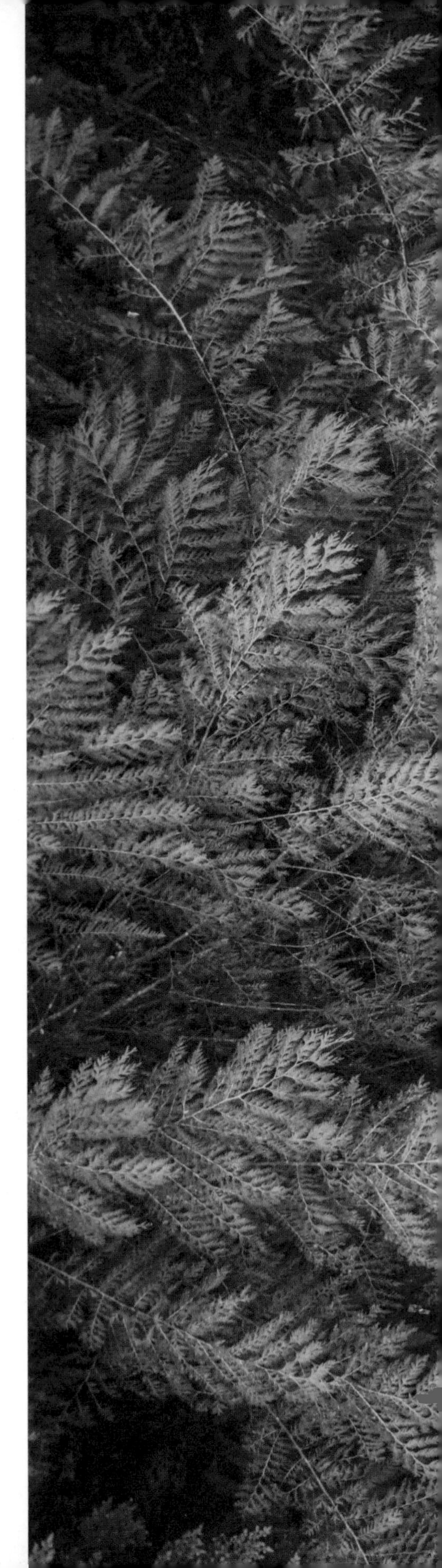

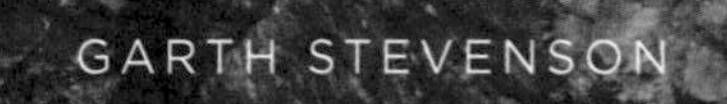
GARTH STEVENSON

distance: the wind coming from miles away then passing through the leaves one hundred feet above my head, the chipmunk twelve feet behind me, the bird up in the tree twenty feet to my left and another bird echoing a quarter mile to my right, the creek a wash of white noise in the gully below me. I listened to the ever-changing rhythm of the elements working together and independently. I found the best way to take it all in was to relax my mind and ears. This was my first experience meditating.

The next step was to pick up my bass and try to play something that fit into the already perfect sonic environment. At first it was almost impossible. Everything I played sounded forced and busy. I tried playing sparsely but it wasn't enough so I created a set of musical rules to follow as an exercise. For example: Play a high plucked harmonic each time the bird to my left sings and play a different note quietly when the bird a quarter mile away sings. Sometimes the birds would leave gaps of ten or twenty seconds between singing. Working within these restrictions helped me redefine my approach to sparseness. I realized in all my years of listening, I had never heard a piece of music with ten seconds of space or silence between notes. How could that be possible? Why not? Another exercise was to bow a note to match the length and volume of the incoming wind. This taught me to play as quietly as I could to match the dimension of the distant wind and brought awareness of how the length of notes could be stretched much further than I was used to.

Over the next ten years, I continued to deepen my practice in nature. I took my bass to the desert in Utah, to the Sierra Mountains, to the barren hills in Tuva just north of Mongolia, to the Falkland Islands, to sea for a month, and to Antarctica. Each location, with its unique set of natural sounds and landscapes, influenced the music in a new way. My interpretation of the thunderous avalanches in Antarctica, the electric-sounding cicadas in Japan, bullfrogs in Massachusetts percussing randomly then spontaneously joining in unison, and the windy hills in Tuva have all worked their way into my recordings. My goal is to create a listening experience similar to that in nature, with sounds moving across the aural spectrum from left ear to right and exploring depth of sound with some elements appearing to be in the foreground while others are in the distance. Occasionally I will incorporate my field recordings from nature into tracks. The sounds of bullfrogs on "Bear Swamp Pond" from the album *Alpine*, crickets on "Dusk" from the album *Flying*, and the ocean off Cape Cod on "Farewell" on my upcoming album.

Hiking into nature with my bass was always done alone until I started the morning meditation hikes at Wanderlust five years ago. As I hiked into the woods with my bass on my back and fifty hikers following close behind, I left the trail and started to improvise a route. It is easier to get lost and meditate in the experience if I'm not following a set route. The journey to the location is half the battle. Once I found a nice place for the group to sit I took my bass out of the case and began to focus on the natural sounds. It always takes me five or ten minutes to settle down and allow my awareness of the surroundings to be at its fullest, and I wanted to give everyone the same opportunity. Once the sound of the melting glacier, the birds singing, the wind overhead, and the flies buzzing started to sound like music instead of just ambient noise, I joined in with my bass. At first the music sounded imposed on the natural sounds, but after a few minutes it settled into a groove. This moment is where the meditation starts for me. If I stay present and continue to allow the moment to unfold, I can sustain the mediation. Many of the hikers came up to me afterward and told me they had reached a place of meditation as well. Chances are, we all found it at a different time. Some could have started on the hike in, others partway through the music, and some may have not meditated but simply enjoyed the experience. My goal isn't to teach others how to meditate, because I can't. All I can do is find my own way and allow others to do the same.

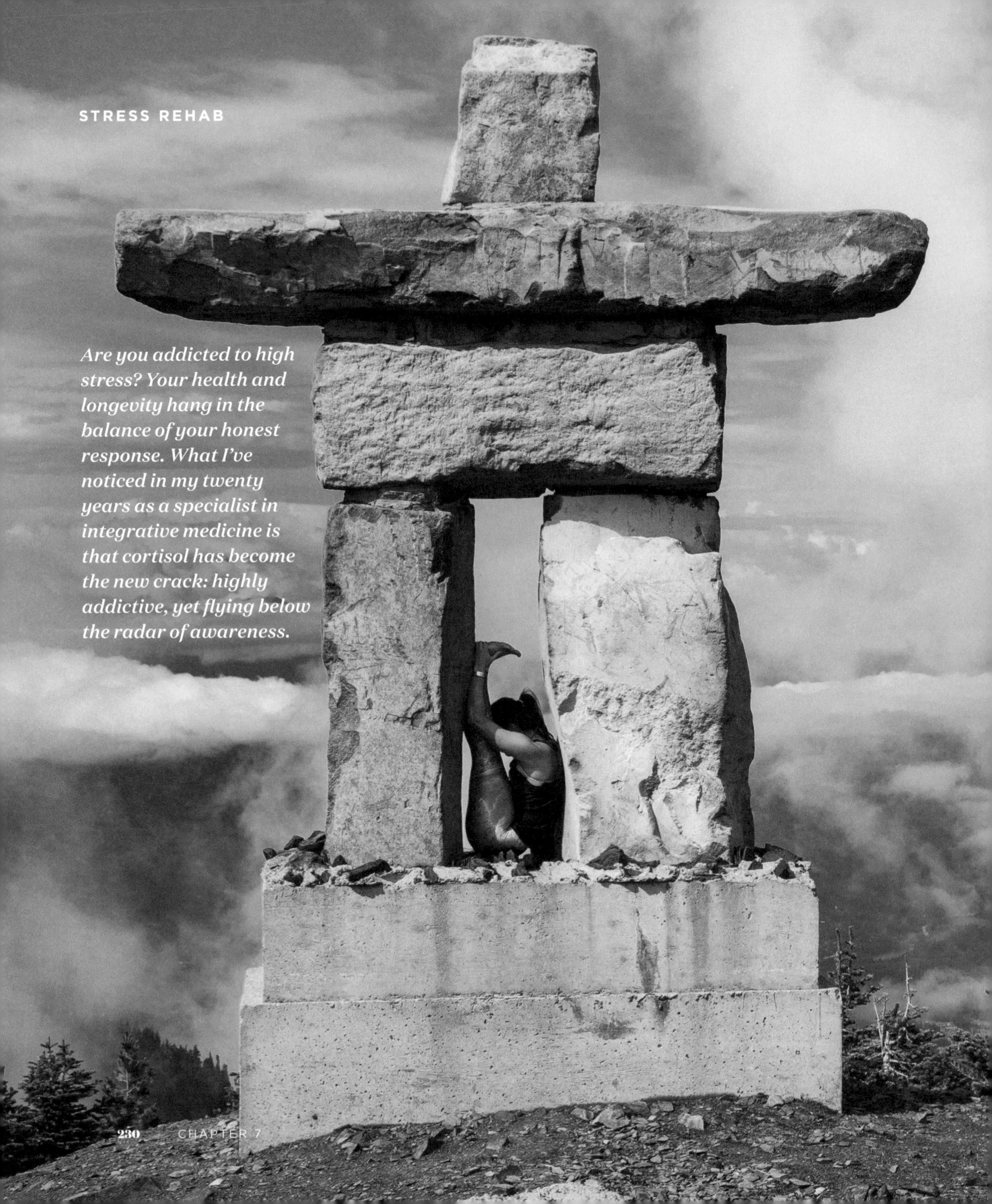

Are you addicted to high stress? Your health and longevity hang in the balance of your honest response. What I've noticed in my twenty years as a specialist in integrative medicine is that cortisol has become the new crack: highly addictive, yet flying below the radar of awareness.

SARA GOTTFRIED, MD

Chronic stress and its hormonal indicator—cortisol—can make you fat, cranky, and inflamed, or at minimum, can cause you to age faster than necessary. Mastering stress as a form of energy, rather than being bullied by it into addictive patterns, is the key to health, prosperity, longer life, and happier days. My mission is to offer novel ways to rehab your rhythm with stress so that there's a playful, hip-hop vibe to it, not the grim march through your twenties, thirties, and forties of racing from one task to the next.

Cortisol is the "fight or flight" hormone and it has a simple job: to get you out of a jam. If a tiger is about to charge you, cortisol raises your blood sugar, heart rate, and blood pressure, sending fresh blood to your muscles so you can either pick up a club and fight the tiger or run like crazy up the nearest tree.

But now many of us live our lives in a near constant state of fight or flight. More than 90 percent of the people who begin their work with me online tell me that cortisol is running the show, and they notice the telltale signs of wear and tear—the to-do list that's a mile long, the second wind at night and lack of sleep, the dependence on coffee, the feeling that they are tired but wired. Even worse, when unaware of the ravages of stress, many wear the busyness like a badge of honor. Our bodies are not set up to tolerate such a high level of unremitting stress. Ultimately, it can become addictive, as high cortisol establishes a new set point in your body, around which you organize the rest of your life.

Put another way, cortisol used to be on our team, and now it's working against us. Not convinced? Here are a few stats to illustrate the role of cortisol as bully:

Got moodiness? Half of people with depression have high cortisol from chronic stress—not surprisingly, high cortisol is associated with low levels of serotonin, the feel-good brain chemical in charge of mood, appetite, and sleep.

Got memory loss or out-of-control emotions? High cortisol shrinks the hippocampus, the part of your brain where you consolidate memory and regulate your emotions.

Got muffin top? High cortisol preferentially makes you store fat at your waistline and causes blood sugar to rise.

Got addictions? The most common ways to crank up cortisol are coffee and alcohol, our favorite psychoactive and addictive drugs.

Just as you can be addicted to meth or heroin, you can be addicted to high cortisol and thereby enable the bully. The signs of addiction are often more subtle than track marks: Perhaps you have workaholism, or just feel chronically depleted from working so hard or giving so much, or you are experiencing wandering attention.

Maybe you have the usual response to your addiction to cortisol: You're in denial. You're thinking, "Yeah, yeah, but I don't have a problem with stress."

Think again. Cortisol is insidious in how it wreaks havoc and creates collateral damage. Beyond feeling tired but wired or getting a second wind at night, here are a few questions to gauge your addiction to cortisol:

Do you have drama in your life—such as your relationship with your partner or your mother or work colleagues? If you have a period of smooth sailing, do you feel bored?

Do you need to exercise to self-regulate? Do you feel out of sorts when you don't get your gym time in?

If you have a day where you are completely unscheduled, do you feel uneasy, maybe anxious—and rush to fill it in?

How's your sex drive? Would you rather get work done than revel in carnal pleasures?

What I learned in my midthirties is that I had to rehabilitate cortisol. I needed to step up to the fact that high cortisol was acting like a mean girl in my body, and to own my part in the various ways, conscious and unconscious, I was feeding my addiction to high-stress living. Unfortunately, when I went to my doctor for help, I was stunned by his lack of insight. I was the woman sitting in the exam room shivering in the pathetic exam gown—explaining to my doctor about how, at thirty-five years of age, I couldn't lose weight, had no sex drive, and was irritable most the time, especially the week before my period. He suggested an antidepressant and a birth control pill, and told me to exercise more, eat less, and reduce stress.

I had a hunch that my doctor's suggestions were completely wrong, and I decided to look for real solutions. My hypothesis was that my problems were hormonal. After all, I'm a gynecologist and think about hormones all day.

Here's the shocking part: When I measured my level of cortisol, the hormone secreted by the adrenal glands, I was stunned to find it was triple what it was supposed to be.

I was addicted to cortisol, and it took me four weeks to kick the habit. I didn't need an antidepressant—I needed the secret sauce of the cortisol rehab. I was a runner, which raises cortisol—and I needed to run differently. I needed adaptive exercise, like yoga and Pilates. I started taking natural supplements to help lower cortisol, like phosphatidylserine.

I hit the pause button, and it worked. If you're addicted to cortisol and need rehab, you can too. It starts with looking at the most important points of leverage in breaking the addiction to cortisol, which involves the way you eat, drink, move, and supplement.

Here are my top five ways to rehab cortisol and get recentered, with cortisol in its sweet spot of not too high and not too low.

1. Start with an easy win: Take phosphatidylserine 400 mg per day.

2. Willpower is strongest in the morning: Institute a morning practice of at least seven minutes' duration and perform diaphragmatic breathing—used in yoga, meditation, and tai chi, and involving the deep inhale of air into your upper and lower lungs while allowing the belly to expand. It's been shown to lower stress and cortisol and raise melatonin, another important hormone of the body's inner clock. My favorites are listed at thehormonecurebook.com/destress.

3. Cut back on the cortisol-raising drinks: anything with caffeine or alcohol. The greatest health benefits come from moderate consumption of green tea (but avoid caffeine if you have sleep issues) and drinking three servings or less of alcohol each week. The irony of caffeine is that it only has short-term benefit; long term, it will make you more tired and addicted to cortisol.

4. Master your sleep. When you're off caffeine, you may sleep an extra hour or two per night, which you need to perform the adrenal repair of high-stress living. Wear a tracker, such as the Up or Fitbit, to track your deep sleep and improve it over time.

5. Enlist your besties. Make a public proclamation to your best friends that you need to be held accountable to your cortisol recovery. No more offers of sugary treats, no more girls' night out for sweet cocktails, no more late nights. Get them on your side to amplify your recovery.

There's a large gap between what conventional medicine offers people who are stressed out and addicted to cortisol, and what they most want and need. Start by getting cortisol into its rightful place—what I call the Goldilocks position of just right for you. High cortisol disrupts your other hormones, including the delicate estrogen/progesterone balance and slows down your thyroid and testosterone production. Once you get cortisol under control—and it doesn't take too long—then start working with the sexier hormones, like thyroid and testosterone.

Don't let cortisol run your show. Unlock your greatness by mastering your navigation of the main stress hormone.

find your center

SCHUYLER GRANT

Your center, your abdomen, separates earth and sky energies (prana and apana). It is the physical point from which you can manifest sublime balance if you tap into equal amounts of effort and grace, strength and surrender (sthiram and sukham).

practice one

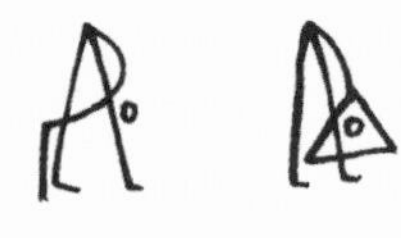

Start in a wide UTTANASANA. *Feet mat distance apart, holding opposite elbow tip.*

WIDE PARSVOTTANASANA *Foot is still outside hand.*

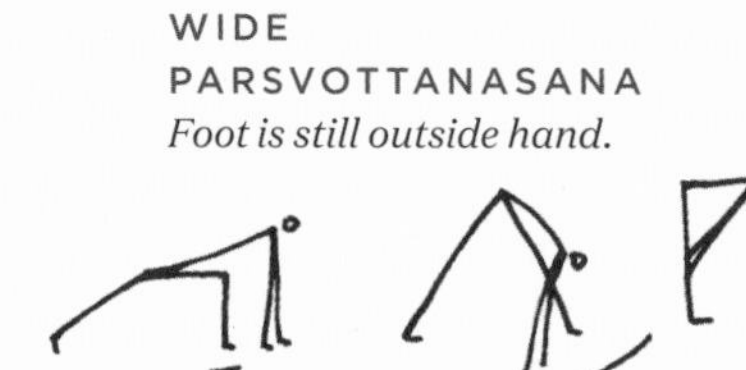

Bring your fingertips to the floor and step your right leg back into a WIDE LUNGE. *Your right foot is outside your right hand.*

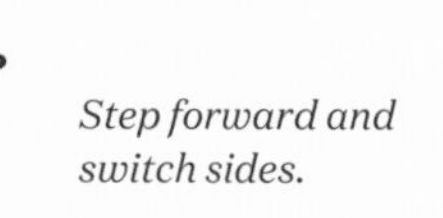

Take 8-16 BREATHS

Step forward and switch sides.

Root up to stand

My power comes from my center.
My receptivity comes from my center.
I am strong. I am soft. I am centered.
Sthira Sukham Asanam.

uddiyana bandha kriya

There are a few important points to remember in the practice of UDDIYANA BANDHA (AUB)*: Perform it only on an empty stomach, and only after an exhalation, never during an inhalation. The first key to practicing this kriya is the ability to completely soften your belly. If you find it impossible to do that, it will be difficult to access the full depth of the practice; you may want to spend some weeks/months opening your abdominal muscles through massage and conscious relaxation.*

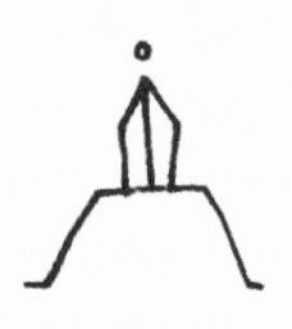

Stand with your feet wider than hip distance, knees bent and turned out over your feet.

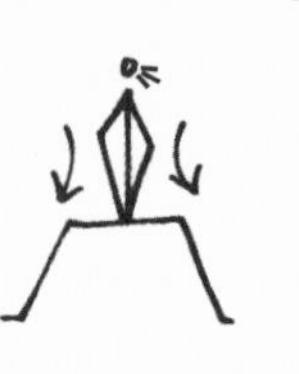

Inhale deeply through your nose, then exhale quickly and forcibly through your nose (or pursed lips), bringing your hands to rest on your thighs. Contract your abdominal muscles fully to push as much air as possible out of your lungs. Then completely relax your abdominals.

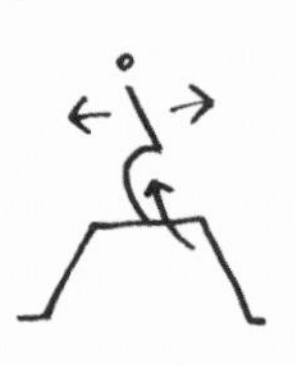

*Perform what's called a "*MOCK INHALATION*"; that is, expand your rib cage (thorax) as if you were inhaling, but don't actually inhale. The expansion of the rib cage (without the inhalation) sucks the abdominal muscles and viscera up into the thorax, creating a deep well in the lower belly.*

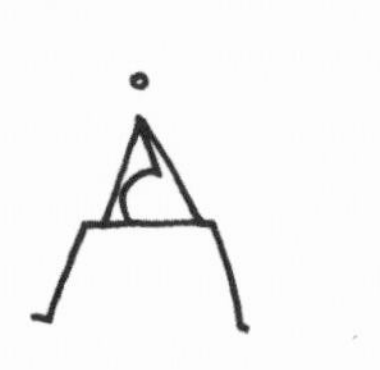

The pelvis may be flexed, tucked, or neutral, but I find a slight tuck to the tailbone is helpful. During the time you retain UDDIYANA BANDHA, *also perform a light* JALANDHARA BANDHA. *Hold the bandha for* 5-15 SECONDS, *or only as long as is comfortable. FIRST, release the action of your ribs and diaphragm and THEN inhale normally, coming up to stand.*

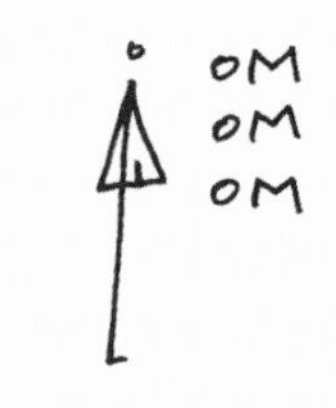

Take a breath or two in between and repeat 8-16 TIMES *total. Chanting of* OM***x3*** *standing in* TADASANA, *feet together, hands in* ANJALI MUDRA.

wave one *I suggest that for the first round, you hold each posture for* 3–8 BREATHS, *then cycle through the sequence as a vinyasa* ***1 or more times.***

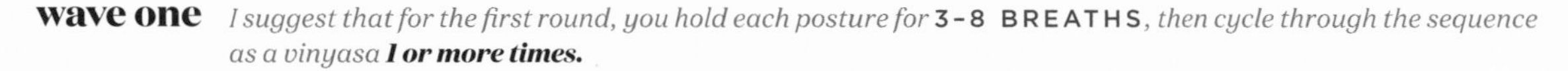

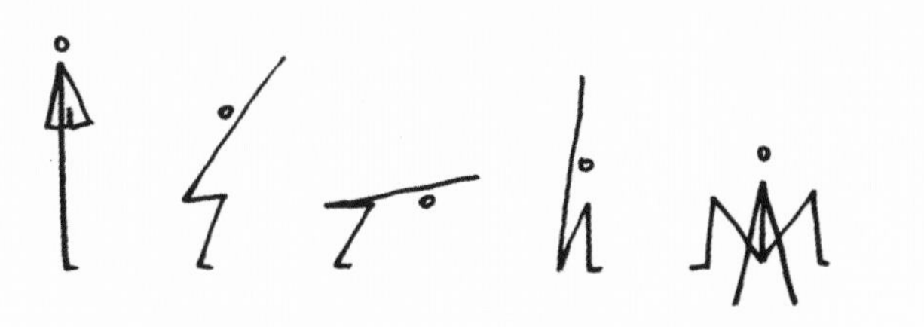

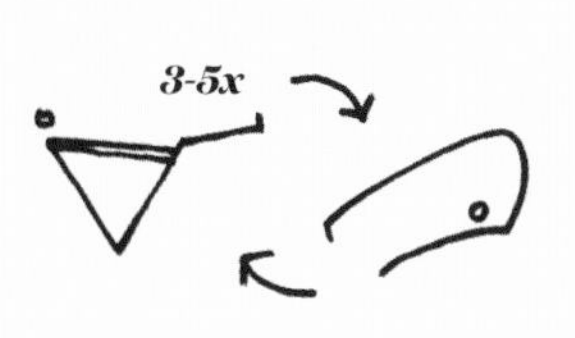

From TADASANA *inhale to* UTKATASANA. *Exhaling, pass through* ARDHA UTKATASANA.

Inhale into MALASANA. *Reach your fingertips on the floor in front of you and relax your neck completely.*

Inhaling, reach your arms strongly straight forward, engage your belly, and, exhaling, slowly lower your sitbones to the floor, coming into BENT KNEE NAVASANA.

Slowly, using your abdominals and the reach forward of your arms to control the transition, roll onto your back and come into a MODIFIED HALASANA. *In this variation, allow your spine to round. You may have your arms on the floor in line with your ears or on the floor facing the front of your mat—whichever will give you more support.*

Feel the ebb and flow of your abdominal muscles in between your thighs.

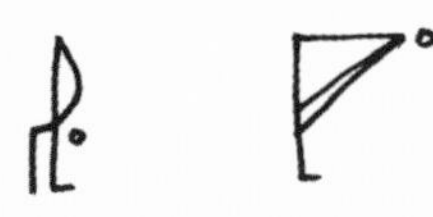

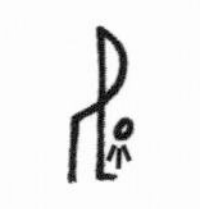

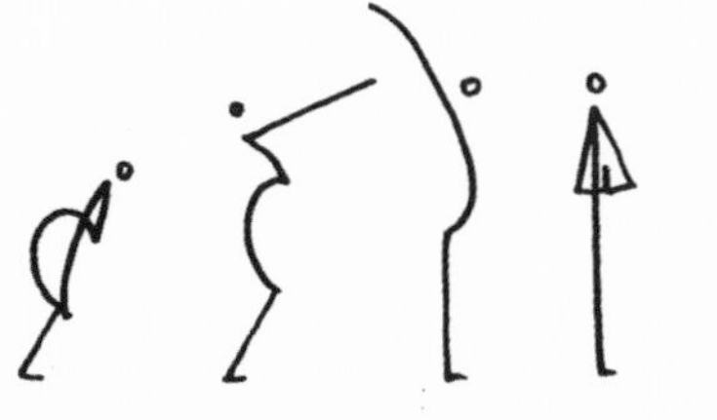

Exhaling, land in TADASANA. *Repeat 1-3x.*

Exhale on your feet in UTTANASANA. *You may find that you need to use your hand on the floor to help you get there at first. Inhale to* ARDHA UTTANASANA. *Exhale completely out the nose or the mouth, coming back to* UTTANASANA.

MOCK INHALE

On the retention empty, engage AUB, *bend your knees generously, and slowly round up to stand, allowing your neck and shoulders to relax completely in this transition. Breathe in when you are about three-quarters of the way upright. Finally arrive in* URDHVA HASTASANA.

wave two *Take* ***3–5 rounds*** *of* SURYA NAMASKA A.

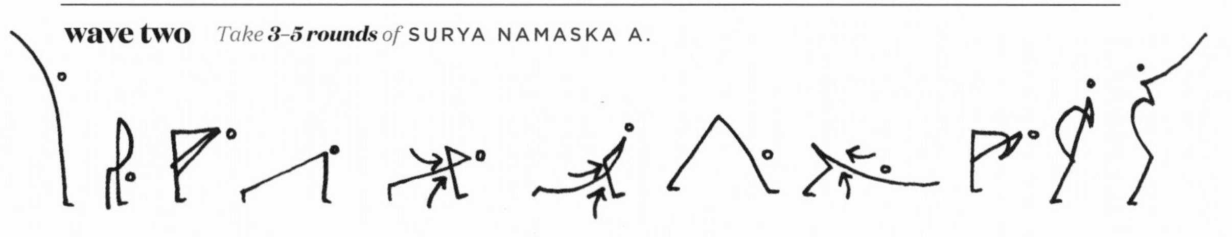

Specific things to remember in this sun salutation practice:

When lowering to CHATURANGA, *remember to hug the abdomen cylindrically and try to maintain as much of that core support as you can when coming into* URDHVA MUKHA SVANASANA.

If you jump forward from ADHO MUKHA SVANASANA *to* UTTANASANA, *try doing so on the retention of your exhalation, with* AUB *engaged. Transition is initiated more from the strength of your belly than the spring off your legs. Focus on using your deeply engaged abdominal to pull your pelvis over your fingernails to lightly land your feet toward your hands.*

Finally, after coming into ARDHA UTTANASANA, *strongly exhale out the nose or mouth, engage* AUB *and HINGE up to stand, on the retention empty, breathing in when you arrive in* URDHVA HASTASANA. *End in* TADASANA.

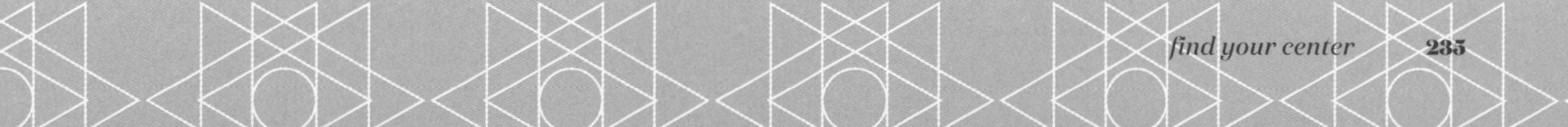

wave three

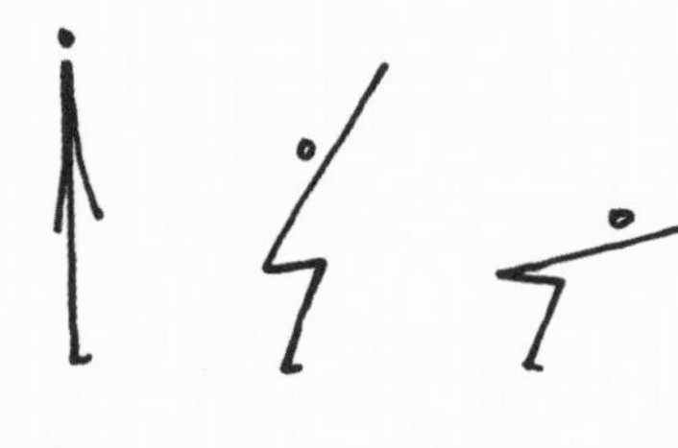

From TADASANA in. to full UTKATASANA

Ex. pass through ARDHA UTKATASANA

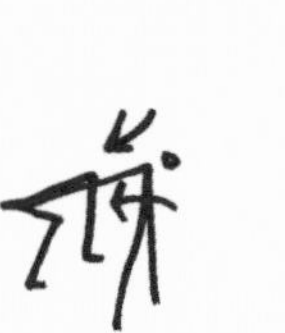

In. transition open your knees shoulder distance apart, lift high on the balls of your feet, hands shoulder distance apart. Ex. prepare for BAKASANA, and on the retention empty, engage AUB and come into the pose.

Express the pose.

In. drop the right foot to the floor a foot or so behind your right wrist and come into ARDHA CHANDRASANA.

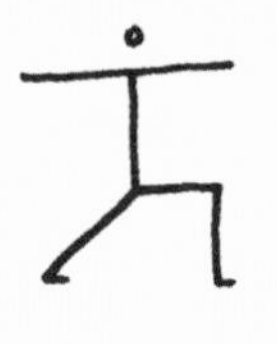

In. / ex. VIRABHADRASANA II

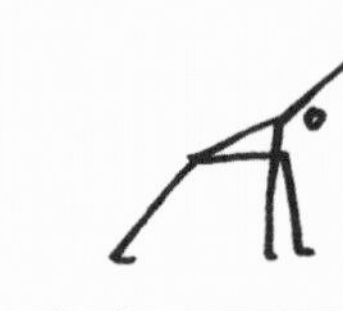

In. / ex. REVERSE TRIKONASANA

In. / ex. UTTHITA PARSVAKONASANA

In. LOW LUNGE

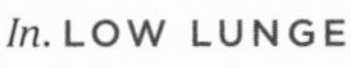

Ex. ANJANEYASNANA

In. / ex. twist to the right in a MODIFIED PARIVRTTA PARSVAKONASANA

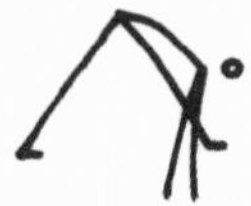

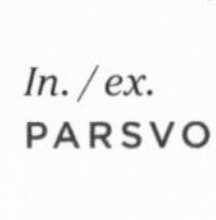

In. / ex. PARSVOTTANASANA

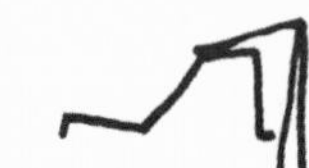

In. through LOW LUNGE

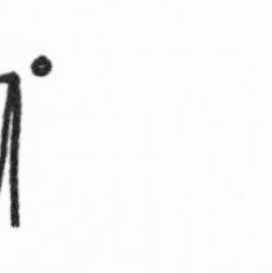

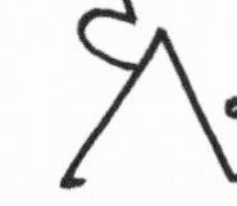

Ex. to DOWN DOG SPLIT

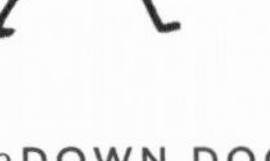

In./ex. bend the right knee and open the hip into a soft backbend (by lifting up onto your right fingertips you will deepen the stretch of your right sidebody).

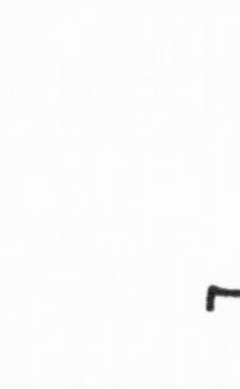

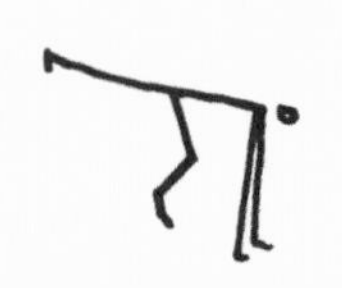

In. step your right foot halfway forward on your mat, landing high on the ball of the foot with the knee bent, lift your left leg in the air, leg straight, hips square.

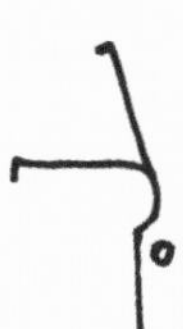

Ex. bring your shoulders way forward out in front of your hands and on the retention empty, engage AUB and come SPLIT HANDSTAND. The final pose should look like a VIRABHADRASNA III on your hands.

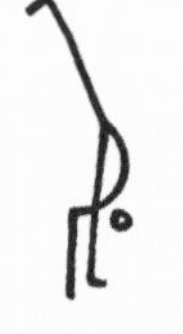

In. land (or lightly hop if you don't catch the split handstand) into a STANDING SPLIT on your right foot. Ex. deepen the forward bend in STANDING SPLIT.

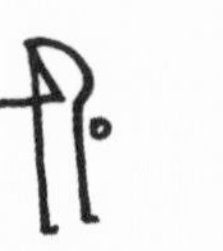

In. tuck your left knee into your nose, lifting onto the ball of your right foot and bending the right knee a little.

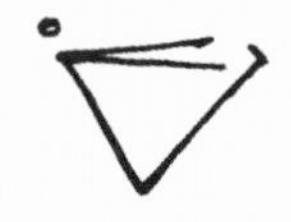

Ex shoot your left leg forward and move toward NAVASANA, this time with your legs straight if that is possible with integrity in your spine.

In. HALASANA, Ex. NAVASANA, knees bent in. back into HALASANA, Ex. all the way on your feet in UTTANASANA.

In. ARDHA UTTANASANA.

Exhale completely back to UTTANASANA.

On the retention empty, catch AUB, and round up to UTKATASANA, inhaling when you arrive. Ex., land in TADASANA. Repeat on the Left side. Take the whole wave three, **2–3 times.**

NOTE: *Remember, when breathing rhythmically—without retention—the inhalation is the slow transition into the asana and the exhalation expresses the pose, but there is nothing static about this practice—think of it more as a series of precise transitions rather than a series of linked postures.*

From standing take UDDIYANA BANDHA KRIYA ***8–16 times*** *(for students familiar with the practices of* AGNI SARA *or* NAULIS*—these may be explored at this time as well).*

Practice Playlist

compiled by Kelly Casey

Holocene (Kyson Mix)—*Bon Iver*

Dream Machine (Kaskade Mix)—*Mark Farina*

Manhattan—*Slow Magic*

Too Much to Lose (Niva Mix)—*Sun Glitters*

Greenland—*Emancipator*

Skyline—*Matt Balzan*

Jetstream—*Luisine*

The Light—*The Album Leaf*

suggested closing postures

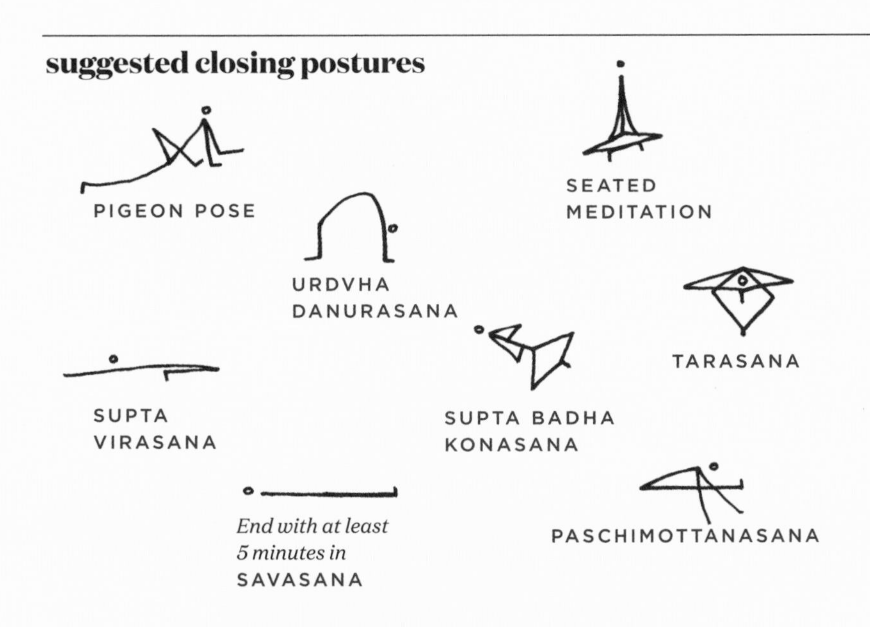

End with at least 5 minutes in SAVASANA

In SAVASANA *if—or should I say when—your mind wanders, take your attention back to the soft, watery quality of your belly. Feel how the breath gently washes your relaxed abdomen around your pelvic bowl and your rib basket. Allow the seat of your emotional heart to be completely open and receptive.* ***3x Chant Om.*** NAMASTE

Always we hope someone has the answer,

Some other place will be better,

Some other time, it will all turn out.

This is it.

No one else has the answer,

No other place will be better

It has already turned out.

At the center of your being you have such answers,

You know who you are.

And you know what you want.

There is no need to run outside for better seeing.

Nor to peer from a window.

Rather, abide at the center of your being.

For the more you leave it, the less you learn.

—LAO TZU

It's time to make your own life mandala, a map of the landscape of your self, and the areas that might still need to be discovered, supported, or reinvented. The ultimate goal is to create a vibrantly and fully colored life mandala representing a balanced lifestyle with an awareness of the interrelationship of all the elements of our lives.

At the center of your being you have the answer; you know who you are and you know what you want.

—Lao Tzu

Your Life Mandala

DURATION:
Thirty minutes

LOCATION:
Quiet place

MINDSET:
Present

TOOLS:
Markers, crayons, colored pencils

1. Write a list of the main aspects of your life. For example, family, health/exercise, work, spirituality, community, romance, home.

2. Next, label one section for each aspect. You can also go online and find some images of basic mandalas to adapt, or create a pattern of connecting shapes that form a larger circle.

3. Take a few minutes to reflect on each topic and write a short paragraph outlining the present state of these aspects of your life.

4. Return to page 239 and choose one color for each area of your life and color in the sections that feel whole and nourished.
5. What areas are still white? Reflect on whether these areas are calling for more attention and energy to bring balance to your life, and write down three things you can do to fill them up. For example, if finance is blank, make a budget, or if family is empty, pick up the phone to call a loved one.
6. Come back to your mandala week after week to color in the empty spaces and fill your mandala, and your life, with vibrancy and color.

7. Once your mandala is complete, write down what changed, and how your day-to-day life is different.

Achieving balance, whether in a yoga pose or in your life, is only accomplished through the perpetual and ceaseless desire and effort to find and maintain it.

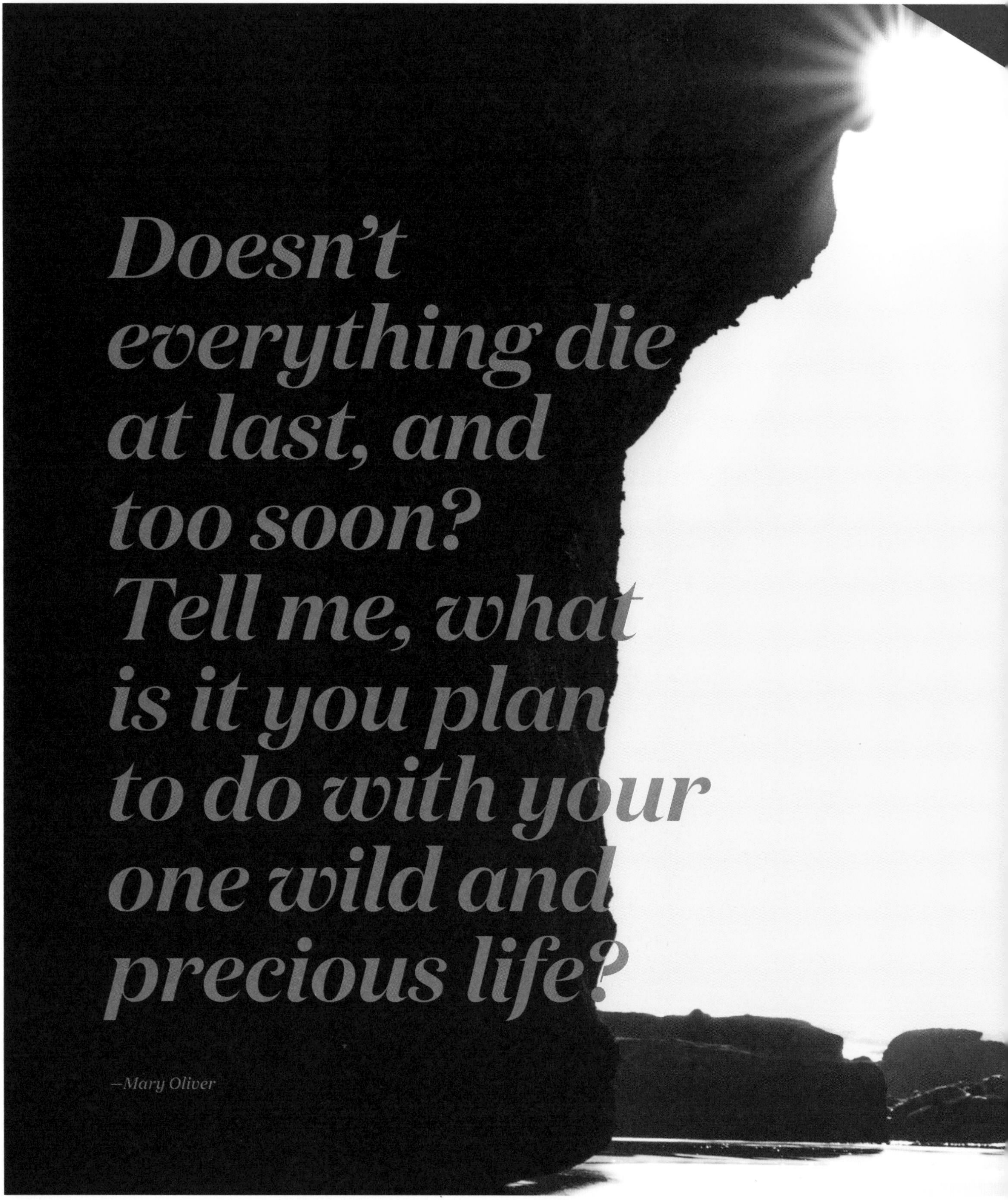

Doesn't everything die at last, and too soon? Tell me, what is it you plan to do with your one wild and precious life?

—Mary Oliver

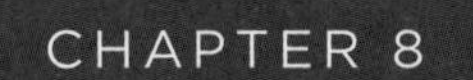

CHAPTER 8

find your true north

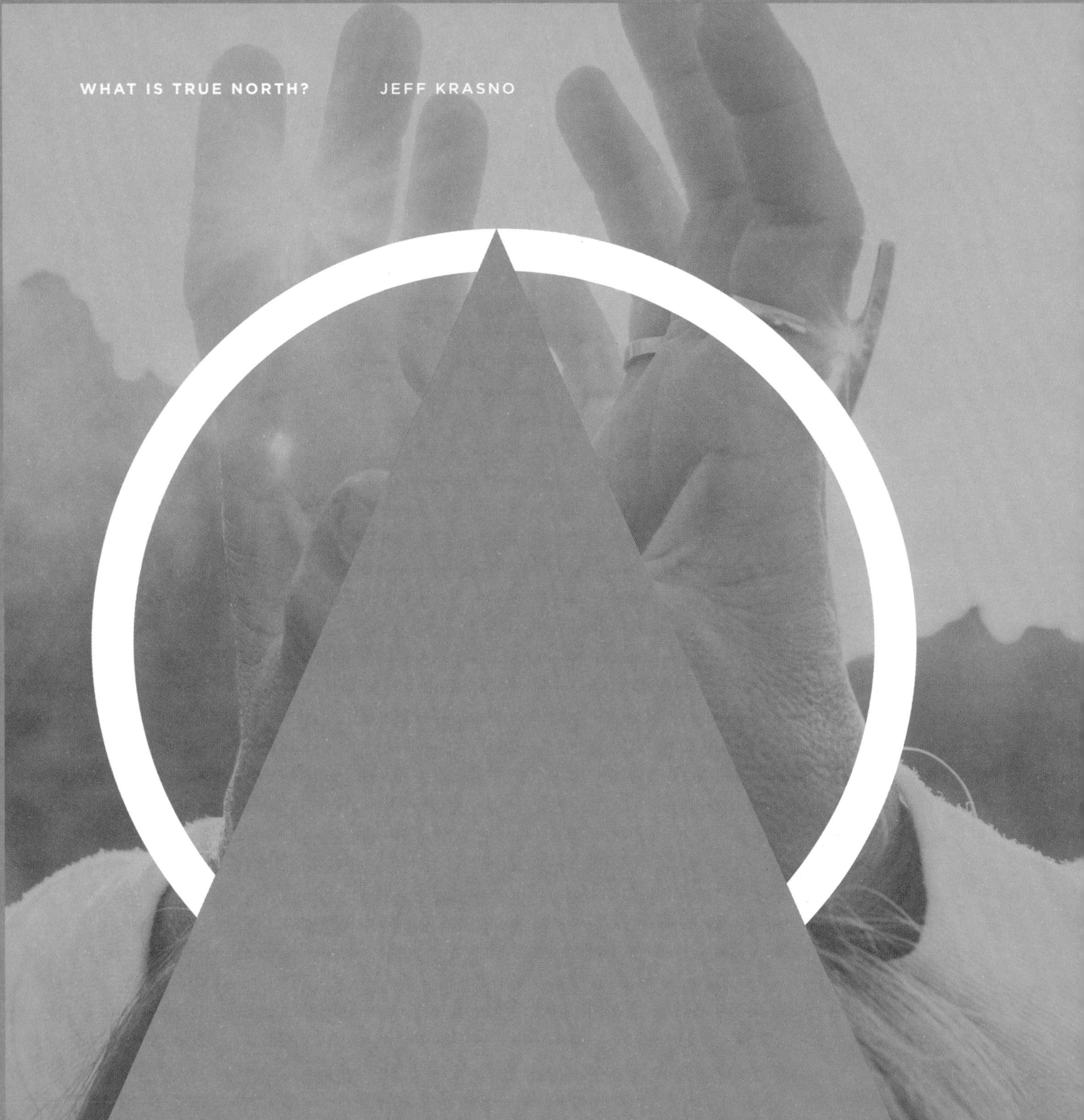

In 2008, amid a heated presidential primary, then-senator Obama delivered one of his most eloquent speeches, focused on the inflammatory issue of race relations in the United States. Obama described the history of the African American struggle from slavery to Jim Crow, from segregation to the civil rights movement, from the voting rights bill to the present day of income stratification.

Through our messy civil rights legacy of debate, tumult, violence, and bravery—the answer to our problems was always there in these words, "We hold these truths to be self-evident, that all men are created equal, that they are endowed by their Creator with certain unalienable rights, that among these are life, liberty, and the pursuit of happiness." Our Declaration of Independence, composed by those who deeply understood the core values of a civil society and who held a passionate vision for what the world could become, set us on the course to become our best selves as a nation. Our founding document gave America its true north.

As individuals, we each have our own Declaration of Independence, a succinct understanding of our core values that shapes our moral compass. Our true north is the continuous practice of these values. True north is not a place. It's a journey, a process for living. Through greed, expediency, ignorance, and carelessness, it is easy to drift off course. A few degrees can drastically alter our trajectory the farther we go, so we continually navigate, resetting our compass. Through our practice, we continue to hone our course.

Our journey outward is mirrored by our search inward. As we explore the world, we look deeper into ourselves to uncover these truths that we hold self-evident, truths that provide the coordinates for our true north. We crystallize the contents of our own personal founding document. You may even want to write it down.

I hope the content of this book provides gems of wisdom that help you (re)discover in some ways what you already know, and that the many visionaries who have contributed provide practices to keep you on course. As with our country, it is the practice of what we already innately know that will lead us toward our best selves, toward an enlightened life characterized by love and compassion.

When it comes your time to die, be not like those whose hearts are filled with the fear of death, so that when their time comes they weep and pray for a little more time to live their lives over again in a different way. Sing your death song and die like a hero going home.

—Tecumseh, Shawnee 1768–1813

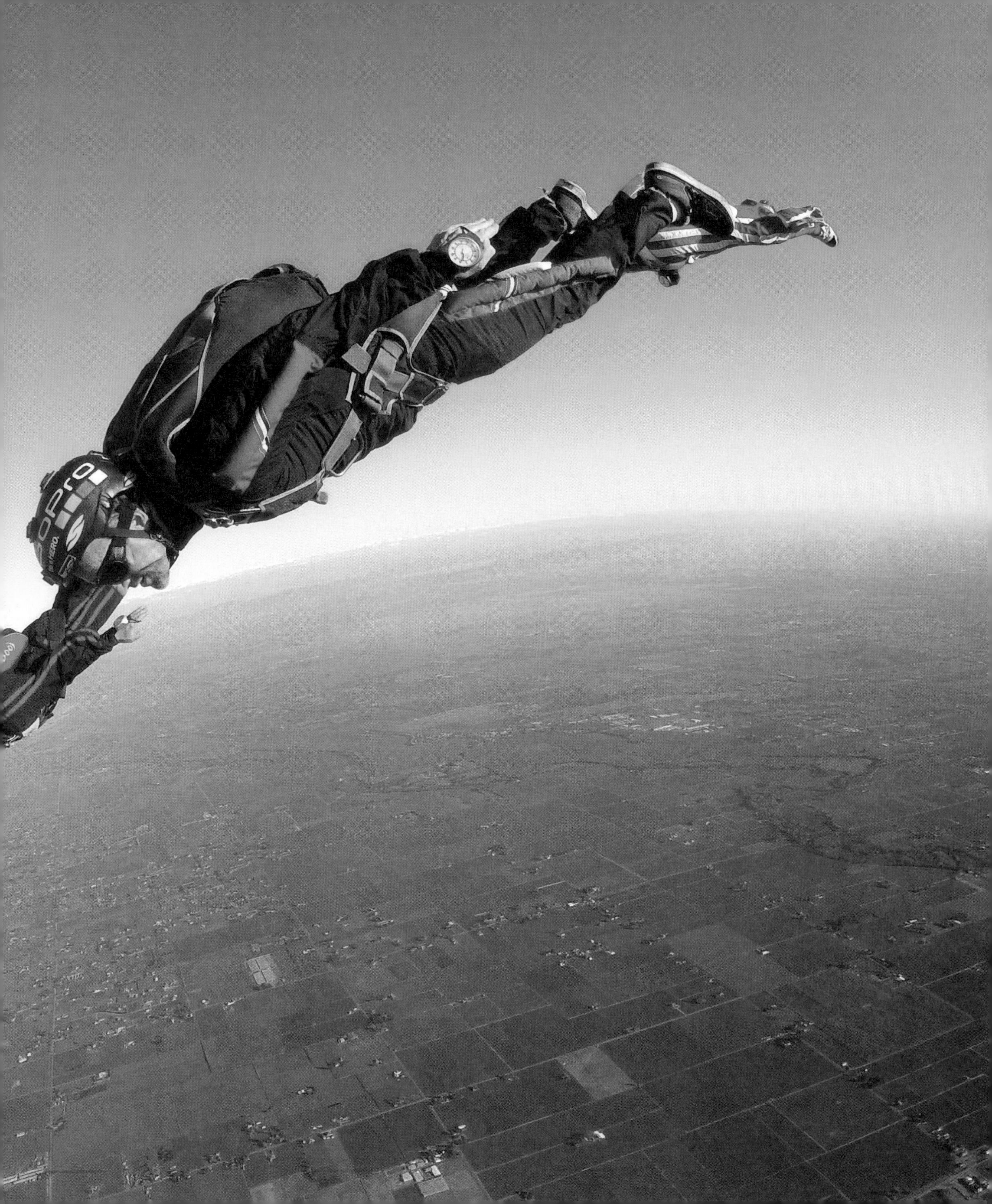

I had a death song. It came to me after I looked down at my arm, mangled, detached from my body, and bleeding. I sang this death song as I reconciled and made peace with dying, thought profoundly of my incredible wife and my three extraordinary children, recalled a truly remarkable life, and prepared to pass. Yet, my death song became the narrative for my living that afternoon.

On a warm, breezy day in October, I was skydiving with two good friends and with the classic three or four discrete things going the wrong way in a sequence, I ended up having to land, downwind, in a vineyard. As I was making my final maneuvers, one of the posts used to support the vines violently took my right arm, and I knelt there alone for fifteen minutes, bleeding out as the great song written by Eddie Vedder, "Just Breathe," came to my mind to help me cope.

The first line of the song is, "Yes, I understand every life must end. As we sit alone, I know someday we must go." My training and experience as a backcountry ranger in Rocky Mountain National Park included many high-angle rescues, each with its own iteration of trauma, and volunteering on a fire and ambulance crew in a very rural part of northwestern Colorado had me sadly seeing and working with more. All of that experience afforded me many things that day, including the plain self-assessment that I was in a very rough patch; that it was unlikely that I would live more than another ten minutes; that making it through the afternoon would bring with it a substantially changed life; that to live would take being at peace with death and reflecting calmly on my life and what I had learned. Yes, in that situation, all of this could be and was accomplished in a very short but torturously long fifteen minutes.

I survived that afternoon. I survived. There's a fair amount of power to those words for me. A fellow skydiver came to me, and I instructed her on how to apply a tourniquet. Over the course of twenty-one surgeries performed by a few very remarkable and talented surgeons, my arm was also saved. Now, four months from that afternoon, two of which were spent in the hospital, my world is physical therapy and work, and is lived with a very consistent sense of true gratitude.

I used that word in the past with such fleeting recognition of what it meant. "Sure, yes, of course I am grateful. . . . " Now, it's become such a powerful, profound, and deep current in my life and my work. In life we can learn how to do things from others—their words, their motion—and who we are can be so profoundly shaped by things that happen to us, people, our surroundings, and who we chose to be.

What was the meaning of all of this? What was the universe offering me?

During a recent press interview on the accident, I was asked, "After dancing with death and surviving, what have been your epiphanies . . . your big life 'ahas'?" This was a fair question to which I had no response. I didn't remember dancing with anyone or anything. For a moment I felt bad . . . like I'd missed a question on a test that I shouldn't have missed. With no forethought whatsoever, I then responded, "I am still surrounded by this. I am only living in the wonderful grace of this very moment. I'll not put away or deny what happened, but I am choosing to live . . . now. Gratitude, in its purest and nonconditioned form, can be so astonishingly powerful. I am alive and so very grateful. That is all I can say as to what I've learned and how this has shaped me."

I put my wife, family, and friends through hell. Very late one night while in the ICU, my oldest son temporarily relieved my wife of her fierce commitment to be with me through every moment and each night. I had multiple IVs in my neck and arm, drainage tubes everywhere it seemed. I was still bleeding from the various donor sites for arteries, muscle, and skin; machines attached to me were always beeping (thankfully!); and I was consistently going from shivering to being overheated. It was truly miserable. My son chose to hold my hand for quite a while, smiled, and then said to me, "You are one tough son of a bitch." He said it with the voice of John Wayne, but with such love and profound gratitude. At that moment, the pain disappeared and I realized how much he and my other two kids meant to me. I'd always loved them, but that very moment came to me a powerful wave of pure love for them, my wife, and my life. A few weeks earlier, I was treasuring their memory; now, I very deeply understood and was so thankful for their presence in my life.

I never really feared dying before this accident; I just never considered it. Now, I consider but don't fear death in any way. Gratitude is a common denominator that can bring us together, regardless of our faith or beliefs. True gratitude can bring freedom and clarity.

I had a death song.

So live your life that the fear of death can never enter your heart. Trouble no one about their religion; respect others in their view, and demand that they respect yours. Love your life, perfect your life, beautify all things in your life. Seek to make your life long and its purpose in the service of your people. Prepare a noble death song for the day when you go over the great divide.

—Tecumseh, Shawnee

One morning in September, I woke up at the crack of dawn, threw on my pantsuit and pumps (for real) and sped in to work. I clocked an eight-minute mile in heels down Madison Avenue, barking into my cell phone and taking everyone out in the process. This morning, in particular, I was on a mission because I had just come off a vacation for my anniversary so I was "fresh," if you can imagine. My storm had some extra power.

This was not unusual for me at the time. I was an overachiever: performing, pleasing, perfecting.

But little did I know that everything was about to change.

One hour into my morning, the first plane hit Tower 2. When I heard the second plane, which was flying abnormally low over the city, I knew that I was about to experience a disruption of epic proportions—I just didn't know how yet.

My stepdad was a fireman but wasn't scheduled to work. However, he had volunteered to work so that he could come out to a family dinner for my anniversary that night. His was the second firehouse to respond to the attacks.

After the attack, we searched for him, we grasped for hope. But he was gone. He died when the first tower collapsed. We recovered recordings of his radio conversations and realized he made it up seventy-eight floors and saved countless people before dying himself.

As you can imagine, everything I knew to be normal and real came crashing down with those towers. I was changed forever. My immediate reaction was to fix the situation, fix something. I gripped onto the part of me that wanted to "make it right" (the arrogance—I actually thought I could fix that moment), but it was all that I knew that could get me through each day. It was my coping mechanism—"when things feel out of control, control them." It wasn't pretty—my family did not like me, my husband was ready to leave me, and I was one breath away from a nervous breakdown.

Enter yoga.

While the city was offering "survivors" everything from therapy to acupuncture to spa treatments to writing workshops to laugh therapy to help us, nothing could crack me. Except yoga. Yoga started as a place just to feel more strong and flexible. But soon, my time on the mat was the ONLY time I was able to feel the full impact of what had happened. The more I moved, the more I was able to unpack the armor and confront the shittiness of that moment, instead of avoiding, fixing, busying. I started to let myself feel on the mat. And it wasn't pretty at first, but I knew it was real. And so I stuck with it.

I discovered that my grief was in my body. There was no way I could have talked or fixed my way into healing. The body was a critical component of my work around 9/11. The practice became for me an oasis, a safe space, to get dark. To confront the horror of that event. The chaos of my life. The crisis in my family. It helped me see clearly my shadow and shift out of my pattern, my armor, my role, and into the truth of what happened. And I learned a lot in that moment of how truth isn't pretty, but essential.

I learned that yoga is a deliberate disruption on every level. It works to disorient the body in a safe space so that you can learn how to ride and navigate the flow. It turns you inside out and upside down so that you can get a new perspective on the world. And in doing this, you build a capacity to cope and respond to the chaos of each moment. In confronting your shit head-on, new pathways toward change reveal themselves. And I think that is what surprised me most . . . that it was not only the profound healing that I discovered through my practice . . . but a huge awakening as well.

Out of that disruption I leapt. I wasn't sure exactly where I was going or what I was going to do, but I knew that as long as I practiced and continued on this path of healing and purpose, I was moving in the right direction. I saw that my life was meant for others, to help and to share.

Once you begin to feel what your true north is, you can use it to serve, to help others and illuminate their paths.

Leadership comes from always orienting around our authentic purpose. When you are in full alignment with your purpose (true north), your expression flows from that place, your actions match your words, and your impact is both significant and sustainable.

This leadership methodology is accessible to ALL who dare to go deep, to uncover the hidden truth, and to courageously live their purpose in the world.

For me, it took the inner hard work of navigating toward my own true north and healing to really begin to serve. But out of that place within, I began to work for Off the Mat, Into the World and help develop the voices of other leaders.

My Story

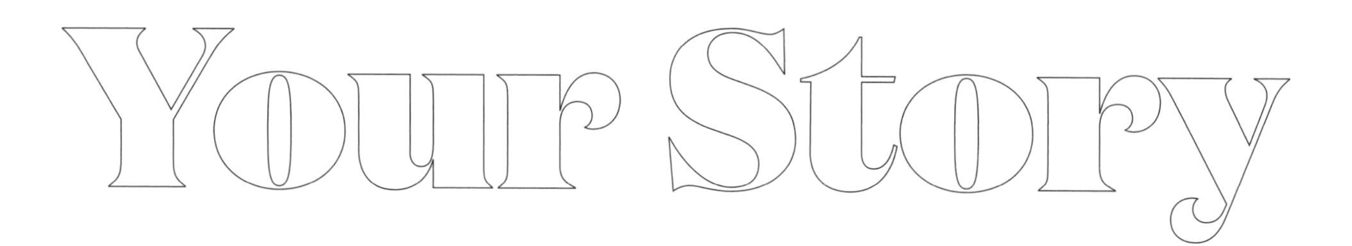

When you embody what is authentic to YOU and what gives you JOY, you move and give and express from a source that is infinite. Your purpose is your power, and if you can learn to live from that place, not only will you serve well, but you will be served.

PURPOSE AS COMPASS

Purpose is not a destination, but a GPS system or a compass. The idea is to maintain a sense of direction, like true north, rather than strive or attach to a specific goal or destination. It is a guiding force that continuously aligns us and our efforts. And when you are clear about your purpose, you can make right decisions about what to say yes to and how to take the next best step. It all comes back to purpose, because at the end of the day, we really can't know what is next, we can only know what is now and who we are. That is what we have to work with. So the more you refine this tool of purpose . . . the more it will lead you into what is next.

What are you GREAT at? Don't be shy. Everyone has a "special sauce."

Good listener

Strategic

Facilitator

Enthusiastic

Motivator

Intuitive

Project manager

Detail oriented

Funny

Intelligent

Storyteller

Receptive

Speaker

Change management

What do you LOVE to do? Seriously . . . the thing you would do for free for the rest of your life.

Dancing

Coaching

Teaching

Writing

Singing

Serving

Parenting

Litigating

Designing

Collaborating

Traveling

Baking

What is your vision for change in the world? Think BIG. What is the world that you want to live in? That you want to leave your children? Does it have to do with restoring our environment? Or reclaiming our food? Does it look like a healthy democracy? How do you want to be a part of making that possible?

Our thoughts limit what we're capable of doing. There are external forces arrayed against us, but there are also internal forces that sabotage us before we even get started. Our mind is good at setting us up for failure and getting us to think small. But I have found that we will do for love that which we don't think is possible. So the question to ask ourselves is "What do I love?"

—Julia Butterfly Hill

I found yoga in my early twenties in an attempt to alleviate my chronic lower-back pain. The practice of healing myself physically has been ever evolving—sometimes frustrating, but never boring—for over two decades. Yoga seduced me early on with arm balancing; this practice came easily to me, and I relished the experience of feeling like a kid frolicking in the grass. But it was in my struggle during the last ten minutes of class, the practices of undoing, that yoga found ME.

I housed the busiest of busy minds, the loudest monkey in the cerebral jungle. My vrittis were so-o-o-o not nirodha! But over time (much time) and practice (so damn much practice), I began to experience a sweetness and quiet connection at the end of class that was more profound than physical healing and more intoxicating than the high of nailing a handstand. And I knew that if I could learn to steep briefly in infinite consciousness during savasana—ANYONE could. I wondered if I could show them how. I set my compass north.

If you're a teacher reading this book, you also probably have a clear memory of what inspired you to make the transition from student to teacher. Things that come easily to you hold a certain seductive charm; but I would bet that you have been most inspired by the parts of the practice (physical, philosophical, spiritual) that have challenged you deeply, healed you, cracked you open. Your greatest frustrations (the injuries, the mind blocks, the heartbreaks) usually become the bedrock of your teaching practice.

If you are still a student, perhaps you are at (or close to) the point where you are so full of enthusiasm for your practice that you feel ready to burst. Most dedicated students arrive here—the moment when you feel that your yoga has given you the tools to navigate this complex, sometimes scary, sometimes heartbreakingly beautiful life. And that you MUST share it with others.

Farmer-poet Wendell Berry says that he doesn't believe in big solutions to big problems—that big problems are solved by a million little solutions. Making the transition from student to teacher can feel like a potent way to express your small part of the solution. The desire to go deeper in your personal practice may result in doing a teacher training, joining a spiritual community for a period of time, dedicating yourself to extended study with one teacher, or any other form of intensive commitment to the "deep dive." Remember Joel Salatin's answer to the question "What can I, just little I, do?" He says, "Consider this. Whatever exists now is a cumulative manifestation of all the individual decisions made by the majority of the people in the culture for a period of time."

After spending the last few decades working with students interested in becoming teachers, I would like to pass along some cautionary advice—as well as what I hope will be simple, applicable questions you might ask yourself along the path.

First of all, after moving deeper into your study, the logical next step is NOT necessarily to become a teacher of the practice that has cracked your heart open. Taking on the role of teacher will inevitably change your relationship to your personal practice—for good and ill. Teaching is deeply enriching, but you also sacrifice something profound when issues like security, money, career goals, and ego enter a relationship you have with yourself that was once intimate and uncluttered.

Remember that the art of teaching, of sharing "the path," can come in many forms. The world needs doctors, bank tellers, politicians, and CPAs who are practicing life from a place of greater awareness and heart. More perhaps than we need an army of asana and mediation teachers! You can be a teacher of yoga in a holistic sense, in every way that you approach your life—to your family, your lovers, your colleagues, the strangers you meet, and perhaps most important, your perceived enemies.

The transition from yoga practitioner to teacher is rarely a straightforward trajectory. People who become physics or history teachers usually have a keen interest in that particular field of study and then set out on a methodical pedagogical path. All yogis start out as students, but most who become teachers never had that in mind until they were well traveled along the path of inquiry. Purity of intention leads many new teachers to feel conflicted about making a living from something they never saw as a business. If you DO become a teacher, it is imperative that you value your time and energy, however that may manifest—as pay, trade, or as an act of loving service. If you can cultivate a clear, honest relationship to the fruits of your labor, everyone feels better about the exchange.

"He who can, does. He who cannot, teaches." But those on the path of mind/body inquiry live in direct refutation to this famous G.B. Shaw adage. Yogic practices have no endgame: There is no product or performance as a fruit of your efforts, just further inquiry. Thus the transition from student to teacher is a muddy one. The honest teacher is a perennial student, which can lead you to question your own credibility. You may ask yourself, "Since I don't have the answers, who am I to teach anyone?" But you must remember that it is simply deep curiosity, a willingness to share, and the skill of communication that make a good teacher.

For those of you who are teachers—or on the path to becoming a teacher (and remember, I use this term broadly)—I offer you a few questions you could regularly ask yourself:

1. Since I am at peace with the fact that I will always be a student first and a teacher second, what is it that I am doing that is feeding my studentship?
2. What is it that inspires me right now (on or off the mat)? How do I articulate and share that (in either a direct or subtle way) with my students/others?
3. What is it that most frustrates/challenges me right now (on or off the mat)? How do I articulate and share that (in either a direct or subtle way) with my students/others?
4. How, on a daily basis, do I bring what I am practicing into my family, my local community, and the larger community?
5. WHY do I teach/offer yoga? What exactly is it feeding?
6. Am I still in love with the practice? Is my compass pointing (more or less) due north? (And remember that an organic trajectory is rarely a direct route.)

Two thousand years ago, Rabbi Hillel asked three questions that remain worth asking: "If I am not for myself, who will I be? If I am only for myself, what am I? And if not now, when?"

One of my favorite passages so clearly explains true surrender: True surrender is not a one-time event or the poof! *that comes at the end of some mental magic. True surrender is a process—the gradual letting go of the small self to the big self in each moment.*

True surrender is the daily dying of our desires, our wants, our expectations, our grievances, and our attachments. It is the release of the thought pattern that tries to get what it wants at any cost. It is the release of the desire to have things our way. It is the release of the habit pattern that sees parts and believes in appearances. It is the release of the expectation that something is wrong if it doesn't go according to our plans.

True surrender requires an opening of the heart to the unknown. We must let go of our preconceptions, assumptions, and expectations, and allow the grace of God to reveal to us our next step and then the next. True surrender is an inner process of transformation that allows us to see with God's eyes, hear with God's ears, speak with God's words, and act with God's grace.

Like the sculptor who chips away to reveal an image in a block of stone, true surrender is an awareness that chips away at that which does not serve us any longer. True surrender is an inner yielding of the soul that frees us to reveal and to accept the perfection of our lives.

To be in a constant state of surrender to our highest self is one of the most divine choices a human being can make. In life we operate from either fear or love. We are either yielding to our fear or stepping into our love in every breath. With every heartbeat we surrender to one or the other. The choice is ours. I choose love. We become that which we choose.

Like a lotus flower unfolding, we are in perpetual bloom. Through our experiences and challenges, we reveal more and more of ourselves. Often we tend to view this process of unveiling fearfully. Instead of surrendering and growing through the challenge, we tend to cling to old patterns and stay stuck in our ego. We don't trust that there is a perfect plan in place and that our life lessons are bringing us back home to our true selves and infinite nature.

At our core we are pure love, light, and wisdom. We are complete and whole, creator and creation. Our worth does not change from our original spark. A hundred-dollar bill comes out of the mint crisp, clean, brand-new, and worth a hundred dollars. Through life that bill gets crumpled up, dirty, squished into pockets, and a bit tired; however, that hundred-dollar bill never loses its value, its worth. However dirty or rumpled, a hundred dollars is still a hundred dollars. We never lose our worth. However crumpled we might get, our value is infinite. As it was in the beginning, so shall it be in the end. How are we going to live through all the breaths between our first and our last? To live in the flow of the divine, we must continually surrender and let go of all the things that keep us small. We must let go of the shore and flow into the ocean of our greatness, our expanded selves. Our wanting to control keeps us in

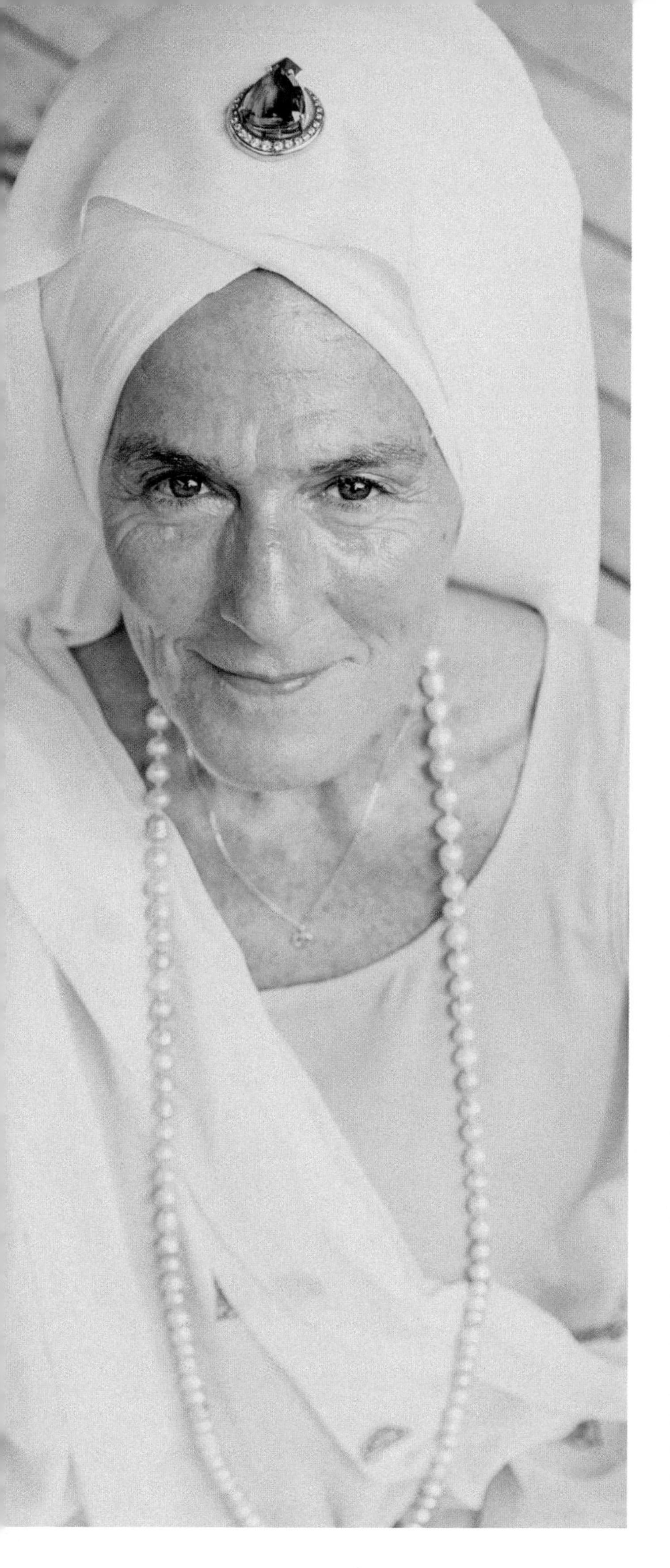

fear. Playing small keeps us seemingly safe within a comfort zone. Surrender to the unknown requires bravery and faith in something bigger than ourselves. Marianne Williamson says that when we allow our light to shine, we unconsciously give permission for others to do the same. By surrendering to the infinite love within ourselves, which is the source of all, our vibration allows new blooms to open, inspiring all to join the current.

Sometimes in this human experience, you may feel that you have to hold on, to keep things close, to cling to possessions, to control situations, and to surrender to what seem to be external pressures; however, that is not the truth. In order for prosperity and abundance to rain down on us, we must give ourselves, let things go, release outcome, and surrender to the internal, which at our core is love. This yielding is an opening of the heart, seeing with eyes of compassion, speaking words of purity, letting go of judgment and need, and replacing both by beaming love through your heart and into your life and the world.

Surrendering to love is truly a choice we must make with every breath. We are constantly challenged by our journey. Each step on the path provides us opportunities to let go and shed a skin. When you make a choice to surrender your will to God's will, a new breath of freedom fills your lungs. You realize that life can be easy. Struggle is not necessary, since the harder you fight, the more constricted you become, limiting your light. There is a way through every obstacle, even if that way doesn't seem clear at the moment. Surrendering the outcome of a situation to prayer allows the play of the universe to unfold your perfect destiny. As the ancient wise ones have taught us: Let go and let God. This allows the flow of the infinite through you. You become the instrument, and life becomes the song that you play through the breath of God and the surrender of will. We have all experienced those moments of pure ecstasy when we are one with all, totally connected, at ease, and complete. These are the moments of pure surrender wherein there is nothing and everything all at once. This is living fully in the now. Achieving this state in every moment as we navigate our lives may prove to be a difficult challenge; however, if we are mindful of the choice of surrender, those experiences of ecstasy will grow until the lotus flower is in illuminated bloom. God's grace runs to you and through you as you surrender, merging your heart with the universe as you come home to the true you ... love.

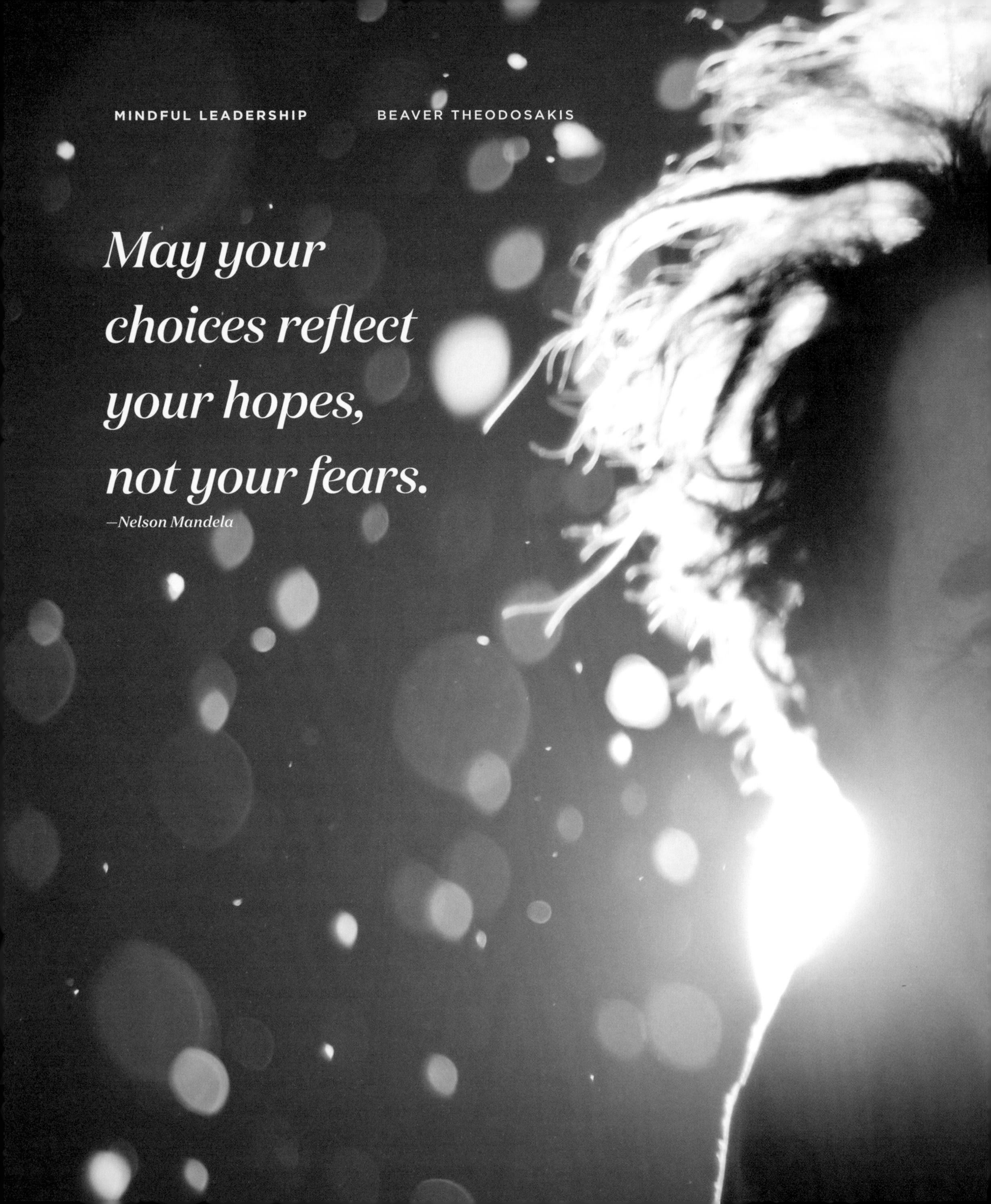

May your choices reflect your hopes, not your fears.

—Nelson Mandela

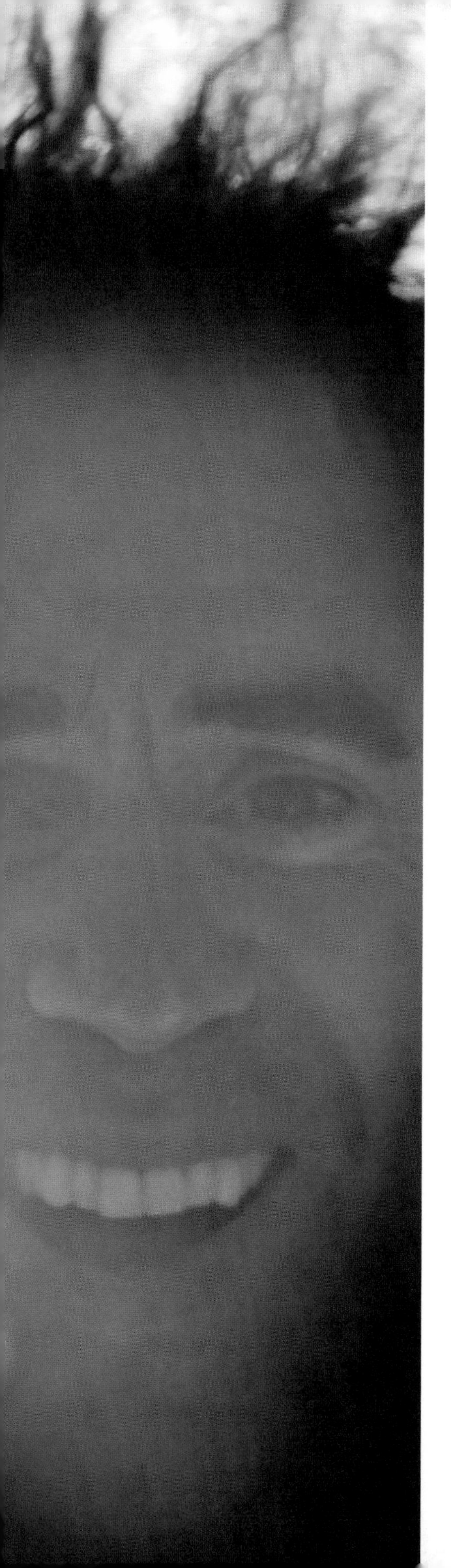

All too often, life just happens. We connect a few dots that seem like good ideas at the time and, BAM, next thing you know, you're stunned, staring blankly at the world around you. Things no longer look familiar and the trip you're on is certainly not your own. This realization can be a rough and rude awakening, an extremely difficult moment that doesn't feel like a moment at all, but an eternity stuck at some lonely crossroad waiting for the light to change.

It seems that we all experience some version of this at some point in life, but that isn't much consolation when you yourself are mired in the muck of more questions than answers. My "moment" came in the early '90s when I lost the friendship of two good buddies and our business together: surf brands *Life's a Beach* and *Bad Boy Club*. We were not communicating well, growing way too fast, got overextended, and it all blew up. It was a wild ride with many glorious moments, but it never felt in balance—it seemed like we were always pushing and forcing things. From the ashes of it all, I began to look inside and inquire about what really mattered to me and, more important, what was going to matter in the years to come.

Of course, at the time, I had no idea that my own individual compass was being redirected toward the ideas, actions, and people that would eventually become prAna.

The crux I had reached seemed strictly personal and well apart from my work and business. And *that* is exactly the point: We can find a life in sync, where there is little or no distinction between the things we are and the things we create.

After more than two decades, prAna is as much a part of me as my left arm or the spirited natures of my children. In many ways, we've all "grown up" together, and there is a definite line distinguishing the events of my life before and after that union.

I do, however, clearly recall the tough questions I forced myself to face and answer all those years ago, and the raw honesty that required some deep digging to reveal. "How did I get on this treadmill? Who am I trying to impress?" Isn't it ironic that people can push themselves to the point where being their true selves can be such hard work? Even more curious is our willingness, however temporary, to follow and even crazily chase random opportunities, trends, money, and relationships, rather than simply lead our lives. No, this is not meant to venture into the territories of self-help and empowerment; I will leave that to more qualified souls and the countless titles available on the subject. Here, the aim is nothing more than to share a personal account of how "leadership of life" directly connects to the effective leadership of people in business. Like many managers, I confess to having tried various styles to inspire, motivate, and direct the folks around me, with mixed results and only one absolute in all of it:

People are much better led by *example* than by power and authority.

So, that puts the onus on you, if you plan to march an army any time soon. You'll need to put your own house in order first, if your leadership is to be authentic. There's no escaping the soul-searching required, and I don't know of any magical method to decode the mystery of what really makes someone tick. What can I do happily for the rest of my life? What do my personal values demand of my professional self? The Q&A might look like this, but is more likely to succeed through trial and error than with any published checklist. Either way, it is a garbage-in-garbage-out exercise relying on truthful admissions of desire and your commitment to achieve them. Living in the modern era requires that money play a part in any vision, or it is likely a lie. Generosity too is essential, if it's going to last in a world revolving around shared thoughts and sentiments. In the leadership of people, this openness includes the conscious practice of offering enthusiasm and value to the ideas of others.

What are the signs of success? When are the traditionally separated aspects of life aligned? From experience, everything becomes much easier instead of more difficult. Timing always seems ideal. Careers become callings, for you and the people around you. In business, all managers love to see luck so clearly favoring the prepared ones around them. You're filled with gratitude at the thought of how seamless life has become, since there is little difference between work and play. Eventually, as if the tides of fortune fully reverse, opportunities flow your way in powerful currents. In short, it is a state of mind and being that you'd wish upon anyone in your life. It is more than merely being in the "flow" or on a winning streak; it is plugging into a current so vast and strong that it all but guarantees a sense of joy and fulfillment for those going for the ride.

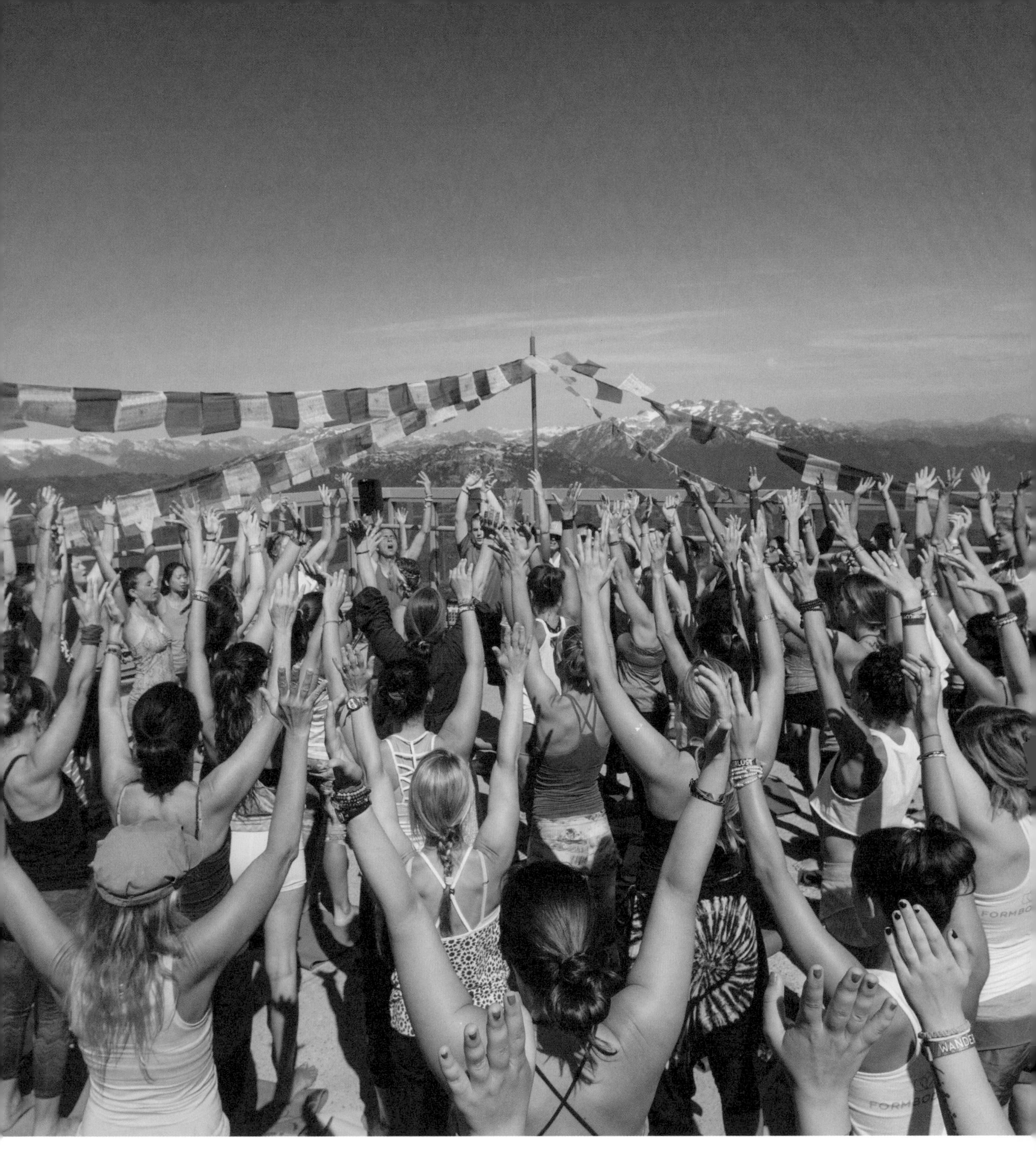

What is my purpose?
Why am I here?

Everyone has a specific and meaningful purpose in this life. Everyone. Here are a few things to consider before you step into your meditation.

INVEST AND INVESTIGATE

The outer world continually barrages us with messages about who we should be and what we should be doing. Add to that the daily assault of honking horns, ringing cell phones, and demanding professional and home lives. There's a lot going on and it can distract us from what is real and beautiful about ourselves and our lives. Through meditation we are able to investigate what our inner voice is offering, and only then will we have the insight to invest in that part of ourselves. To ***invest*** *means to "endow with authority." On your own authority, embrace any self-knowledge you gain through meditation with great esteem—what your heart calls for is on purpose and valuable—let your actions and your choices reflect that.*

TOLERATE DOUBT

We all long for fulfilling and inspiring work. We want to believe that what we are doing with our lives matters, that our actions will have a positive impact on the world. Perhaps most of all we want the feeling of knowing. Knowing that we are doing what we are meant to do. Well, it turns out that indecision and doubt are insidious and crafty companions on this journey. They don't need to be absent in order to move forward with your great work—they only need to be dealt with properly. Try to eradicate doubt. Good luck! It comes with the human condition. Instead of being intolerant of doubt, make friends with it, keep it in its place. Allow doubt a seat on the ride—just not in the driver's seat. Tolerate doubt skillfully. Rinse it with the clarity of the heart mind so that you can see it for what it is—this way it cannot override reasonable perspective.

TRUST

In the beginning, trusting your inner voice may take some practice. It may require pausing several times throughout the day to check in and notice if your actions are congruent with your heart calling. The feeling of congruency should be YES, this feels right, I belong here. This doesn't mean right action is exempt from challenge, confusion, or even multiple failures, but when you are able to step back and observe yourself in the work, it should feel like home. Over time, I assure you that trusting yourself will become an intuitive boon to your interface with the world.

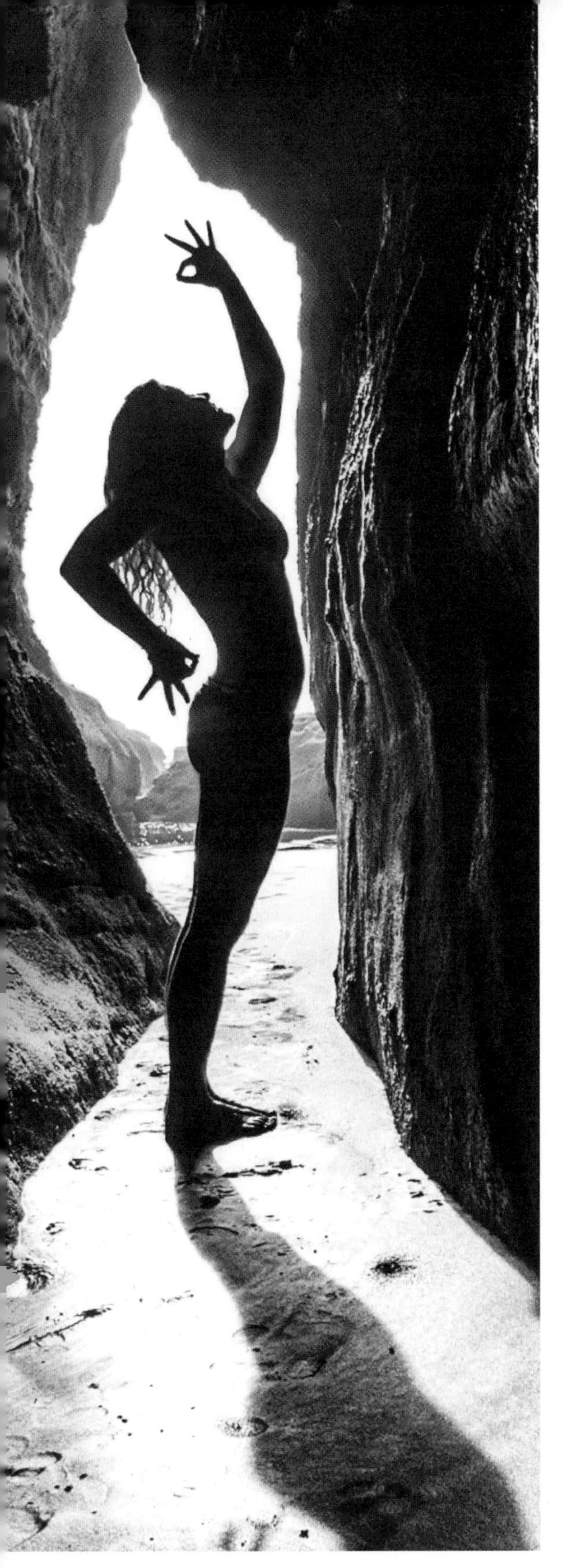

MEDITATION

Find a quiet place free from distraction. Sit comfortably either on the floor or in a chair with sit bones firmly supported and spine vertical. Take several easy deep breaths, clearing out all that has come before this moment.

Close your eyes.

Turn your gaze inward toward your spiritual heart at the center of your chest. Imagine yourself seated there at the altar of your heart. There is a fire burning, the fire of the innermost self. Pause and observe the fire. Take the next step with courage and without inhibition. Offer into the fire all of the ideas you hold about your outer self. Offer all of the ways you identify your outer self, i.e., husband, mother, lawyer, teacher, male, female, etc. Avoid becoming rigid—just let the descriptions float into the fire. Pause. Next offer all of the attributes of your personality that you are attached to, good and bad. For instance, you may consider yourself nice, jealous, smart, arrogant, angry, generous, compassionate, strong, weak, etc. Be honest and offer all of it. This is the time to LET GO.

Once you have offered everything you can think of, keep your gaze on the fire. Observe the fire transform from a blaze into a single flame that burns undisturbed as if in a windless cave. Sit by the flame and wait. Listen. Going deeper still into the knowing and wisdom of the innermost self, rest your mind on the flame that burns in the cave of the heart. Spend several minutes in this phase of the meditation; listen and watch the thoughts. Over time, you will become more skillful at discerning the difference between the thoughts that come from the neurotic mind (which are influenced by the outer world) and the thoughts that come from your heart mind (which are not influenced by the outer world).

Be patient. Some thoughts will be old fears and conditions that will burn off if you let them. Some thoughts will be jewels of wisdom offered from deep within. Do not color your observation of the inner voice by analyzing. Be the patient witness as the fire of the heart cooks the questions into answers. The final stage of the meditation is returning to ground resource. Still visualizing your seat at the fire, establish that you are being supported there, stable and steady. Then slowly zoom out, floating awareness back into the physical body, sensing that the outer seat is a reflection of the inner seat. Feel your sit bones on the support of the floor or chair and, keeping the eyes closed, become keenly aware of the outer world. Spend a moment here. Notice that you are connected to both the inner and outer experiences simultaneously. Finally, bring your hands together in front of your heart. Feel both unburdened and grounded.

To close your meditation and open the channels of gratitude and reception repeat this mantra three times: "THANK YOU FOR THIS BODY, THANK YOU FOR THIS LIFE."

MAKING PEACE WITH THE END; A SHORT REFLECTION ON SAVASANA, OM, AND NAMASTE

The penultimate pose in any yoga class is usually savasana, followed by a seated chant of OM and a shared namaste. For the few years that I was practicing hatha yoga, these closing practices were my most challenging. Savasana, in my mind, translated from the Sanskrit to roughly "time to lie around and obsess about things left undone—or things done I wish I could change." My OM was a froggy croak, which I did my best to muffle under the enthusiastic chanters around me. The final exchange of namaste felt awkward; I don't come from a religious background, and the gesture of prayer at my heart struck me as intuitively sweet but somehow like fakery.

I clearly remember the class when a teacher mentioned that *sava* means corpse (and I knew that *asana* meant pose); that we should put a rolled-up blanket under our legs and set up for corpse pose. "How macabre," I thought. But it wasn't long before I began to relish the idea that day after day we were preparing for a conscious death, acknowledging that dying is all around us and is our inevitable end. In a culture that closets aging and death within hospitals and institutions, how poignant to make practicing death a sacred part of your day. And that the emergence out of the pose, every time, represents the possibility of a more keenly observed and cherished life.

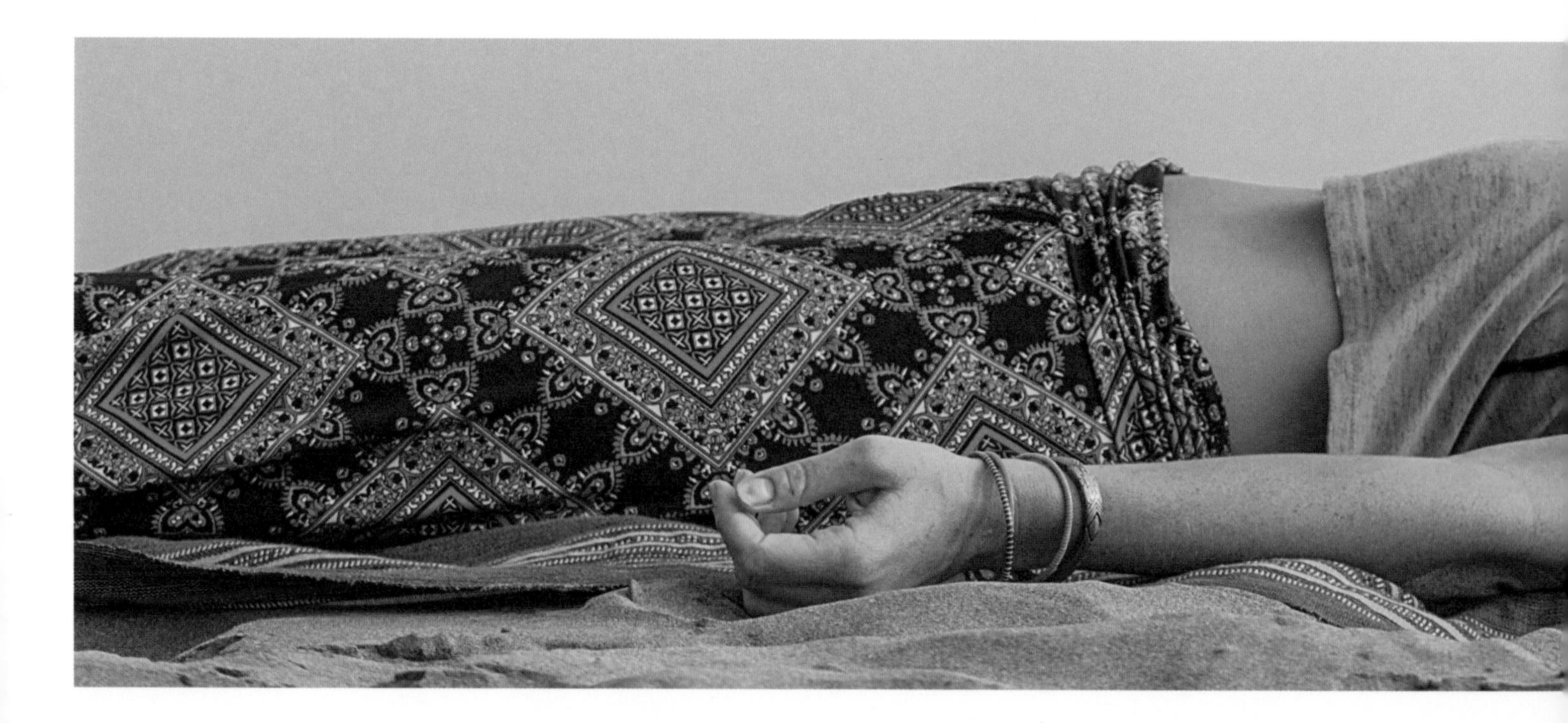

The experience of savasana changed completely for me over time. This isn't to say that I don't struggle with a mind that careens wildly between past and future at the end of class, but I also occasionally taste the nectar of the true meaning of yoga during corpse pose—the unification of my consciousness, the merging of my individual limitation, with something greater than myself.

My OM will always be a little off pitch and ragged, but I have finally released the tightness in my chest enough to be able sound my heart through my throat with my community. What sweet release to be able to sing in public. (And even lead the chant in public—perfect pitch be damned!) The only other place you'll find me doing that is late night at a bar.

The first step in demystifying *namaste* was when I discovered that it's the Southeast Asia version of *aloha*—an everyday greeting when people meet and a farewell when they part, often expressed without words by the gesture of folded palms before the heart and a bow of the head to indicate at once friendship, respect, and humility. Decoding the Sanskrit roots of the word deepened my regard for this deceptively simple gesture: *Nama* means "bow," *as* means "I," and *te* means "you." "I bow to you." I can do that! The word *namaha* can also be literally interpreted as "na ma"—not mine—which has the significance of relinquishing one's ego in the presence of another. Relinquish my ego?! That's harder. But I can aspire.

In a spiritual sense, namaste is taken to mean "I bow to the divine in you"; that there is a divine spark within each of us that is located in the heart center. In a classroom context, for a teacher and students, namaste sets a tone wherein individuals come together energetically in a place of true connection, free of ego. The myriad ways of interpreting namaste are much like the flexibility of the yoga practice as a whole. Complex and simple at once, perfectly suited for students to inhabit at the level at which they feel comfortable, flexible but challenging, and infinitely expandable.

Don't underestimate the power of those last ten minutes of class. Every time you practice or teach savasana, you might ask, "When I die, what do I want to be able to say about how I lived?" When you sound OM and namaste, it is your opportunity to pour your heart through your throat and hands—to connect to the students around you, to your teachers and their teachers, and to the great unknown.

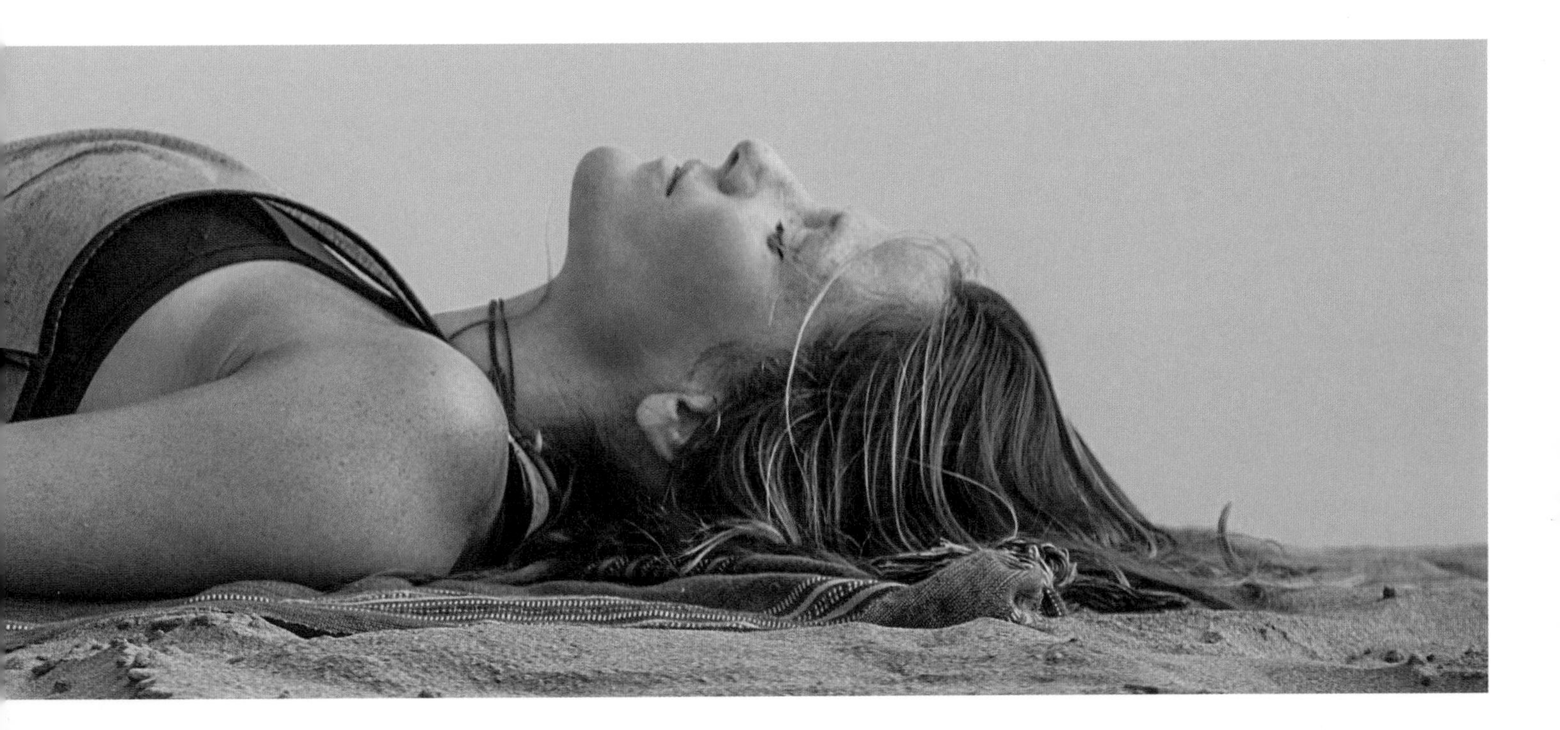

find your true north

MC YOGI AND AMANDA GIACOMINI

Years ago, I was talking with a close friend who was going through a difficult and confusing time. "It's a terrible thing not to know your own heart," she said. These words struck a deep chord and helped me remember what a gift it is to truly know what our hearts are longing for. Practicing yoga can be a wonderful way to silence the surface chatter of the mind in order to drop in and discover what your pure heart's desire is. From this place of clarity, we can begin to craft, design, and direct our lives in a way that is in alignment with this highest truth. This awareness and ability to keep checking in with our inner compass just might be our best chance of finding our true north and the secret to lasting happiness.

wave one *centering + shoulder and neck stretches*

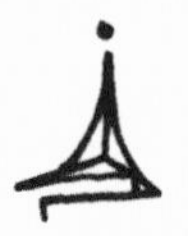

Take a few minutes to breathe and listen to what your heart has to say.

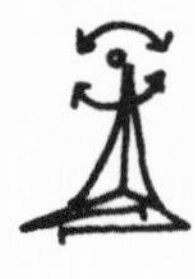

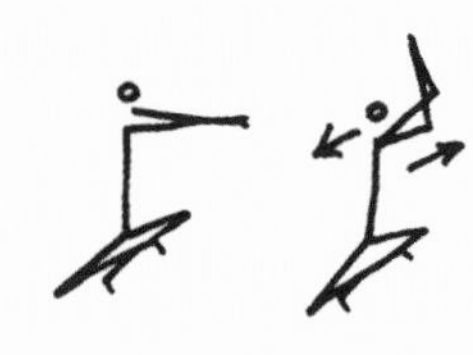

SUKASANA *Sit for a moment on your mat. Be still. Listen to your breath.*

NECK ROLLS *Slowly drop your chin to your chest and roll your chin gradually to the right. Pause and take 5 breaths. Come back to center and roll your chin to the left, pause and take 5 deep breaths.*

GARUDASANA ARMS *Take the arms to the left and look to the right. Bring arms back to center. Uncross. Switch sides.*

wave two *hips and hamstrings*

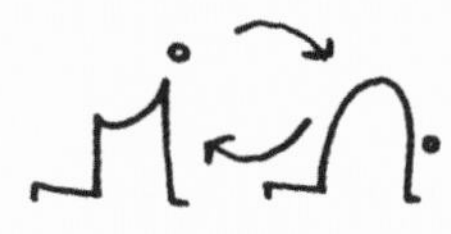

CHAKRAVAKASANA (CAT COW) *Warm your spine with simple wavelike motion.*

ONE LEGGED DOG *Bend knee, rotate hip open.*

LOW LUNGE *Take* 5 BREATHS *fingertips on blocks or the floor, then* 5 BREATHS *hands to hips.*

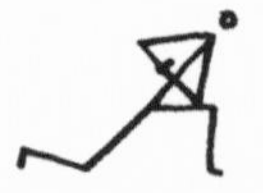

LOW LUNGE TWIST

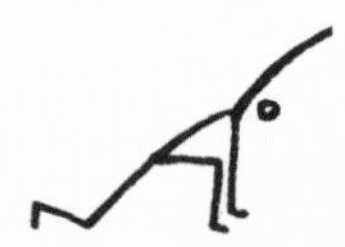

SIDE STRETCH *in* LOW LUNGE *Reach right arm over your head and bend whole torso to the left.*

HAMSTRING STRETCH (ARDHA HANUMANASANA)

Return to all fours. Take CAT COW *again to clear the path and realign the spine. Repeat on left side.*

Practice Playlist

compiled by Kelly Casey

Far Nearer—*Jamie xx*

Mind Eye—*Nightmares on Wax*

Sweet Disposition—*The Temper Trap*

Anything Could Happen—*Ellie Goulding*

Days to Come—*Bonobo*

Galapagos—*Emancipator*

Lucy Dub—*Loscil*

wave three *opening to compass pose*

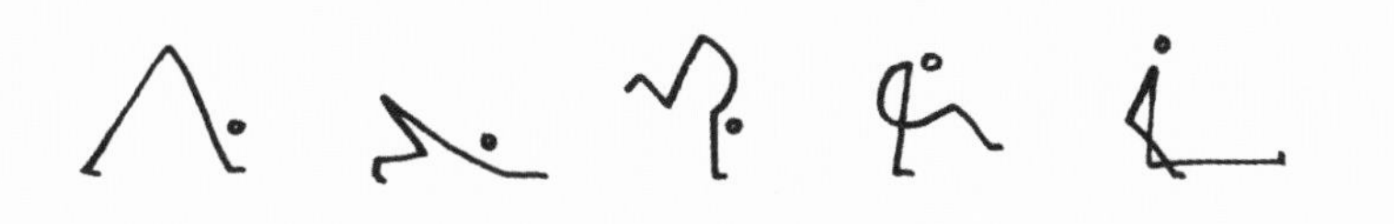

DOWN DOG

Jump through to sit.

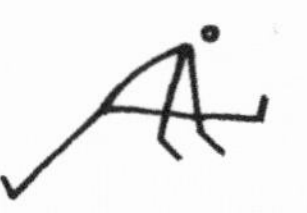

UPTAVISTA KONASANA *Chill out here for 2–3 minutes. Just let your hips and hamstrings open up. Be patient. Walk your fingertips forward after the first minute.*

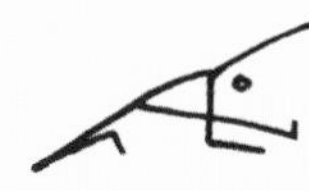

PARIVRITA JANU SIRSASANA. *Fold right foot in. Take left arm to the inside of left leg. Extend right arm up and over, keep right hip grounded, and breathe deeply as tension and stress release from the side body. Repeat on left side.*

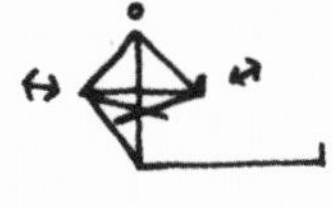

ROCK THE BABY *with right leg. Cradle knee in right arm crease and either put your foot in the left arm crease or modify and put foot in left hand. Gently rock the leg back and forth.*

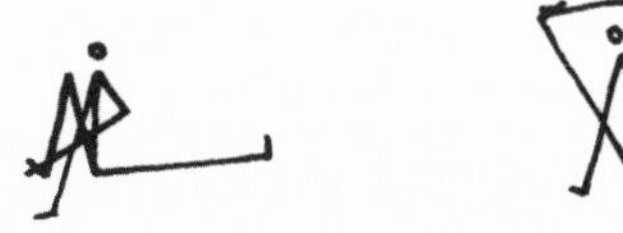

PARIVRITA SURYA YANTRASANA (COMPASS POSE) *Seated version of this pose. Hook right leg over upper right arm. With left hand, grab the outside edge of the right foot. Slowly extend the right leg.*

As your leg straightens, bring your right hand to the floor to support yourself. Draw chest forward until your head comes in front of your arms, then rotate chest and head to the left. Breathe deep.

wave four *unwind and relax*

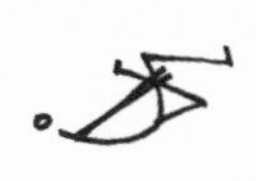

THREAD THE NEEDLE

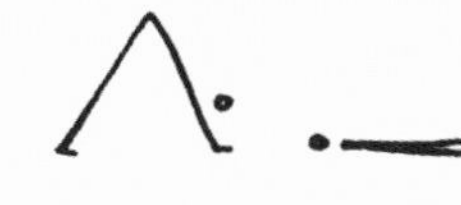

DOWN DOG TO LYING DOWN ON BACK

HUG KNEES TO CHEST

RECLINING TWIST

SHAVASANA *Relax and trust you will find your way.*

A surefire way to know you found your true north is to use the measuring stick: Does it benefit everybody involved, do I wake up In the morning enthused and excited to continue on this path, is it making me a kinder and more compassionate person? Yoga helps us connect with the center of our inner compass so that we can become more skillful at navigating our life in a way that brings more reverence, gratitude, and love.

The greater the distance you travel, the closer to home you become. This is the beautiful paradox of traveling, of yoga, and of finding your true north: Everything is already inside you. You have all of the answers and tools you need to actualize your dreams.

No one saves us but ourselves. No one can and no one may. We ourselves must walk the path.

—Buddha

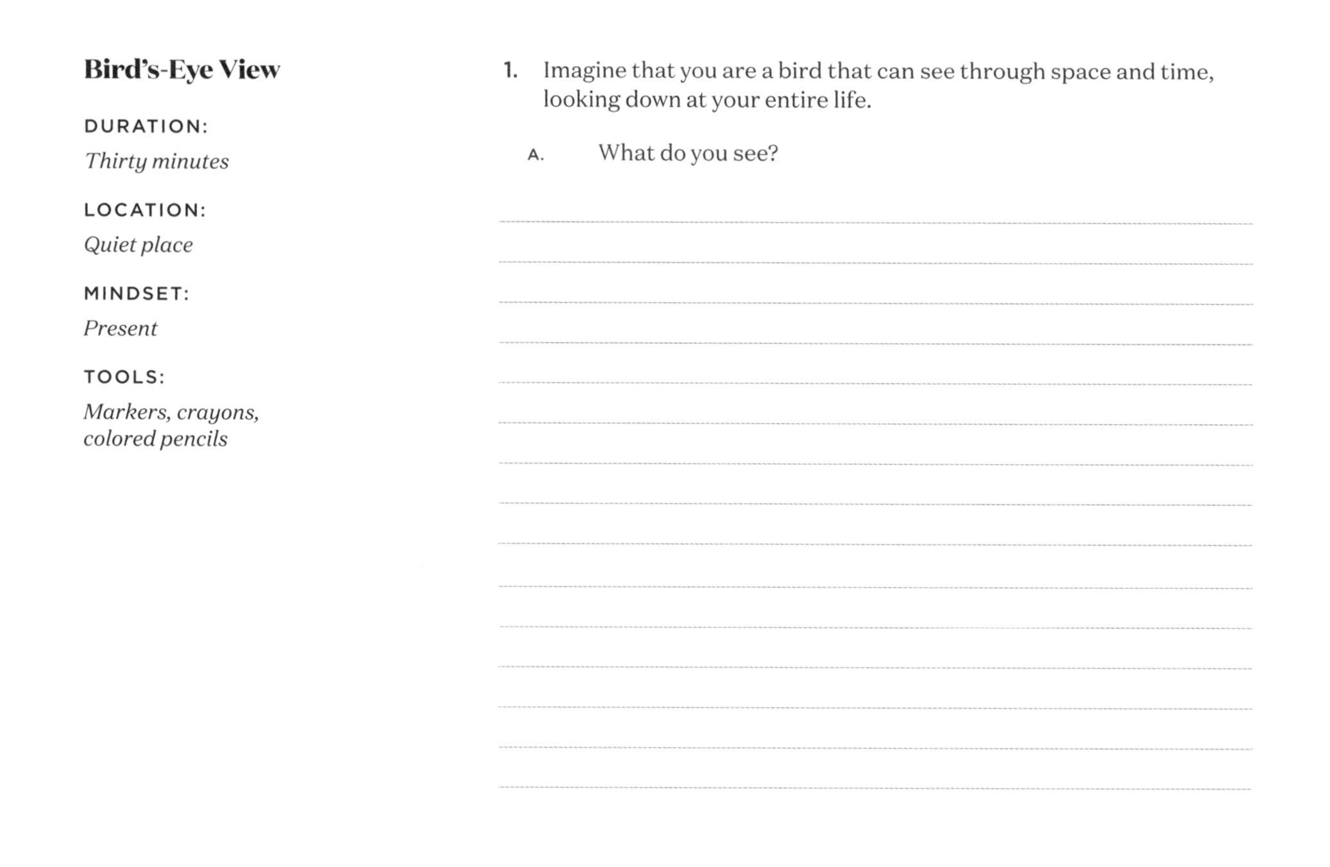

Bird's-Eye View

DURATION:
Thirty minutes

LOCATION:
Quiet place

MINDSET:
Present

TOOLS:
Markers, crayons, colored pencils

1. Imagine that you are a bird that can see through space and time, looking down at your entire life.

   A. What do you see?

2. Write down your history so far: your successes, your struggles, your fears and your regrets.
   A. What would you repeat?
   B. What would you do differently?
   C. Take a good look at the present.
   D. Who are you now?
   E. What does your life look like from the outside?
   F. What about this do you like?
   G. What do you want to change?
   H. Soar into the future.
   I. What are people saying about you?
   J. What have you accomplished?
   K. What impact do your actions have?
   L. What kinds of relationships do you have?
   M. Where have you gone and what type of person have you become?

You might be at the end of this book, but this is only the beginning of your journey. Now, fully live it. You are stronger, brighter, braver than you know!

Through our asana practice, our form has grown stronger and more flexible. Through eating what is ripe and local, our bodies are healthier. Through our breathing, we have learned to reduce stress. Through meditation, we have found a deeper knowledge of self and the world around us.

We are evolving.

We used to see only shadows on the wall of the cave. Perhaps we thought our path to happiness was in the future acquisition of material objects. Or maybe we just lived that way. But now we are turning toward the fire and seeing things for what they truly are. We have a clearer vision for how to live, what to eat, how to love.

Before enlightenment,
chop wood,
carry water.
After enlightenment
chop wood,
carry water.

—Zen Proverb

Sorry to say, though, that the train has no terminus. The conductor never says, "You have arrived at true north. Everyone please move toward the exits. This is the last stop." We end where we started . . . with practice, chopping wood, and carrying water.

Finding your true north is a process. By focusing on the process of our lives, we unwittingly discover happiness. When we are deeply in process, we cultivate our truest essence. Have you ever been working on a project, or playing a sport, or making a painting and time just disappears? This flow is the inspiration behind the saying, "Do what you love, and you will never work a day in your life."

If the train trip represents process, it is helpful to see stops along the way as milestones of our evolution. These stops may be self-imposed tests, moments where we confront our fears. For example, I have a gift for public speaking and I am also extremely fearful of it. I try to apply mindfulness training to overcome this fear, and every six months or so, put myself in a situation where I have to speak in front of a lot of people. I observe myself in these instances. How am I dealing with the stress? Am I present in the moment? As we heal ourselves, we can then focus on healing the world.

Finding your true north is bringing your best self into the world where you are right now. And again where you are right now.

Acknowledgments

JEFF KRASNO WOULD LIKE TO THANK . . .

My partner, Sean, and my wife, Schuyler, for embarking on the Wanderlust journey and for creating the ability to live one life, where work and play are seamless.

My coconspirators, Nicole Lindstrom and Sarah Herrington, for seeing this immense project through. Our brilliant designer, Erica Jago, and to all of the amazing photographers, particularly Ali Kaukas and Sasha Juliard.

All of the contributors who generously shared their wisdom in this book.

The Wanderlust team, too many to name, for your creativity, love, and devotion to your work and our common mission.

My daughters, Phoebe, Lolli, and Micah; my parents, Richard and Jean, who have always stood by me; and my brother, Eric.

My dedicated agent, Kitty Cowles, and all the folks at Rodale, in particular, my editor, Ursula Cary, Jeff Batzli, Rae Ann Spitzenberger, Jess Fromm, Hope Clarke, and Sara Cox.

My personal mentors, including Michael Lazarus, Jeff Walker, Beaver Theodosakis, Chip Conley, Shiva Rea, and Dave Kennedy.

Elena Brower for your inspiration and Seane Corn for your relentless leadership. Nick and Amanda for your creative spirit. Tim Ryan for being a proud voice of a mindful movement.

All the yogis who have wandered to a festival or into a studio.

The inspiring community of teachers, musicians, lecturers, expedition leaders, athletes, organic chefs, conscious entrepreneurs, and spiritual leaders. All the partners, big and small, who have supported us.

C3, Starr Hill, and Raine, who believed in our vision, including Charlie Walker, Coran Capshaw, Jordan Zachary, Pat O'Connor, and Pete Amaro.

All of our Wayfarers, our studio partners, and our Wanderlust studio pioneers in Austin, Montreal, and Squaw Valley. The Spence family and Jo Kutchey.

All of our resort partners, who have given us incredible canvases on which to paint, in particular, Andy Wirth, who contributed to this book and has been so generous to us.

Michael Coyle, the Houssian family, and Skip Taylor. Jimmy Brinkeroff, for your passion.

Our cocreators at lululemon: Rachel, Mila, Alli, Lauren, Amanda, Lindsay, Jessica, Carolyn, Aly, Brenda, Laurent, Eric, and so many others.

The Kula yoga community in New York for providing inspiration and community at home.

Our production and operations teams over the years who have toiled in the spirit of creating a unique and inspiring experience, particularly Judd Kleinman and Scott Nichols at All Phases.

Bree.

Lastly, thank you to my grandfather, Arthur Kaplan, who looks down upon me. I measure my success every day against the example he set for me.

SARAH WOULD LIKE TO THANK . . .

Thank you to Jeff Krasno and Nicole Lindstrom, for being the best partners in creation-crime. Thank you to the entire Wanderlust team for joining effort with intention to make conscious adventures real. Deep gratitude to my yoga teachers and writing mentors for encouraging me to move and speak from the heart. And thank you to my family, for the roots from which to rise.

NICOLE WOULD LIKE TO THANK . . .

I would like to thank each and every contributor to *Wanderlust*. Thank you for your words of insight, wisdom, and aching beauty. It is you who have made this book the work of brilliance that it is.

I would like to thank each and every Wanderlust employee. Thank you for your endless hours of dedication in heart and strength; every hour with you has made every hour worth it.

And lastly, I would like to thank each and every person I have met at a Wanderlust festival. Thank you for your vibrancy and for your vulnerability. This one's for you.

Glossary

Ahimsa—Nonharming. A foundational practice in yoga and the first yama, or social guideline, in the yoga sutras.

Ananda—Bliss.

Aparigraha—Nonhoarding, one of the yamas.

Asana—Seat, or yoga pose.

Ashram—Traditional retreat center, hermitage, place for spiritual practice.

Asteya—Nonstealing, one of the yamas.

Atman—Inner self, or soul, in Hinduism.

Avidya—Ignorance, the opposite of vidya.

Bandha—Energy locks sometimes used in yoga practice. The three main bandhas are *mula bandha* (root lock), *uddiyana bandha* (abdominal lock, a "flying up" lock), and *jalandhara bandha* (throat lock). Bandhas help the yoga practitioner contain and redirect energy within. When all three are activated, it's called *maha bandha*, or great lock.

Bhagavad Gita—Hindu text from around 200 BCE, telling a story of peaceful warriorship, selfless action, and yoga.

Bhakti yoga—*Bhakti* translates to "devotion." Bhakti yoga is devotional yoga, focusing on connection to the divine through chanting, kirtan, prayer, and mantra practice.

Brahmacharya—Responsible use of sexual and creative energy. One of the yamas.

Chakras—Translates to wheel, or centers of energy in the human body. There are seven basic centers of energy, commonly referred to as chakras: root, sacral, solar plexus, heart, throat, third eye, and crown. Each governs a particular part of the body and emotional/mental/spiritual consciousness. Chakras are often referred to as being in balance or out of balance.

Chin mudra—Hand position made by bringing the thumb and index finger to touch, closing a circuit of energy.

Chitta vritti—Mind chatter, or fluctuations of the mind. Yoga practice aids in calming this activity. The saying *Yoga chitta vritti nirodha* (from the yoga sutras) means: "When in a state of yoga, there is a calming of the fluctuations of the mind."

Dhyana—State of meditation, one's attention being absorbed in one thing.

Drishti—Soft yet focused gaze, or the gazing point itself, used in yoga practice.

Dukkha—Suffering, stress. Often relates to being attached to things that are impermanent.

Enlightenment—Self-realization, realization of interconnectedness of all things. Having the "light turned on" to truth.

Gunas—Three qualities or states of being that exist in all of nature, including people! They are: tamas (heaviness), rajas (agitation), and sattva (harmony).

Guru—"Dispeller of darkness." This term is usually used for a teacher who guides the student on the path of yoga. Many also say, "The one true guru is in the center of your own heart."

Hatha yoga—Ha (sun) and tha (moon) in Sanskrit, with yoga (union). Hatha yoga refers to the union of dualities. Today, it is often used to describe a gentle asana practice.

Japa—Discipline of repeating a mantra, often with mala beads used to aid counting. This practice helps to connect the heart, mind, and intentions to that which is being repeated, in deep focus.

Karma—Action, or the sum of one's actions.

Kirtan—Devotional signing, often in a call-and-response format. From the Sanskrit word for praise.

Kosha—Sheath or layer. In Vendantic philosophy, there are five sheaths, visualized as layers of an onion:
 Annamaya kosha = physical sheath
 Pranamaya kosha = energy sheath
 Manomaya kosha = mental sheath
 Vijnanamaya kosha = wisdom sheath
 Anandamaya kosha = bliss sheath

Leela—Play, spontaneous creativity.

Mantra—Word or phrase repeated with intention. Said to aid in crossing over from one state of thoughts to another.

Mauna—Silence. A practice in which a yogi keeps silent to listen within.

Maya—Illusion.

Mudra—Seal. Often shows up in hand positions used in yoga practice.

Nadis—Channels for the flow of energy, or consciousness, through the body. Main nadis referenced include:
 Sushumna nadi (running from the base to crown chakra)
 Pingala nadi (associated with solar/masculine energy, it runs up the right side of the body)
 Ida nadi (associated with lunar/feminine energy, it runs up the left side of the body)

Namaste—Greeting meaning "the light in me recognizes the light in you."

Niyamas—Guidelines for actions and beliefs toward one's self:
 Saucha (cleanliness)
 Santosha (being content and happy with what you have)
 Tapas (working hard and with enthusiasm; discipline)
 Svadhyaya (studying yourself)
 Isvara pranidhana (being devoted, or surrendering our efforts to the greater good)

OM—One-syllable mantra representing unity. Many define it as "the sound of the universe." Also spelled as AUM.

Patanjali—Sage who wrote down the yoga sutras.

Prana—Life energy, vitality.

Pranayama—Prana (energy) and yama (control); the extension of prana (life force); often relates to breathing exercises that affect our energy.

Rājas—State of agitation or overactivity, one of the three gunas.

Sacrum—Large triangular bone in the lower back made of five fused vertebrae. Located above the tailbone and in between both hip bones.

Samādhī—Translates to "make firm." A state in which the individual experiences union with the universe. Often considered the highest state of meditation in yogic philosophy.

Sanskrit—Ancient language of India, used often in naming yoga poses and practices and in chanting. Considered to carry meaning in both the sound and definitions of words, it is also referred to as Devanagari, or language of the gods.

Santosa—Contentment.

Sattva—State or quality of harmony, clarity, lightness. One of the three gunas.

Sattvic—Adjective describing things with a state of balance, lightness, and harmony. A sattvic diet refers to foods that are gentle and harmonizing to body, mind, and energy.

Satya—Truth, truthfulness, honesty. One of the yamas.

Saucha—Cleanliness. One of the niyamas.

Savasana—Corpse pose. Often the final resting pose in a series, it allows the body, mind, and spirit to integrate all the poses that came before.

Sukha—Ease, happiness.

Surya Namaskar—Sun Salutations. A set vinyasa, or flow of poses.

Sutra—Translates as "thread" from the Sanskrit, a precept or maxim; the sutras are collections or threads of lessons and discourses.

Tamas—Quality of sluggishness or heaviness, one of the three gunas.

Tapas—Discipline or heat.

Ujjayi—Type of breathing often used through yoga asana practice to create heat in the body and calm in the mind; translates to "victorious" breath. Inhalation and exhalation are both done through the nose. The "ocean" sound is a result of the throat being narrowed. Inhalations and exhalations are even in length, contributing to the evenness of mind.

Vidya—Correct knowledge, clarity; the opposite of avidya.

Vinyasa—Flow of poses, one into the next, with no stopping in between. This practice generates heat in the body, encourages focus and coordination.

Viveka—Discrimination. Discerning between the real and unreal, the real meaning as that which is permanent and the unreal as that which is temporary.

Yamas—Guidelines for one's behavior toward others in the external world. Patanjali laid out the yamas, or social contracts, in his eight limbs of yoga:

Ahimsa (nonviolence; no harm)
Satya (honesty; truth)
Asteya (nonstealing)
Brahmacharya (using creative and sexual energy wisely)
Aparigraha (nonhoarding)

Yoga—Translates to "union" or "yoke" in Sanskrit, meaning yoking the mind, body, and spirit. Yoga is an umbrella term for many practices, but commonly describes poses, breath work, meditation, and ways of living and being in the world promoting well-being, truth, and peace. Yoga is about being unified and connected with one's self and the world.

Yoga sutras—Foundational text of yoga, written down by Patanjali.

Yogi—Person who practices yoga (sometimes *yogini* for females).

Yogic—Of or relating to all things yoga! (See above definition of yoga for how big that small word is.)

Contributors

Yoga teacher, founder of Farm to Yoga, co-owner of Growing Heart Farm, and local food advocate, **ABBY PALOMA** has been teaching about yoga and food since 2007. Abby's work is to connect people to the source of their nourishment. You can find Abby teaching yoga, nurturing her medicinal herb garden, or studying for her master's in Chinese medicine in New York City.

AMANDA GIACOMINI is a yoga teacher, illustrator, and fine artist. She owns Yoga Toes Studio in Point Reyes, California, and travels and teaches all over the world with her husband, MC Yogi. She is currently working on a project to paint ten thousand Buddhas.

ANAND MEHROTRA, founder of Sattva yoga, is a visionary yoga master and community leader. Born and raised in Rishikesh, India—the birthplace of yoga—Anand combines the ancient wisdom of his upbringing with a lighthearted rebelliousness to support the transcendence of the individual and the collective. He is the founder of Sattva Retreat Centre and Sattva Yoga Academy based in Rishikesh, leads the Khushi Charitable Society and Sattva Foundation, has launched several businesses based on community collaboration, and is featured in the documentary *The Highest Pass* based on his teachings.

ANDY WIRTH is the president and chief executive officer of Squaw Valley | Alpine Meadows ski resorts. He is also active in his community as an environmental advocate and activist and philanthropist.

BEAVER THEODOSAKIS is the cofounder (with his wife, Pam) of the apparel company prAna. He cofounded Spy Optics, Life's a Beach, and Bad Boy Club action sports brands.

BROOK COSBY directed the meditation program at Kula Yoga Project Williamsburg in Brooklyn from 2011 to 2014. She has studied, practiced, and taught yoga and meditation for more than ten years, and she is the co-owner/codirector of Hyde, a line of organic cotton yoga apparel.

EKABHUMI CHARLES ELLIK is a poet, artist, and instructor by trade. His work has been widely published, and his *Shakti Coloring Book* from Sounds True Press will be available in 2015. When not writing, painting, or sitting at the feet of his teacher, he can be found in the garden learning directly from nature.

Hospitality guru, world traveler, and bestselling author, **CHIP CONLEY** built America's most unique boutique hotel company, Joie de Vivre, with one mission: to create joy. From Bali to Burning Man, he experienced the transformative power of festivals and launched Fest300.com because "the more virtual we get, the more ritual we need." And as head of Global Hospitality & Strategy at Airbnb, he's bridging cultural barriers in more than two hundred countries.

DAVE ROMANELLI has pioneered the art of fusing ancient Eastern practices with modern passions like exotic chocolate and fine wine. He has written two books: *Yeah Dave's Guide to Livin' the Moment* (Broadway Books, 2009) and *Happy Is the New Healthy* (Skyhorse Publishing, 2015).

DEV AUJLA is the CEO of Catalog, where he recruits for and advises companies that make money and do good. He is the coauthor of *Making Good: Finding Meaning, Money, and Community in a Changing World* (Rodale, 2012).

Legendary yoga teacher **SRI DHARMA MITTRA** first encountered yoga as a teenager before meeting his guru in 1964 and beginning his training in earnest. He founded one of the early independent schools of yoga in New York City in 1975 and has taught hundreds of thousands the world over in the years since. Sri Dharma is the model and creator of the "Master Yoga Chart of 908 Postures" and the author of *Asanas: 608 Yoga Poses,* and he has released two DVDs to date: *Maha Sadhana* levels I and II.

DJ DREZ blends yesterday's roots with the innovative urban beats of today. His trailblazing, genre-bending body of work has made him a prominent figure in the yoga with music movement around the globe.

ELENA BROWER is a mama and teacher of yoga and meditation. She is a producer of *On Meditation,* which takes a personal look into the practices and lives of meditators, and teaches international trainings and retreats. Her book *Art of Attention* has been translated into several languages and has been number one in book design in both the United States and France. Practice with Elena on YogaGlo.

ERICA JAGO is an accomplished graphic designer, teacher, and artist who designed *Wanderlust* and coauthored and designed the groundbreaking yoga workbook *Art of Attention.* She is known in her local classes in Hawaii and on her global retreats for incorporating design concepts into artful and spiritual class experiences. Trained in Vinyasa and Kundalini yoga, Erica teaches us how to master a profound love in our attitudes, emotional experiences, and relationships to our bodies.

Collectively known as the Haiku Guys, **ERICK SZENTMIKLOSY** and **DANIEL ZALTSMAN** are traveling poets who improvise haiku on typewriters at social gatherings. Their mission is to write haiku for everyone.

GABRIELLE BERNSTEIN has been named "a new thought leader" by Oprah Winfrey. She appears regularly as an expert on NBC's *Today* and was named "a new role model" by the *New York Times.* Gabrielle is the *New York Times* best-selling author of the books *May Cause Miracles* and *Miracles Now.* In 2014, Gabrielle cohosted the Guinness Book of World Records' largest group meditation gathering with Deepak Chopra.

GARTH STEVENSON is a Brooklyn-based film composer and double bassist. Raised in the mountains of western Canada, nature became his primary inspiration and the common thread between his life and music.

GERRY LOPEZ is a surfer who believes that surfing may be a path to a higher consciousness.

GINA CAPUTO is the founder and director of the Colorado School of Yoga, based in Boulder, where she teaches inspired, informed, and lively Integrated Vinyasa classes. She is also the creatrix of On The Loose Goods and a champion of getting out into nature and hiking as moving meditation.

GURMUKH KAUR KHALSA is the director of Golden Bridge Yoga with centers in Santa Monica and New York City. Since being baptized forty-four years ago with the spiritual name that means "one who helps people across the world ocean," Gurmukh has dedicated her life to fulfilling her namesake. As the world's leading Kundalini yoga teacher, she and her husband, Gurushabd, travel worldwide, bringing this vast technology and teacher training programs to students globally.

JANET STONE practices and teaches yoga in San Francisco and around the world. Through her teaching, writing, training, and online offerings, she shares the message of yoga as a lifelong practice of healing, fostering community, and waking up to the profound gift of this life.

JOEL SALATIN is a pastured livestock farmer, author of nine books, conference speaker, and ardent supporter of local foods and food freedom. His family owns and operates Polyface Farm in Virginia's Shenandoah Valley.

JONINA TURZI is a doctor of physical therapy and movement educator specializing in core strength and yoga. She is the founder of West End Yoga Studio in Lancaster, Pennsylvania. Her mission is to facilitate healing by integrating Eastern and Western modalities.

JOSEPH GIACONA is a doctor of acupuncture, a practitioner of naturopathic medicine, a longtime Buddhist meditation teacher, and an entrepreneur involved in many personal and community-based projects. He is the founder of Neighborhood Natural Medicine in Brooklyn.

KERRI KELLY is a recovering corporate executive and athlete turned renowned yoga teacher, coach, and changemaker. She has been instrumental in bridging mindfulness and social change and is currently the founder and president of CTZNWELL, a movement to mobilize communities around programs and policies that bring about the well-being of all.

KEVIN COURTNEY is known for his innovative and authentic teaching style. Based in New York City, he leads teacher trainings, workshops, and retreats around the globe and trains high-level executives in philosophy and meditation. He is also cocreator of the yoga music project Nada Sadhana.

KIA MILLER is one of the most well-known Kundalini teachers in the West, with an ability to translate the subtle teachings of Kundalini yoga in a highly accessible way. She teaches workshops, retreats, and teacher trainings throughout the world.

KRISHNA DAS is a Grammy nominee in the New Age category for his album *Live Ananda* released in 2012. Regarded as the bestselling Western chant artist of all time, he travels worldwide sharing this practice and conducting workshops, discussing how we can integrate chanting into our everyday lives.

MANOJ CHALAM presents workshops on symbolisms of Hindu and Buddhist deities at yoga studios, festivals, ashrams, and universities. An Indian-born scientist with a PhD from Cornell University, Manoj helps individuals find their archetypes in yogic deities.

MANORAMA, founder of Luminous Soul and Sanskrit Studies Methods, guides students in how to bridge their everyday experiences with the meaningful spiritual and to unlock the keys to authentic happiness.

MARA MUNRO is a writer, yoga teacher, and archaeologist of the spirit. She is currently digging up ancient and modern healing rituals from around the world for her first book.

MATT GIORDANO and **CHELSEY KORUS** met in 2009 and immediately started their acrobatic partnership. Six months later, they had their first performance at the first annual AcroYoga festival. In 2012, they were featured as performers and teachers on national television and have been touring internationally as an acrobatic duo ever since.

MC YOGI is an internationally recognized musician and yoga teacher, best known for blending his knowledge of yoga culture with hip-hop, reggae, and electronic music.

MEGGAN WATTERSON is the author of *Reveal: A Sacred Manual for Getting Spiritually Naked* and the coauthor of *How to Love Yourself (And Sometimes Other People).*

MICHAEL RADPARVAR is a cofounder at Holstee, which he started with his brother David and friend Fabian Pfortmüller. What began as a values-driven T-shirt line has evolved into a global movement, ignited by the mantra they wrote when they first started. To this day, Holstee exists to help us remember what matters through the thoughtful design of experiences and products.

MOBY was born in New York City but grew up in Connecticut, where he started making music when he was nine years old. He has toured extensively, playing well over three thousand concerts in his career. He has also had his music used in hundreds of films, including *Heat, Any Given Sunday, Tomorrow Never Dies,* and *The Beach,* among others. Moby released his first single, "Go," in 1991 (listed as one of *Rolling Stones*' best records of all time) and has been making albums ever since. His own records have sold more than twenty million copies worldwide, and he's produced and remixed scores of other artists, including David Bowie, Metallica, the Beastie Boys, Public Enemy, among others. Moby also works closely with different charities, including the Humane Society and the Institute for Music and Neurologic Function.

NICOLE LINDSTROM is a writer and traveler based in New York City. She is the creator and editor of the online travel guide GLDMNE and producer of the Wanderlust Festival Speakeasy Lecture Series. When not traveling with the festival, Nicole continues to travel the globe.

ROLF GATES is an industry leader who conducts 200 hour/300 hour Vinyasa teacher trainings around the country and online. He is a cofounder of the Yoga, Meditation, and Recovery Conference and advisor to Mindful Yoga Therapy Veterans Program. A former US Army Ranger and social worker, he is also the author of the acclaimed book on yogic philosophy, *Meditations from the Mat: Daily Reflections on the Path of Yoga.*

RONALD A. ALEXANDER, PhD, executive director of the OpenMind Training Institute in Santa Monica, teaches mindfulness meditation worldwide and is an executive and transformational leadership coach. He is the author of *Wise Mind, Open Mind* and regularly blogs for *Huffington Post* and *Psychology Today* on mindfulness, creativity, and communication.

SARA GOTTFRIED, MD, is a Harvard-educated physician, natural hormone expert, speaker, yoga teacher, and author of the *New York Times* bestselling book, *The Hormone Cure: Reclaim Balance, Sleep, Sex Drive, and Vitality with the Gottfried Protocol* (Scribner, 2014).

SARA ELIZABETH IVANHOE is an MA candidate in Loyola Marymount University's inaugural yoga philosophy program. She is the yoga spokesperson for Weight Watchers and holds an undergraduate degree from New York University as well as a yoga and ecology degree from the Green Yoga Association. She is celebrating her twentieth year of teaching and, for most of it, has called Yoga Works in Santa Monica her home.

SARAH COPELAND is food expert, cookbook author, and curator of good living, and she's currently the food director at *Real Simple* magazine. She is a frequent guest expert on television and the Web, and her recipes and articles have appeared in numerous national magazines. Sarah is the author of *Feast: Generous Vegetarian Meals for Any Eater and Every Appetite* (Chronicle Books, 2013) and *The Newlywed Cookbook: Fresh Ideas and Modern Recipes for Cooking with and for Each Other* (Chronicle Books, 2011). An active gardener and nutrition educator, Sarah lives in New York City and upstate New York with her young family.

SARAH HERRINGTON is a writer, editor, and yogi living in New York. Her writing has appeared in the *New York Times, San Francisco Chronicle,* and *Poets and Writers,* and she was named a "poet to watch" by *Oprah* magazine. She has written several books about asana practice and facilitates OM Schooled teacher trainings for youth yoga. She has major Wanderlust.

SARAH NEUFELD is a violinist, composer, yoga instructor, and co-owner of Modo Yoga NYC. Best known for her work in the rock group Arcade Fire, she is a founding member of Montreal's Bell Orchestre, and she released her critically acclaimed debut solo album *Hero Brother* in 2013.

SCHUYLER GRANT is the cofounder of the festival that inspired this book. Wanderlusting aside, she is the director of Kula Yoga Project, a teacher of intelligent alignment-based Vinyasa classes and teacher trainings, and mother to three girls with her husband, Jeff, in Williamsburg, Brooklyn.

SEANE CORN is an internationally renowned yoga teacher and spiritual activist who teaches self-empowerment, self-actualization, and purpose. Featured in commercials and magazines and on NPR and Oprah.com, Seane now utilizes her national platform to bring awareness to global humanitarian issues. Since 2007, she has been training leaders of activism and fundraising for communities in need through her cofounded organization Off the Mat, Into the World, which has collectively raised nearly $4.5 million.

SHAKTI SUNFIRE is an internationally recognized movement guide and an advocate of the Earth. She blends her deep love of conscious dance, classical Tantra, yoga, mythology, and the study of many nature-based traditions into inspiring thematic explorations of soul, all designed to coax the essential self to the frontier of our life conversation.

SHARON SALZBERG is the cofounder of the Insight Meditation Society in Barre, Massachusetts, and the author of nine books. These include *Lovingkindness,* the *New York Times* bestseller *Real Happiness,* and *Real Happiness at Work.*

SHIVA REA, global yoga teacher, energy activist, and movement alchemist, collaborates with musicians, DJs, and movers and shakers from around the world for positive change. As the founder of Prana Vinyasa and Samdura Global School for Living Yoga, she offers online practices, retreats, and trainings for living flow.

STEPH DAVIS is a professional climber, BASE jumper, and wing-suit pilot. She is the author of *High Infatuation* and *Learning to Fly* and blogs at highinfatuation.com about climbing, flying, veganism, fear, and simple living.

STEPHANIE SNYDER teaches Vinyasa yoga all over the world and is known for combining sophisticated alignment with a mature understanding of yogic philosophy. She is the creator of the Yoga Journal DVD *Strength and Toning* and is one of the original core YogaGlo teachers. Stephanie used the platform of TED to talk about her experience and deepest struggles and how yoga can pull any of us up and into the flow of empowerment.

SUZANNE STERLING is a dedicated musician, yogi, activist, and social innovator who has been performing and teaching transformational workshops for more than twenty years. She is a leading expert in sound and consciousness; a cofounder of Off the Mat, Into the World; and the founder of Voice of Change.

TASHA BLANK is a DJ, music producer, and founder of The Get Down. Her events and sounds disrupt the status quo by injecting incredible beats with the intention to let wild our most liberated badassery. She loves you like crazy.

THOMAS DROGE is the author of the forthcoming book *Elemental Bodywork*. He has been practicing qi gong, tai ji, and Chinese healing arts for the past twenty-five years. He teaches workshops throughout the world and is the founder of the Droge Clinic for Transformational Healing in New York City.

An international yoga teacher, author, and health and wellness expert, **TIFFANY CRUIKSHANK** is known as a teacher's teacher and has written for and graced the cover of many prominent publications. She is internationally acclaimed due to her ability to combine more than two decades of teaching yoga and studying holistic medicine with over a decade working with patients to create Yoga Medicine—an effective method that trains teachers to use yoga as medicine.

TIM RYAN represents Ohio's Thirteenth District, which includes Akron, Youngstown, Warren, and Kent. He was first elected to the US House of Representatives in 2002 and sworn in on January 7, 2003. Successfully reelected six times, he is now serving his seventh term. He is the author of *A Mindful Nation: How a Simple Practice Can Help Us Reduce Stress, Improve Performance, and Recapture the American Spirit* and *The Real Food Revolution: Healthy Eating, Green Groceries, and the Return of the American Family Farm.*

TRAVIS ROBINSON has spent the last two decades working at the intersection of sustainability, finance, and philanthropy as a business builder, innovative operator, and impact investor in early-stage business and social enterprise. He has founded, operated, advised, or invested in several companies and nonprofits, including Bloom Energy, Brightsource Energy, Twitter, Ourstage, Elephant Journal, H2 Energy, and most recently The Kitchen Community with Kimbal Musk, creating the Learning Garden and outreach campaigns to connect kids and parents to real food in schools and communities across the country.

TRINITY DOMINO is an interior designer and the owner of Domino Designs in Petaluma, California, since 1984. She also owns Altar Your Reality, a production company that has been providing sacred décor and altars on the West Coast and internationally to music festivals for more than a decade.

Photo Credits

PAGE / PHOTOGRAPHER / LOCATION

i / Ali Kaukus / Turtle Bay, Oahu
ii–iii / Milou & Olin Photography / Squaw Valley, CA
iv–v / Ali Kaukus / Squaw Valley, CA
vii / Ali Kaukus / Copper, CO
viii–ix / Christen Vidanovic / Turtle Bay, Oahu
x–xi / Jon Chiang / Whistler, BC
xii–xiii / Ali / Whistler, BC
xiv–1 / Chris McLennan / Snowshoe, VT
2–3 / Jake Laub / Squaw Valley, CA
6–7 / Sasha Juliard / Great Sand Dunes National Park, CO
10–11 / Ali Kaukus / Stratton, VT
12–13 / Sasha Juliard / Aspen, CO
14–15 / Sasha Juliard / Aspen, CO
17 / Charles Ekabhumi
18–19 / Sasha Juliard / Evergreen, CO
20–21 / Sasha Juliard / Evergreen, CO
22–23 / Ali Kaukus / Squaw Valley, CA
28–29 / Sasha Juliard / Great Sand Dunes National Park, CO
33 / Ali Kaukus / Whistler, BC
34–35 / Sasha Juliard / Old Saybrook, CT
37 / Ali Kaukus / Manchester, Vermont
44–45 / Sasha Juliard / Whistler, BC
46–47 / Raffaella Dice / Whistler, BC
49 / Sasha Juliard / Old Saybrook, CT
50–51 / Sasha Juliard / Old Saybrook, CT
52–53 / Sasha Juliard / Old Saybrook, CT
55 / Daniel Craig / Squaw Valley, CA
56–57 / Daniel Craig / Squaw Valley, CA
58 / Daniel Craig / Squaw Valley, CA
60–61 / Sasha Juliard / Great Sand Dunes National Park, CO
70–71 / Sasha Juliard / Old Saybrook, CT
72–73 / Sasha Juliard / Old Saybrook, CT
76 / Ali Kaukus / Whistler, BC
78 / The Holstee Manifesto © 2009 / Design by Rachael Beresh
81 / Ali Kaukus / Costa Rica
83 / Sasha Juliard / Old Saybrook, CT
84 / Sasha Juliard / Old Saybrook, CT
86–87 / Christen Vidanovic / Squaw Valley, CA
88–89 / Sasha Juliard / Old Saybrook, CT
91 / Sasha Juliard / Old Saybrook, CT
92 / Sasha Juliard / Old Saybrook, CT
95 / Sasha Juliard / Old Saybrook, CT
104–105 / Eric Ward / Whistler, BC
106 / Ali Kaukus / Tremblant, QC
110–111 / Amanda Bjorn / Turtle Bay, Oahu
112 / Jake Laub / Squaw Valley, CA
114–115 / Chris McLennan / Snowshoe, VT
116–117 / Ali Kaukus / Vancouver Island
119 / Chip Conley / Fes, Morocco
120–121 / Art Gimbel / Oaxaca, Mexico
124–125 / Ali Kaukus / Stratton, VT
126–127 / Jon Chiang / Whistler, BC
128 / Ali Kaukus / Santa Teresa, Costa Rica
138–139 / Connie Grisley / Tremblant, QC
140 / Raffaella Dice / Whistler, BC
142–143 / Ali Kaukas / Squaw Valley, CA
144–145 / Mario Covic / Squaw Valley, CA
146–147 / Sasha Juliard / Corfu, Greece
149 / Ali Kaukas / Whistler, BC
150–151 / Matt Peyton / Haiti
152 / Casey Meade / Growing Heart Farm, Pawling NY
154–155 / Casey Meade / Growing Heart Farm, Pawling NY
157 / Casey Meade / Growing Heart Farm, Pawling NY
159 / Max Landerman / Copper, CO
160–161 / Ali Kaukas / Squaw Valley, CA
162–163 / Ali Kaukas / Squaw Valley, CA
165 / Laurie Smith / Los Angeles, CA
169 / Jake Laub / Copper, CO
174–175 / Ali Kaukas / Copper, CO
176 / Ali Kaukas / Squaw Valley, CA
179 / Eric Ward / Whistler, BC
180 / Sasha Juliard / Old Saybrook, CT
183 / Sasha Juliard / Old Saybrook, CT
184–185 / Christen Vidanovic / Los Angeles, CA
187 / Ali Kaukas / Whistler, BC
188 / Ali Kaukas / Squaw Valley, CA
192–193 / Amanda Giacomini / "10,000 Buddha Project"
194 / Amanda Giacomini / "10,000 Buddha Project"
195 / Ali Kaukus / Whistler, BC
196–197 / Sasha Juliard / Old Saybrook, CT
198–199 / Erica Jago / Oahu
208–209 / Ali Kaukas / Tulum, Mexico
210–211 / Ali Kaukas / Santa Teresa, Costa Rica
217 / Ali Kaukas / Tulum Mexico
218–219 / Ali Kaukas / Tulum Mexico
220–221 / Jake Laub / Turtle Bay, Oahu
223 / Ali Kaukas / New York City
224–225 / Ali Kaukas / Tulum Mexico
226–227 / Jake Laub / Tremblent, QC
228–229 / Ali Kaukas / Vancouver, Canada
230–231 / Sasha Juilard / Old Saybrook, CT
242–243 / Ali Kaukas / El Zonte, El Salvador
244–245 / Ali Kaukas / Santa Teresa Costa Rica
246–247 / Charles Bryan / California
250–251 / Ali Kaukas / New York City
253 / Ali Kaukas / Santa Teresa Costa Rica
256–257 / Patty Cousins Stratton, VT
258–259 / Christen Vidanovic / Squaw Valley, CA
260–261 / Boone Speed / Crested Butte, CO
263 /Boone Speed / Crested Butte, CO
264–265 / Ali Kaukas / El Zonte El Salvador
266–267 / Ali Kaukas / Vancouver Island
274–275 / Ali Kaukas / Whistler, BC
276–277 / Leah Martin / Whistler, BC
286 / Christen Vidanovic / Los Angeles, CA
290 / Ali Kaukas / Tremblant, QC

Index

Underscored page references indicate sidebars. **Boldface** references indicate illustrations and photographs.

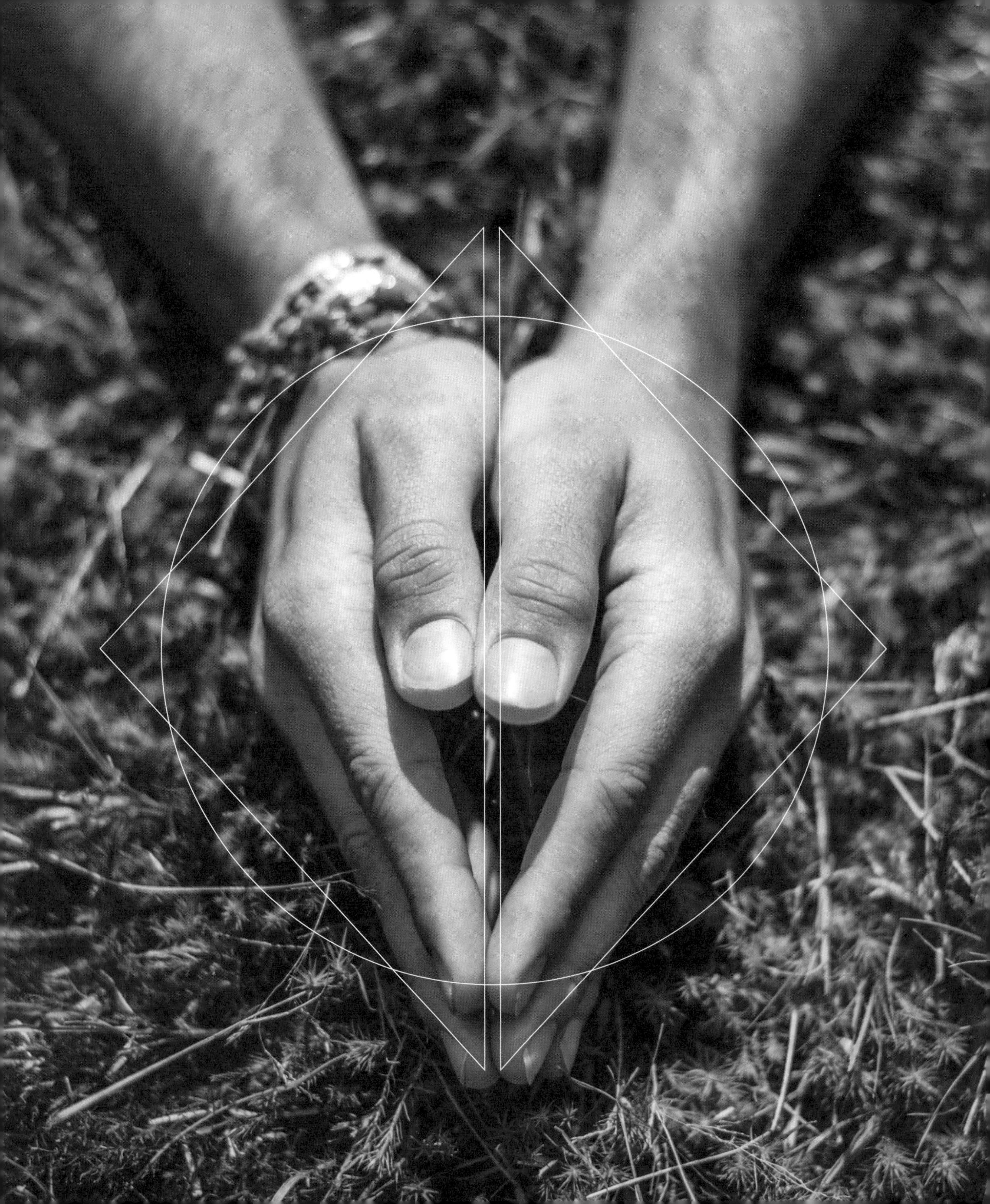